D0002144

ILLUSTRATED

Dental Embryology, Histology, AND Anatomy

SECOND EDITION

MARY BATH-BALOGH, BA, BS, MS

Faculty, Department Coordinator
Department of Biological Sciences
Pierce College, Lakewood, Washington

MARGARET J. FEHRENBACH, RDH, MS

Oral Biologist and Dental Hygienist
Adjunct Faculty Position, Marquette University, Milwaukee, Wisconsin
Educational Consultant and Private Practice, Seattle, Washington

Illustrated by

PAT THOMAS, CMI

Certified Medical Illustrator, AMI
Oak Park, Illinois

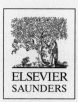

ELSEVIER
SAUNDERS

ELSEVIER
SAUNDERS

11830 Westline Industrial Drive
St. Louis, Missouri 63146

ILLUSTRATED DENTAL EMBRYOLOGY, HISTOLOGY,
AND ANATOMY
Copyright © 2006, Elsevier Inc.

All rights reserved. No part of this publication may be reproduced or transmitted in any form or by any means, electronic or mechanical, including photocopying, recording, or any information storage and retrieval system, without permission in writing from the publisher.
Permissions may be sought directly from Elsevier's Health Sciences Rights Department in Philadelphia, PA, USA: phone: (+1) 215 239 3804, fax: (+1) 215 239 3805, e-mail: healthpermissions@elsevier.com. You may also complete your request on-line via the Elsevier homepage (http://www.elsevier.com), by selecting 'Customer Support' and then 'Obtaining Permissions'.

Notice

Neither the Publisher nor the Authors assume any responsibility for any loss or injury and/or damage to persons or property arising out of or related to any use of the material contained in this book. It is the responsibility of the treating practitioner, relying on independent expertise and knowledge of the patient, to determine the best treatment and method of application for the patient.

The Publisher

Previous edition copyrighted 1997

ISBN-13: 978-1-4160-2499-6
ISBN-10: 1-4160-2499-9

Publishing Director: Linda Duncan
Executive Editor: Penny Rudolph
Developmental Editor: Courtney Sprehe
Publishing Services Manager: Melissa Lastarria
Project Manager: Ellen Kunkelmann
Designer: Teresa McBryan

Printed in the United States of America

Last digit is the print number: 9 8 7 6 5 4 3

Working together to grow
libraries in developing countries

www.elsevier.com | www.bookaid.org | www.sabre.org

ELSEVIER   BOOK AID International   Sabre Foundation

Preface

OVERVIEW

This textbook provides an extensive background for the dental professionals in the area of oral biology, as well as graduates of dental professional programs that need to take competency examinations or update their background knowledge in this area. It is divided into four units: Introduction to Dental Structures, Dental Embryology, Dental Histology, and Dental Anatomy. The textbook was organized into units to accommodate differing curriculum.

FEATURES

Each of the four units of this textbook consists of several chapters, with each chapter building on the preceding ones. Each chapter begins with an outline, objectives, and key terms (with a pronunciation guide when needed). The chapters contain both microscopic and clinical photographs as well as useful tables. Within each chapter are discussions of clinical and developmental considerations, which allow for an increased integration of the material into everyday practice for the dental professional. Within each chapter, there may be references to other chapters so that the reader can review or investigate interrelated subjects. The content of this edition incorporates additional input from students and educators.

The textbook concludes with a bibliography, complete glossary of terms (with pronunciation guide when needed), and appendices that contain a review of anatomical nomenclature, units of measurement, tooth measurements, and developmental information.

A separate workbook is available for student use. The workbook features activities such as structure identification exercises, glossary exercises, tooth drawing exercises, and case studies. An Evolve site is also available for both the student and instructor, featuring discussion questions, supplemental considerations, and content updates. Instructors can also obtain an instructor's manual to accompany the text, featuring a testbank and transparency masters.

This textbook is coordinated with the *Illustrated Anatomy of the Head and Neck* by Margaret J. Fehrenbach and Susan W. Herring, and as such can be considered a companion textbook to complete the curriculum in oral biology.

Mary Bath-Balogh

Margaret J. Fehrenbach

Acknowledgments

We would like to thank Editors Penny Rudolph and Courtney Sprehe and the staff at Elsevier for making this textbook possible. In addition, we would like to thank Heidi Schlei, RDH, MS, Instructor, Waukesha County Technical College, Milwaukee, Wisconsin, for reviewing the textbook; Susan Herring, PhD, Professor of Orthodontics, School of Dentistry, University of Washington, Seattle, Washington, for reviewing the embryology unit; Patricia L. Toma, RDH, BS, of Grosse Pointe, Michigan, for her clinical expertise; and the late Herbert K. Kashiwa, PhD, Associate Professor, Department of Biological Structure, University of Washington, Seattle, Washington, for his histological micrographs.

Also used in the compilation of this text was information on occlusion from Dr. Major M. Ash, DDS, MS, Professor, University of Michigan, School of Dentistry, Ann Arbor, Michigan and Dr. Dona M. Seely, DDS, MSD, Orthodontic Associates, Bellevue, Washington. Many of the elegant microscopic sections are from the Dr. Bernhard Gottlieb Collection, courtesy of Dr. James E. McIntosh, PhD, Assistant Professor, Department of Biomedical Sciences, Baylor College of Dentistry, Dallas, Texas. Finally, we would like to thank our families, students, and colleagues.

Mary Bath-Balogh

Margaret J. Fehrenbach

Table of Contents

INTRODUCTION TO DENTAL STRUCTURES

CHAPTER 1

Face and Neck Regions

This chapter discusses the following topics:

- Regions of the face
  - Frontal, orbital, and nasal regions
  - Infraorbital and zygomatic regions
  - Buccal region
- Oral region
- Mental region
- Regions of the neck

After studying this chapter, the reader should be able to:

1. Define and pronounce the key terms in this chapter.
2. Locate and identify the regions and associated surface landmarks of the face and neck on a diagram and on a patient.
3. Integrate the knowledge of surface anatomy of the face and neck into the clinical practice of patient examination and the understanding of the developmental aspects of these regions.

Key Terms

Ala (a-lah) (plural, alae [a-lay])
Angle of the mandible
Buccal region (buk-al)
Coronoid notch, process (kor-ah-noid)
Condyle (kon-dyl), articulating surface (ar-tik-you-late-ing), mandible
External nose
Frontal region (frun-tal)
Golden Proportions
Hyoid bone (hi-oid)
Infraorbital region (in-frah-or-bit-al)
Labial commissure (kom-i-shoor)
Larynx (lare-inks)
Lymph nodes (limf)

Mandible (man-di-bl)
Mandibular symphysis (sim-fi-sis)
Masseter muscle (mass-et-er)
Mental region (men-tal)
Naris (nay-ris) (plural, nares [nay-rees])
Nasal (nay-zil) region, septum (sep-tum)
Nose, apex, root
Oral region
Orbit
Orbital region (or-bit-al)
Parathyroid glands (par-ah-thy-roid)
Parotid salivary gland (pah-rot-id)
Philtrum (fil-trum)
Ramus (ray-mus)

Regions of the face, neck
Sternocleidomastoid muscle (stir-no-klii-do-mass-toid)
Sublingual salivary gland (sub-ling-gwal)
Submandibular salivary gland (sub-man-dib-you-lar)
Temporomandibular joint (tem-poh-ro-man-dib-you-lar)
Thyroid cartilage, gland (thy-roid)
Tubercle of the upper lip (too-ber-kl)
Vermilion border, zone (ver-mil-yon)
Vertical dimension of the face
Zygomatic arch, region (zy-go-mat-ik)

Dental professionals must be thoroughly familiar with the surface anatomy of the face and neck as discussed in this introduction to **Unit I.** The superficial features of the face and neck provide essential landmarks for many of the deeper anatomical structures. Dental professionals may need to review these underlying structures in a head and neck anatomy textbook before continuing further in the study of orofacial embryology and histology as well as dental anatomy.

Examination of these accessible features by visualization and palpation can give information about the health of deeper tissues. Any changes or deviations from normal noted in these surface features must be recorded by the examining dental professional. Some degree of variation in surface features can be considered within a normal range. However, a change in a surface feature in a given person may signal a condition of clinical significance. Thus it is not the variations among individuals that should be noted but the changes in a particular individual.

Some of these surface changes in the features of the face and neck may be due to underlying developmental disturbances. Knowledge of the surface features of the face and neck also helps dental professionals to understand the developmental pattern of these tissues. *Unit II* in this textbook describes the development of the face and neck and any developmental disturbances. Other surface changes may be due to underlying histological reasons. *Unit III* describes the histology of the face and neck that gives them many of their characteristic surface features.

The study of the face and neck begins with the division of the surface into regions. Within each region are certain surface landmarks. Practice finding these landmarks in each region on yourself in a mirror to improve the skills of examination, and then locate them on peers and then on patients in a clinical setting.

REGIONS OF THE FACE

The **regions of the face** include the frontal, orbital, nasal, infraorbital, zygomatic, buccal, oral, and mental regions (Figure 1-1). **Lymph nodes** are located in certain areas of the face and head and when palpable should be noted (Figure 1-2, *A* and *B*).

Frontal, Orbital, and Nasal Regions

The **frontal region** of the face includes the forehead and the area above the eyes (Figure 1-3). In the **orbital region** of the face, the eyeball and all its supporting structures are contained in the bony socket called the **orbit.**

The main feature of the **nasal region** of the face is the **external nose** (Figure 1-4). The **root of the nose** is

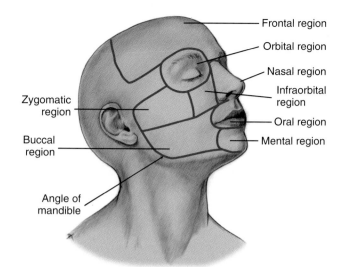

FIGURE 1-1 Regions of the face: frontal, orbital, infraorbital, nasal, zygomatic, buccal, oral, and mental. (Adapted from Fehrenbach MJ, Herring SW. *Illustrated Anatomy of the Head and Neck,* ed 2. WB Saunders, Philadelphia, 2002.)

located between the eyes, and the tip is the **apex of the nose.** Inferior to the apex on each side of the nose is a nostril, or **naris.** The nares are separated by the midline **nasal septum.** The nares are bounded laterally by winglike cartilaginous structures, the **ala** of the nose.

Infraorbital and Zygomatic Regions

The **infraorbital region** of the face is located inferior to the orbital region and lateral to the nasal region (see Figure 1-3). Farther laterally is the **zygomatic region,** which overlies the bony support for the cheek, the **zygomatic arch.** The zygomatic arch extends from just below the lateral margin of the eye toward the middle part of the ear.

Inferior to the zygomatic arch and just anterior to the external ear is the **temporomandibular joint (TMJ).** This is where the upper skull forms a joint with the lower jaw (see Chapter 19 for more discussion). The movements of the joint occur when a person opens and closes the mouth or moves the lower jaw to the right or left. One way to feel the lower jaw moving at the temporomandibular joint is to place a finger into the external ear canal.

Buccal Region

The **buccal region** of the face is composed of the soft tissues of the cheek (see Figure 1-3). The cheek forms the side of the face and is a broad area of the face between the nose, mouth, and ear. Most of the upper cheek is fleshy, mainly formed by a mass of fat and

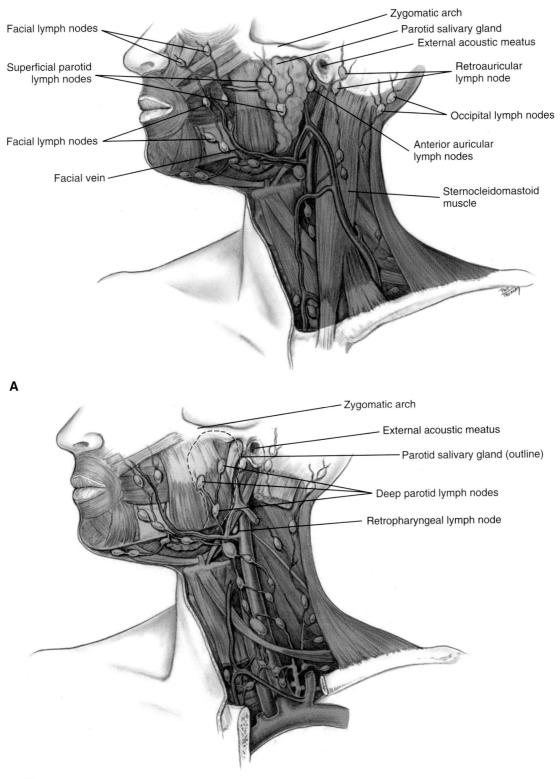

A

B

FIGURE 1-2 Location of the lymph nodes of the head and associated structures.
A: Superficial nodes of the head. **B:** Deep nodes of the head. (From Fehrenbach MJ, Herring SW. *Illustrated Anatomy of the Head and Neck*, ed 2. WB Saunders, Philadelphia, 2002.)

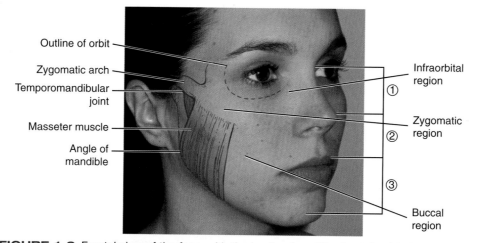

FIGURE 1-3 Frontal view of the face, with the landmarks of the frontal, orbital, infraorbital, zygomatic, buccal, and mental regions noted. Also noted is the vertical dimension of the face. (From Fehrenbach MJ, Herring SW. *Illustrated Anatomy of the Head and Neck*, ed 3. WB Saunders, St Louis, 2007.)

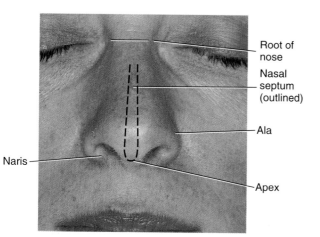

FIGURE 1-4 View of the face, with the landmarks of the nasal region noted. (From Fehrenbach MJ, Herring SW. *Illustrated Anatomy of the Head and Neck*, ed 2. WB Saunders, Philadelphia, 2002.)

muscles. One of these muscles forming the cheek is the strong **masseter muscle,** which is felt when a patient clenches the teeth together. The sharp angle of the lower jaw inferior to the earlobe is termed the **angle of the mandible.**

The **parotid salivary gland,** a major salivary gland, has a small portion that can be palpated in the buccal region as well as in the zygomatic region (Figure 1-5). Thus the parotid gland is located irregularly from the zygomatic arch down to the posterior border of the lower jaw.

Oral Region

The **oral region** of the face has many structures within it, such as the lips and oral cavity. The oral cavity is discussed further in Chapter 2 (Figure 1-6). The lips are fleshy folds that mark the gateway of the oral cavity

proper. Each lip's **vermilion zone** has a darker appearance than the surrounding skin. The lips are outlined from the surrounding skin by a transition zone, the **vermilion border.**

On the midline of the upper lip, extending downward from the nasal septum, is a vertical groove called the **philtrum.** The philtrum terminates in a thicker area of the midline of the upper lip, the **tubercle of the upper lip.** The upper and lower lips meet at each corner of the mouth, or the **labial commissure.**

Clinical Considerations with the Lips

Any loss of the vermilion border is very important to note. With this loss, it is hard to determine the border between the lips and the surrounding skin (Figure 1-7). This loss may be due to scar tissue from past traumatic incidents, developmental disturbances, changes resulting from solar damage, or cellular changes in the tissues. These changes may represent a serious condition and may be associated with cancer. Only with biopsy of the tissues can cancerous changes in the cells be verified. If loss of the vermilion border is due to solar damage, protection of the lips with sunscreen is important because sun exposure increases the risk of cancerous changes (as do alcohol consumption and smoking).

Loss of the vermilion border caused by a traumatic incident is important to note given that the rest of the oral cavity may be affected. If loss of the vermilion border is part of a developmental disorder such as cleft lip, this also needs to be noted because of its impact on dental treatment.

Mental Region

The chin is the major feature of the **mental region** of the face. The bone underlying the mental region is the **mandible,** or lower jaw bone. The midline is marked by the **mandibular symphysis.**

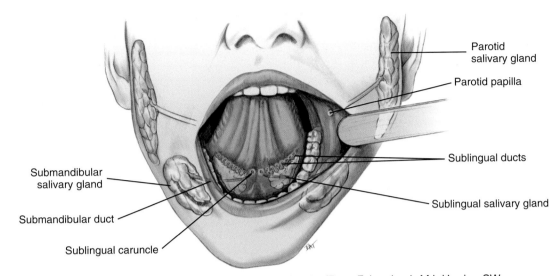

FIGURE 1-5 Location of the major salivary glands. (From Fehrenbach MJ, Herring SW. *Illustrated Anatomy of the Head and Neck*, ed 2. WB Saunders, Philadelphia, 2002.)

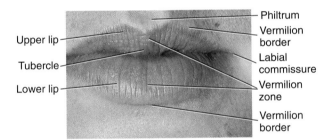

FIGURE 1-6 Frontal view of the lips within the oral region. A normal vermilion border. (From Fehrenbach MJ, Herring SW. *Illustrated Anatomy of the Head and Neck*, ed 2. WB Saunders, Philadelphia, 2002.)

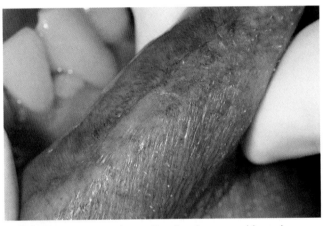

FIGURE 1-7 Loss of vermilion border caused by solar damage.

On the lateral aspect of the mandible, the stout, flat plate of the **ramus** extends upward and backward from the body of the mandible on each side (Figures 1-8 and 1-9). At the anterior border of the ramus is a thin, sharp margin that terminates in the **coronoid process.** The main portion of the anterior border of the ramus forms a concave forward curve called the **coronoid notch.**

 Clinical Considerations of Facial Dimensions

The face is sometimes thought of as divided into thirds, and this perspective is called the **vertical dimension of the face.** A discussion of vertical dimension allows a comparison of the three portions of the face for functional and aesthetic purposes using the **Golden Proportions,** a set of guidelines (Figure 1-10). Loss of height in the lower third, which contains the teeth and jaws, can occur in certain circumstances (see Chapters 14 and 20 for more discussion).

The posterior border of the ramus is thickened and extends from the angle of the mandible to a projection, the **condyle of the mandible,** with its neck. The **articulating surface of the condyle** is an oval head involved in the temporomandibular joint. Between the coronoid process and the condyle is a depression, the mandibular notch.

REGIONS OF THE NECK

The **regions of the neck** extend from the skull and lower jaw down to the clavicles and sternum (Figure 1-11). Lymph nodes are located in certain areas of the neck and, when palpable, should be recorded (Figure 1-12, *A* and *B*). The regions of the neck can be divided into different cervical triangles on the basis of the large

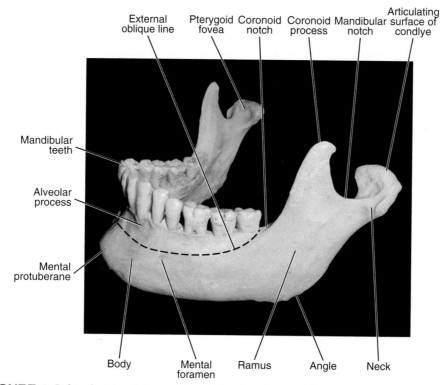

FIGURE 1-8 Landmarks of the facial and lateral surfaces of the mandible. (From Fehrenbach MJ, Herring SW. *Illustrated Anatomy of the Head and Neck*, ed 3. WB Saunders, St Louis, 2007.)

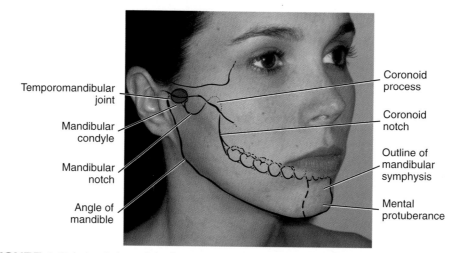

FIGURE 1-9 Lateral view of the face showing the landmarks of the mandible. (From Fehrenbach MJ, Herring SW. *Illustrated Anatomy of the Head and Neck*, ed 3. WB Saunders, St Louis, 2007.)

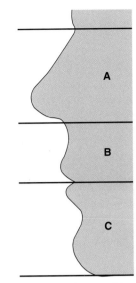

FIGURE 1-10 The Golden Proportions can be used to discuss aesthetic concerns of the vertical dimension of the face. With these guidelines the nasal height (A) is related to the maxillary height (B) as 1.000 : 0.618. The sum of nasal height and maxillary height (A + B) are related to the mandibular height (C) as 1.618 : 1.000. The mandibular height (C) is related to the maxillary height (B) as 1.000 : 0.618. The orofacial height (B + C) is related to the nasal height (A) as 1.618 : 1.000. Note that each ratio is 1.618, which is integral in these guidelines.

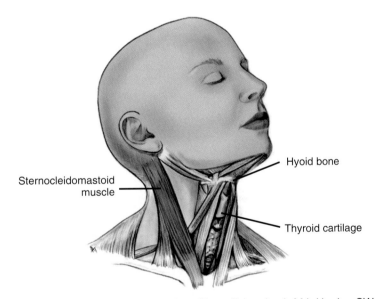

FIGURE 1-11 Landmarks in the neck region. (From Fehrenbach MJ, Herring SW. *Illustrated Anatomy of the Head and Neck*, ed 2. WB Saunders, Philadelphia, 2002.)

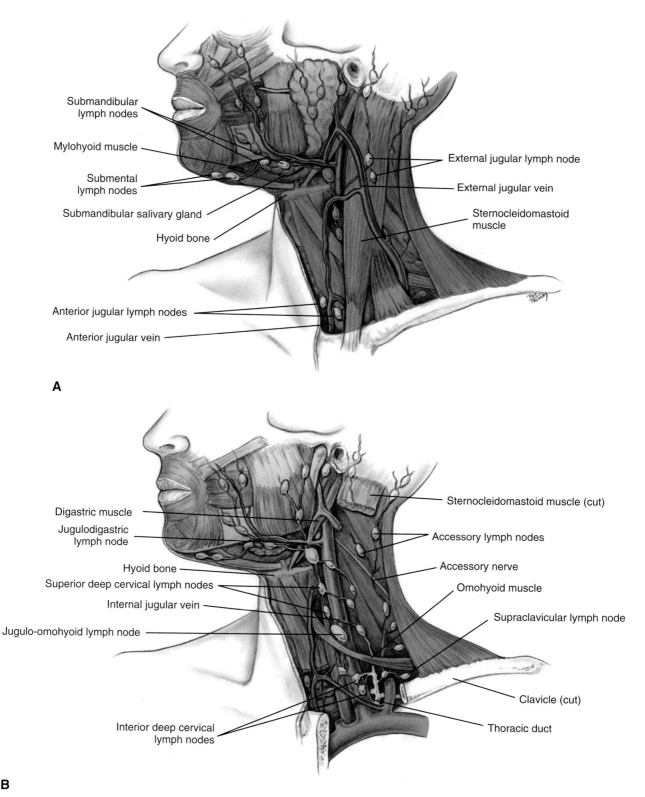

A

B

FIGURE 1-12 Location of the lymph nodes of the neck and associated structure.
A: Superficial cervical nodes. **B:** Deep cervical nodes. (From Fehrenbach MJ, Herring SW. *Illustrated Anatomy of the Head and Neck*, ed 2. WB Saunders, Philadelphia, 2002.)

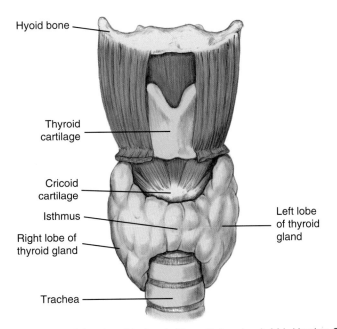

Hyoid bone

Thyroid
cartilage

Cricoid
cartilage

Isthmus

Right lobe of
thyroid gland

Left lobe
of thyroid
gland

Trachea

FIGURE 1-13 Location of the thyroid gland. (From Fehrenbach MJ, Herring SW. *Illustrated Anatomy of the Head and Neck*, ed 2. WB Saunders, Philadelphia, 2002.)

bones and muscles in the area (see a head and neck anatomy text for more information).

The large strap muscle, the **sternocleidomastoid muscle (SCM)**, is located on each side of the neck (see Figure 1-11). At the anterior midline is the **hyoid bone**, which is suspended in the neck. Many muscles attach to the hyoid bone, which controls the position of the base of the tongue. Also found in the anterior midline, inferior to the hyoid bone, is the **thyroid cartilage**, which is the prominence of the "voice box," or **larynx**. The vocal cords, or ligaments of the larynx, are attached to the posterior surface of the thyroid cartilage.

The **thyroid gland,** an endocrine gland, can also be palpated within the midline cervical area (Figure 1-13). Thus the thyroid gland is located inferior to the thyroid cartilage, at the junction of the larynx and the trachea. The **parathyroid glands** are located close to or within the posterior aspect of the thyroid gland and cannot be palpated. The major salivary glands, the **submandibular salivary gland** and the **sublingual salivary gland**, can also be palpated in the neck region (see Figure 1-5).

Oral Cavity and Pharynx

■ ■ ■

This chapter discusses the following topics:

- Divisions of the oral cavity
  - Oral vestibules
  - Jaws, alveolar processes, and teeth
- Oral cavity proper
- Divisions of the pharynx

■ ■ ■

After studying this chapter, the reader should be able to:

1. Define and pronounce the key terms in this chapter.
2. Locate and identify the divisions and associated surface landmarks of the oral cavity on a diagram and on a patient.
3. Describe the divisions of the pharynx.
4. Integrate the knowledge of the oral cavity and pharynx into the clinical practice of patient care and later into the understanding of the developmental aspects of this region.

■ ■ ■

Key Terms

Alveolar mucosa, processes (al-**ve**-o-lar)
Alveolus (al-**vee**-oh-lus) (plural, alveoli [al-**vee**-oh-lie])
Anterior faucial pillar (faw-shawl)
Anterior teeth
Buccal (buk-al)
Buccal fat pad
Canine eminence (kay-nine em-i-nins)
Canines (kay-nines)
Cementum (see-**men**-tum)
Circumvallate lingual papillae (serk-um-**val**-ate)
Dental arch
Dentin (den-tin)
Ducts: parotid, sublingual, submandibular (sub-man-**dib**-you-lar)
Enamel (ih-**nam**-l)
Exostoses (eks-ox-**toe**-seez)
Facial (fay-shal)

Fauces (faw-seez)
Filiform lingual papillae (fil-i-form)
Foliate lingual papillae (fo-le-ate)
Foramen cecum (for-ay-men se-kum)
Fordyce's spots (for-die-seez)
Fungiform lingual papillae (fun-ji-form)
Gingiva (jin-ji-vah): attached, interdental (in-ter-den-tal), marginal
Gingival sulcus (sul-kus)
Incisive papilla (in-sy-ziv pah-pil-ah)
Incisors (in-sigh-zers)
Labial (lay-be-al), frenum (free-num)
Laryngopharynx (lah-ring-gah-fare-inks)
Linea alba (lin-ee-ah al-bah)
Lingual (ling-gwal), papillae (pah-pil-ay), tonsil, frenum (free-num)

Mandible (man-di-bl), body
Mandibular teeth (man-**dib**-you-lar), torus (tore-us) (plural, tori [tore-eye])
Mastication (mass-ti-**kay**-shin)
Maxilla (mak-sil-ah)
Maxillary (mak-si-lare-ee) sinuses (sy-nuses), teeth, tuberosity (too-beh-**ros**-i-tee)
Median lingual sulcus
Median palatine raphe (pal-ah-tine ra-fe)
Melanin pigmentation (mel-a-nin)
Molars (mo-lerz)
Mucobuccal fold (mu-ko-buk-al)
Mucogingival junction (mu-ko-jin-ji-val)
Mucosa (mu-ko-sah): buccal, labial, oral
Nasopharynx (nay-zo-fare-inks)
Oral cavity proper

Oropharynx (or-o-fare-inks)
Palatal (pal-ah-tal), torus (tore-us)
Palate (pal-it): hard, soft
Palatine tonsils (pal-ah-tine ton-sils),
   rugae (ru-ge)
Parotid papilla (pah-**rot**-id pah-**pil**-ah),
   salivary gland
Periodontal ligament
   (pare-ee-o-**don**-tl)
Permanent teeth
Plica fimbriata (pli-kah
   fim-bree-**ay**-tah) (plural, **plicae**

fimbriatae, pli-kay
   fim-bree-**ay**-tay)
Posterior teeth and faucial pillar
Premolars (pre-**mo**-lerz)
Primary teeth
Pterygomandibular fold (teh-ri-go-
   man-**dib**-yule-lar)
Pulp
Retromolar pad
   (re-tro-**mo**-ler)
Submandibular salivary glands
   (sub-man-**dib**-you-lar)

Sublingual salivary glands, fold,
   caruncle (kar-unk-kl)
Sulcus terminalis (**sul**-kus ter-mi-
   nal-is)
Taste buds
Tongue apex, base, body, dorsal,
   lateral, ventral
Uvula of the palate (u-vu-lah)
Vestibular fornix (ves-**tib**-u-lar
   fore-niks)
Vestibules (ves-ti-bules)

A dental professional must be exceptionally knowledgeable, genuinely enthusiastic, and totally committed to improving the oral health of each and every patient. In order to accomplish this, dental professionals must be particularly knowledgeable about their chief area of focus, the oral cavity. To visualize this area of focus successfully, it is important to know the boundaries, terminology, and divisions of the oral cavity and the adjacent throat or pharynx. *Unit II* in this textbook describes the development of these oral tissues and related developmental disturbances. *Unit III* describes the underlying histology of these oral tissues that gives them many of their characteristic surface features.

Any changes in the tissues of the oral cavity and visible portions of the pharynx must be recorded by the dental professional. Some degree of variation in tissues of the oral cavity and pharynx is within a normal range. However, a change in any tissue in a given person may signal a condition of clinical significance. Thus it is not the variations among individuals that should be noted but the changes in a particular individual.

DIVISIONS OF THE ORAL CAVITY

The oral cavity is divided into the vestibules, jaws and alveolar processes, teeth, and oral cavity proper. Within each part of the oral cavity are certain surface landmarks. Practice finding these landmarks in your own oral cavity to improve your knowledge of this very important area.

An understanding of the divisions of the oral cavity is aided by an appreciation of its boundaries. Many tissues of the face and oral cavity mark the boundaries of the oral cavity (Figure 2-1). The lips of the face mark the anterior boundary of the oral cavity, and the pharynx or throat is the posterior boundary. The cheeks of the face mark the lateral boundaries, and the palate marks the superior boundary. The floor of the mouth is the inferior border of the oral cavity.

Many oral structures are identified with orientational terms based on their relationship to other orofacial structures, such as the facial surface, lips, cheek,

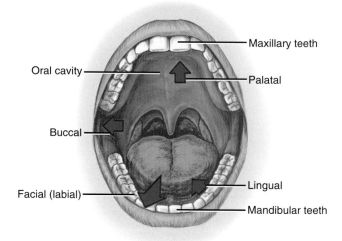

FIGURE 2-1 Oral cavity and the jaws, with the designation of the orientational terms *facial, labial, buccal, palatal,* and *lingual* within the oral cavity. (From Fehrenbach MJ, Herring SW. *Illustrated Anatomy of the Head and Neck,* ed 2. WB Saunders, Philadelphia, 2002.)

palate, and tongue (see Figure 2-1). Those structures closest to the facial surface or lips are termed **facial** or **labial.** Those structures close to the inner cheek are considered **buccal.** Those structures closest to the palate are termed **palatal.** Those structures closest to the tongue are termed **lingual.**

Oral Vestibules

The upper and lower horseshoe-shaped spaces in the oral cavity between the lips and cheeks anteriorly and laterally and the teeth and gums medially and posteriorly are called the maxillary and mandibular **vestibules** (Figure 2-2). These oral vestibules are lined by a mucous membrane, or **oral mucosa.** The inner portions of the lips are lined by a pink **labial mucosa.** The labial mucosa is continuous with the equally pink **buccal mucosa** that lines the inner cheek. Both the labial and buccal mucosa may vary in coloration, as do other areas of the oral mucosa, in individuals with pigmented skin (see Chapter 9).

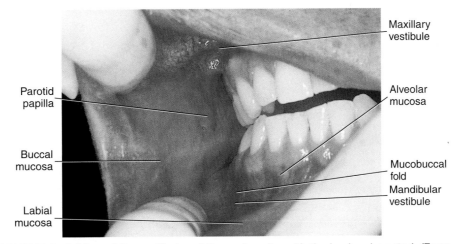

Maxillary vestibule

Alveolar mucosa

Mucobuccal fold

Mandibular vestibule

Parotid papilla

Buccal mucosa

Labial mucosa

FIGURE 2-2 View of the vestibules of the oral cavity, with the landmarks noted. (From Fehrenbach MJ, Herring SW. *Illustrated Anatomy of the Head and Neck,* ed 2. WB Saunders, Philadelphia, 2002.)

The buccal mucosa covers a dense pad of underlying fat tissue at the posterior portion of each vestibule, the **buccal fat pad.** The buccal fat pad acts as a protective cushion during **mastication,** or chewing.

On the inner portion of the buccal mucosa, just opposite the maxillary second molar, is a small elevation of tissue called the **parotid papilla.** The parotid papilla protects the opening of the **parotid duct** (or Stenson's duct) of the **parotid salivary gland** (see Chapters 1 and 11 for more information).

Deep within each vestibule is the **vestibular fornix,** where the pink labial mucosa or buccal mucosa meets the redder **alveolar mucosa** at the **mucobuccal fold.** The **labial frenum** is a fold of tissue located at the midline between the labial mucosa and the alveolar mucosa on the upper and lower arches.

 Clinical Considerations with Oral Mucosa

Sometimes noted on the surface of the labial and buccal mucosa is a normal variation, **Fordyce's spots** or granules (Figure 2-3, A). These are visible as small, yellowish elevations on the mucosa. They are deeper deposits of sebum from trapped or misplaced sebaceous gland tissue that are usually associated with hair follicles. Most of the population has these harmless spots, and they are more prominent in older individuals than in children or young adults.

Another normal variation noted on the buccal mucosa is the **linea alba** (Figure 2-3, B). This is a white ridge of raised callused tissue that extends horizontally at the level where the maxillary and mandibular teeth come together and occlude. The histology of these changes is discussed in Chapter 9. These oral habits are discussed further in Chapter 20. Similar ridges of white raised tissue can sometimes be noted on the perimeter of the tongue.

Jaws, Alveolar Processes, and Teeth

The jaws are deep to the lips and within the oral cavity (Figure 2-4). Underlying the upper lip is the upper jaw, or **maxilla.** The bone underlying the lower lip is the lower jaw, or **mandible.**

The maxilla consists of two maxillary bones that are sutured together. The maxilla has a nonmovable articulation with many facial and skull bones, and each maxillary bone includes a body and four processes. Each body of the maxilla is superior to the teeth and contains the **maxillary sinuses.**

In contrast, the mandible is a single bone with a movable articulation with the temporal bones at each temporomandibular joint. The heavy horizontal portion of the lower jaw inferior to the teeth is called the **body of the mandible.**

The **alveolar processes,** or alveolar bones, are the bony extensions of the maxilla and mandible that contain the tooth sockets of the teeth (see Figure 2-4 and Figure 2-5). Each tooth socket is called an **alveolus.** The facial portion of the alveolus of the canine, the vertically placed **canine eminence,** is especially prominent on the maxilla. All the teeth are attached to the bony surface of the alveoli by the fibrous **periodontal ligament (PDL),** which allows some slight tooth movement within the alveolus while supporting the tooth.

Each of the mature and fully erupted teeth consists of a crown and root (see Figure 2-5 and Figure 2-6). The crown of the tooth is composed of the hard outer **enamel** layer and the moderately hard inner **dentin** layer overlying the **pulp** of the tooth. The pulp is the soft innermost layer in the tooth. The moderately hard dentin continues to cover the soft tissue of the pulp of the tooth in the root, but the outermost layer of the root is composed of **cementum.** The bonelike cementum is the portion of the tooth that attaches to the periodontal ligament, which then attaches to the alveoli of bone.

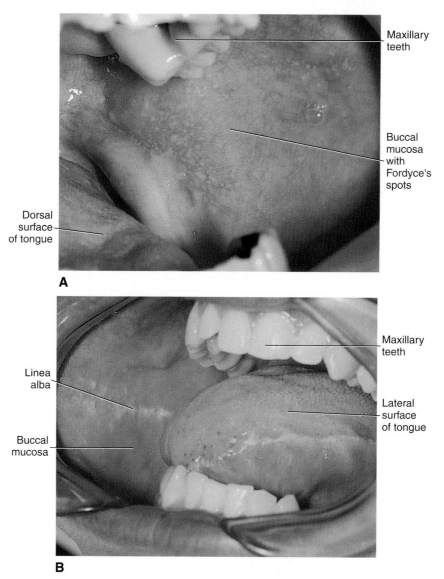

Maxillary teeth

Buccal mucosa with Fordyce's spots

Dorsal surface of tongue

A

Maxillary teeth

Linea alba

Lateral surface of tongue

Buccal mucosa

B

FIGURE 2-3 Close-up views of the buccal and labial mucosa of the oral cavity, with normal variations noted. **A:** Fordyce's spots visible as small, yellowish elevations on the mucosa. **B:** Linea alba noted on the mucosa as a white ridge of raised tissue that extends horizontally at the level where the teeth occlude. Note a similar white ridge on the perimeter of the lateral surface of the tongue.

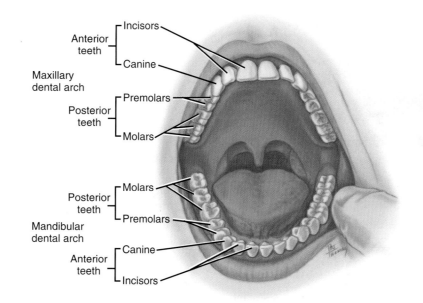

Incisors

Anterior teeth

Canine

Maxillary dental arch

Premolars

Posterior teeth

Molars

Molars

Posterior teeth

Premolars

Mandibular dental arch

Canine

Anterior teeth

Incisors

FIGURE 2-4 The alveolar processes and teeth, with the landmarks noted.

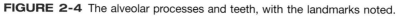

DENTAL ARCHES

The alveolar processes with the teeth in the alveoli are also called **dental arches,** maxillary and mandibular (see Figure 2-4). The teeth in the maxillary arch are the **maxillary teeth,** and the teeth in the mandibular arch are the **mandibular teeth.**

Just distal to the last tooth of the maxillary arch is a tissue-covered elevation of the bone called the **maxillary tuberosity.** Similarly, on the lower jaw, just distal to the last tooth of the mandibular arch, is a dense pad of tissue, the **retromolar pad.** The tooth types in both arches of the teeth of children, or **primary teeth,** include **incisors, canines,** and **molars.**

Adult teeth, or **permanent teeth,** also include all the same teeth as the primary teeth, as well as **premolars.** The teeth in the front of the mouth, the incisors and canines, are considered **anterior teeth.** The teeth located toward the back of the mouth, molars, and premolars, if present, are considered **posterior teeth.**

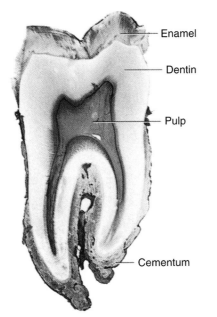

— Enamel

— Dentin

— Pulp

— Cementum

FIGURE 2-5 Section showing the distribution of the tissue of the tooth. (From Nanci A. *Ten Cate's Oral Histology*, ed 6. Mosby, St. Louis, 2003.)

Clinical Considerations with Alveolar Process

A normal variation noted usually on the facial surface of the alveolar process of the maxilla is **exostoses,** which are localized developmental growths of normal bone with a hereditary etiology (Figure 2-7). They may be single, multiple, unilateral, or bilateral raised hard areas, usually in the premolar to molar region. They are covered by normal oral tissue and may appear radiographically as radiopaque (light) areas. Exostoses may interfere with restorative and periodontal therapy and thus must be noted on a patient's chart.

Another normal variation noted on the lingual aspect of the mandibular arch is the **mandibular torus** (plural, **tori**) (Figure 2-8). Each one is a developmental growth of normal bone with a hereditary etiology, similar to exostoses. These tori are usually present bilaterally in the area of the premolars and can appear lobulated or nodular or even fused together.

These mandibular tori are covered in normal oral tissue and vary in size. They are slow growing and asymptomatic and also may be seen on radiographs as radiopaque (light) masses. They may interfere with oral hygiene procedures, radiographic placement, and denture therapy considerations. The patient may require reassurance. This normal variation must be noted on a patient's chart.

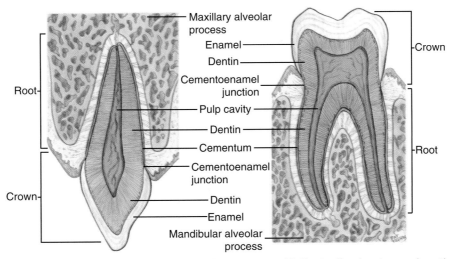

Maxillary alveolar process

Enamel

Dentin

Cementoenamel junction

Pulp cavity

Dentin

Cementum

Cementoenamel junction

Dentin

Enamel

Mandibular alveolar process

Crown

Root

Root

Crown

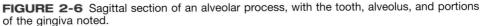

FIGURE 2-6 Sagittal section of an alveolar process, with the tooth, alveolus, and portions of the gingiva noted.

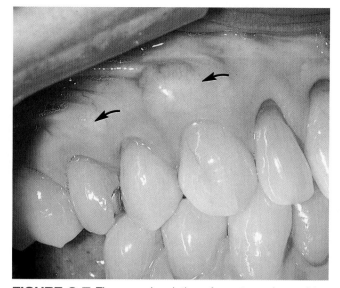

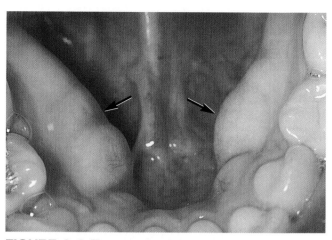

FIGURE 2-8 The normal variation of bilateral mandibular tori (*arrows*) is noted on the lingual surface of the mandible at the floor of the mouth.

FIGURE 2-7 The normal variation of exostoses (*arrows*) is noted on the facial surface of the maxilla.

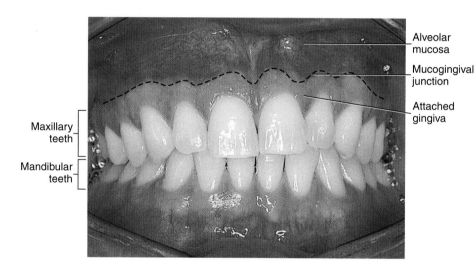

FIGURE 2-9 The gingiva and its landmarks. (From Fehrenbach MJ, Herring SW. *Illustrated Anatomy of the Head and Neck,* ed 2. WB Saunders, Philadelphia, 2002.)

The anterior maxillary teeth are supplied by the anterior superior alveolar artery and the maxillary posterior teeth by the posterior superior alveolar artery. The mandibular teeth are supplied by branches of the inferior alveolar artery. The maxillary teeth are drained by the posterior superior alveolar vein and mandibular teeth by the inferior alveolar vein.

GINGIVA

Surrounding the maxillary and mandibular teeth in the alveoli and covering the alveolar processes are the gums, or **gingiva,** composed of a firm pink mucosa (Figure 2-9). The gingiva that tightly adheres to the bone around the roots of the teeth is the **attached gingiva.** The attached gingiva may have areas of **melanin pigmentation.** The line of demarcation

between the firmer and pinker attached gingiva and the movable and redder alveolar mucosa is the scallop-shaped **mucogingival junction.**

At the gingival margin of each tooth is the **marginal gingiva,** or free gingiva, which forms a cuff above the neck of the tooth (Figure 2-10). The inner surface of the gingiva faces a space, the **gingival sulcus.** The gingiva between adjacent teeth is an extension of attached gingiva and is called the **interdental gingiva,** or interdental papilla.

Oral Cavity Proper

The inside of the mouth is known as the **oral cavity proper** (Figure 2-11). This is a space that is enclosed anteriorly by the maxillary and mandibular arches. Posteriorly, the opening from the oral cavity proper into the pharynx or throat is the **fauces.**

The fauces are formed laterally by the **anterior faucial pillar** and the **posterior faucial pillar** on each side. The **palatine tonsils** are located between these folds of tissue created by underlying muscles (see Chapter 11 for more information) and are what patients call their "tonsils." Included within the oral cavity proper are the palate, tongue, and floor of the mouth.

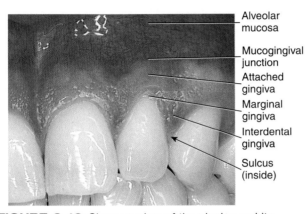

FIGURE 2-10 Close-up view of the gingiva and its associated landmarks. (From Fehrenbach MJ, Herring SW. *Illustrated Anatomy of the Head and Neck*, ed 2. WB Saunders, Philadelphia, 2002.)

PALATE

Within the oral cavity proper is the roof of the mouth or **palate** (see Chapters 5 and 11 for more discussion). The palate separates the oral cavity from the nasal cavity. The palate has two parts, an anterior portion and posterior portion (Figure 2-12). The firmer anterior portion is called the **hard palate.**

A midline ridge of tissue on the hard palate is the **median palatine raphe,** which overlies the bony fusion of the palate. A small bulge of tissue at the most anterior portion of the hard palate, lingual to the anterior teeth, is the **incisive papilla.** Directly posterior to this papilla are **palatine rugae,** which are firm, irregular ridges of tissue radiating from the papilla and raphe.

The looser posterior portion of the palate is called the **soft palate** (see Figure 2-12). A midline muscular structure, the **uvula of the palate**, hangs down from the posterior margin of the soft palate. The **pterygomandibular fold** extends from the junction of hard and soft palates down to the mandible, just behind the most distal mandibular tooth, and stretches when the mouth is opened wider. This fold covers a deeper fibrous structure and separates the cheek from the throat.

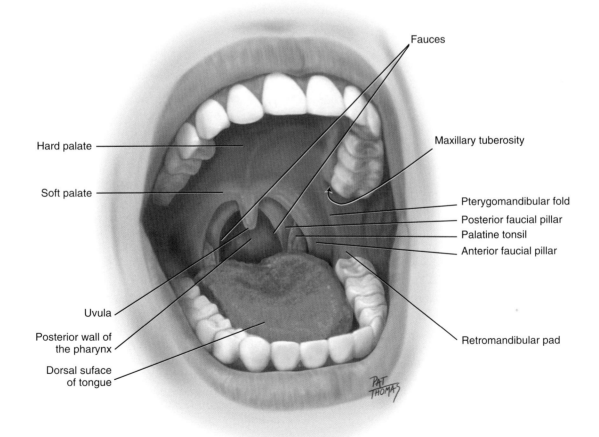

FIGURE 2-11 The oral cavity proper and the landmarks that form its boundaries. (From Fehrenbach MJ, Herring, GW. *Illustrated Anatomy of the Head and Neck*, ed 2. WB Saunders, Philadelphia, 2002.)

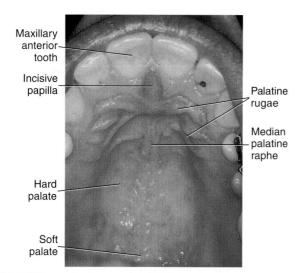

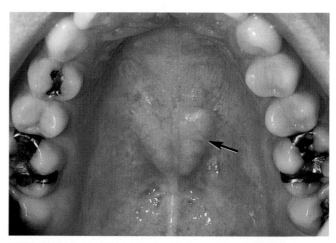

FIGURE 2-12 The palate and its landmarks. (From Fehrenbach MJ, Herring SW. *Illustrated Anatomy of the Head and Neck,* ed 2. WB Saunders, Philadelphia, 2002.)

FIGURE 2-13 The normal variation of the palatal torus (*arrow*) is noted on the midline of the hard palate.

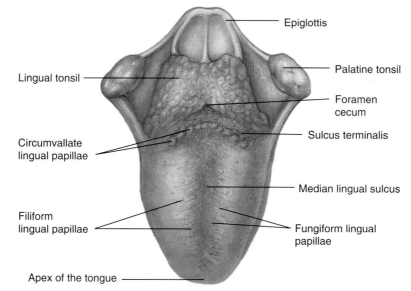

FIGURE 2-14 Dorsal view of the tongue, with its landmarks noted. (Adapted from Fehrenbach MJ, Herring SW. *Illustrated Anatomy of the Head and Neck,* ed 2. WB Saunders, Philadelphia, 2002.)

Clinical Considerations with the Palate

A normal variation noted on the midline of the hard palate is the **palatal torus** (Figure 2-13), similar to the mandibular tori. These are developmental growths of normal bone with a hereditary etiology. These tori vary in size, are slow growing and asymptomatic, and may be seen on radiographs. They interfere only when denture therapy is considered. Patients may need to be reassured. This variation must be noted on the patient's chart.

TONGUE

The tongue is a prominent feature of the oral cavity proper (Figure 2-14; see Chapters 5 and 11 for more information). The posterior third is the pharyngeal portion of the tongue, or **base of the tongue.** The base of the tongue attaches to the floor of the mouth. The base of the tongue does not lie within the oral cavity proper but within the oral part of the throat (discussed later in this chapter). The anterior two thirds of the tongue, termed the **body of the tongue,** lies within the oral cavity proper. The tip of the tongue is the **apex of the tongue.**

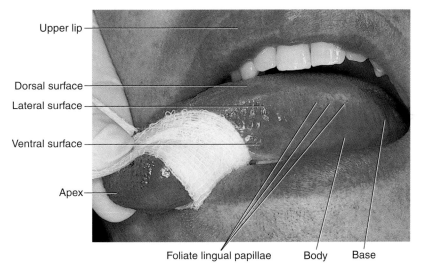

FIGURE 2-15 Lateral view of the tongue, with its portions and landmarks noted. (From Fehrenbach MJ, Herring SW. *Illustrated Anatomy of the Head and Neck,* ed 2. WB Saunders, Philadelphia, 2002.)

Certain surfaces of the tongue have small elevated structures of specialized mucosa called **lingual papillae,** some of which are associated with **taste buds.** Taste buds are the specialized organs of taste.

The top, or **dorsal surface of the tongue,** has a midline depression, the **median lingual sulcus,** corresponding to the position of a midline fibrous structure deeper in the tongue and fusion tissue area. The dorsal surface of the tongue also has many lingual papillae. The slender, threadlike, whitish lingual papillae are the **filiform lingual papillae,** which give the dorsal surface its velvety texture. The reddish, smaller, mushroom-shaped dots on the dorsal surface are called **fungiform lingual papillae.** Farther posteriorly on the dorsal surface of the tongue and more difficult to see clinically is an inverted V-shaped groove, the **sulcus terminalis.** The sulcus terminalis separates the base from the body of the tongue, demarcating a line of fusion of tissue in the tongue's development. Where the sulcus terminalis points backward toward the throat is a small, pitlike depression called the **foramen cecum.** The 10 to 14 large mushroom-shaped lingual papillae, the **circumvallate lingual papillae,** line up along the anterior side of the sulcus terminalis on the body. Even farther posteriorly on the dorsal surface of the base of the tongue is an irregular mass of tissue, the **lingual tonsil** (discussed further in Chapter 11).

The side or **lateral surface of the tongue** is noted for its vertical ridges of lingual papillae, called **foliate lingual papillae** (Figure 2-15).

The underside, or **ventral surface of the tongue,** is noted for its visible large blood vessels, the deep lingual veins, which pass close to the surface (Figure 2-16). Lateral to each deep lingual vein is the **plica fimbriata** with fringelike projections.

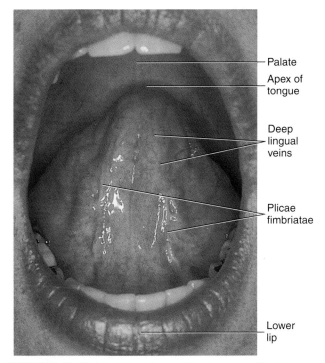

FIGURE 2-16 Ventral surface of the tongue, with its landmarks noted. (From Fehrenbach MJ, Herring SW. *Illustrated Anatomy of the Head and Neck,* ed 2. WB Saunders, Philadelphia, 2002.)

FLOOR OF THE MOUTH

The floor of the mouth is located in the oral cavity proper, inferior to the ventral surface of the tongue (Figure 2-17). The **lingual frenum** is a midline fold of tissue between the ventral surface of the tongue and the floor of the mouth.

A ridge of tissue on each side of the floor of the mouth, the **sublingual fold,** joins in a V-shaped

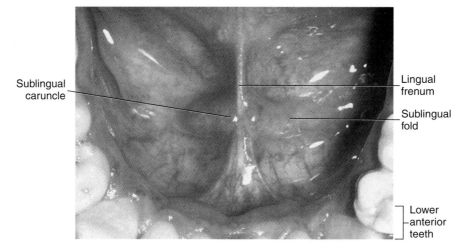

FIGURE 2-17 View of the floor of the mouth, with its landmarks noted. (From Fehrenbach MJ, Herring SW. *Illustrated Anatomy of the Head and Neck*, ed 2. WB Saunders, Philadelphia, 2002.)

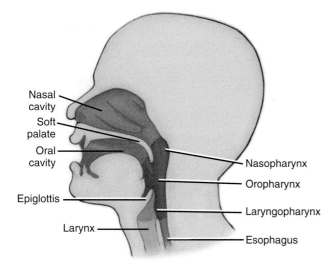

FIGURE 2-18 Midsagittal section of the head, with the divisions of the pharynx noted. (From Fehrenbach MJ, Herring SW. *Illustrated Anatomy of the Head and Neck*, ed 2. WB Saunders, Philadelphia, 2002.)

configuration extending from the lingual frenum to the base of the tongue. The sublingual folds contain openings of the sublingual duct from the **sublingual salivary gland** (see Chapters 1 and 11 for more information on salivary glands). The small papilla, or **sublingual caruncle,** at the anterior end of each sublingual fold contains openings of the **submandibular and sublingual ducts** (or Wharton's duct and Bartholin's duct, respectively) from both the **submandibular salivary gland** and sublingual salivary gland.

DIVISIONS OF THE PHARYNX

The oral cavity proper provides the entrance into the throat, or **pharynx.** The pharynx is a muscular tube that serves both the respiratory and digestive systems. It has three divisions: the nasopharynx, the oropharynx, and the laryngopharynx (Figure 2-18).

The division of the pharynx that is superior to the level of the soft palate is the **nasopharynx,** which is continuous with the nasal cavity. The division that is between the soft palate and the opening of the larynx is the **oropharynx,** which is the oral portion of the pharynx. The fauces, discussed earlier, marks the boundary between the oropharynx and the oral cavity proper. Only portions of the nasopharynx and oropharynx are visible on an intraoral examination (see Figure 2-11). The **laryngopharynx** is more inferior, close to the laryngeal opening, and thus is not visible on an intraoral examination.

DENTAL EMBRYOLOGY

CHAPTER 3

Overview of Prenatal Development

■ ■ ■

This chapter discusses the following topics:

- Prenatal development
- Preimplantation period
- Embryonic period
  - Second week
- Third week
- Fourth week
- Fetal period

■ ■ ■

After studying this chapter, the reader should be able to:

1. Define and pronounce the key terms in this chapter.
2. Discuss the periods of prenatal development, especially the major events that occur during the early weeks.
3. Integrate a background on prenatal development into the development of the face, neck, and oral structures and developmental disturbances related to these structures.

■ ■ ■

Key Terms

Amniocentesis (am-nee-o-sen-**tee**-sis)
Amniotic cavity (am-nee-**ot**-ik)
Bilaminar embryonic disc (by-**lam**-i-nar)
Bilateral symmetry
Blastocyst (**blas**-tah-sist)
Caudal end (**kaw**-dal)
Cephalic end (se-**fal**-ik)
Central nervous system
Cleavage (**kleve**-ij)
Cloacal membrane (klo-**ay**-kal)
Congenital malformations (kon-**jen**-i-til mal-for-**may**-shins)
Cytodifferentiation (site-oh-dif-er-en-she-**ay**-shun)
Differentiation (dif-er-en-she-**ay**-shun)
Down syndrome
Ectoderm (**ek**-toe-derm)
Ectodermal dysplasia (**ek**-toe-derm dis-**play**-ze-ah)
Ectopic pregnancy (ek-**top**-ik)

Embryo (**em**-bre-oh)
Embryoblast layer (**em**-bre-oh-blast)
Embryology (em-bre-**ol**-ah-jee)
Embryonic cell layers (em-bre-**on**-ik), folding, period of prenatal development
Endoderm (**en**-doe-derm)
Epiblast layer (**ep**-i-blast)
Fertilization (fur-til-uh-**zay**-shun)
Fetal alcohol syndrome
Fetal period of prenatal development (**fete**-il)
Fetus (**fete**-is)
Foregut (**fore**-gut)
Fusion (**fu**-zhin)
Growth: appositional (ap-oh-**zish**-in-al), interstitial (in-ter-**stish**-il)
Hindgut (**hind**-gut)
Histodifferentiation (his-toe-dif-er-en-she-**ay**-shun)

Hypoblast layer (**hi**-po-blast)
Implantation (im-plan-**ta**-shin)
Induction (in-**duk**-shin)
Karyotype (**kare**-e-oh-tipe)
Maturation (ma-cher-**ray**-shin)
Meiosis (my-**oh**-sis)
Mesenchyme (**mes**-eng-kime)
Mesoderm (**mes**-oh-derm)
Midgut (**mid**-gut)
Mitosis (my-**toe**-sis)
Morphodifferentiation (mor-foe-dif-er-en-she-**ay**-shun)
Morphogenesis (mor-fo-**jen**-is·is)
Morphology (mor-**fol**-ah-je)
Neural crest cells (**noor**-al), folds, groove, plate, tube
Neuroectoderm (noor-oh-**ek**-toe-derm)
Oropharyngeal membrane (or-oh-fah-**rin**-je-al)
Ovum (**oh**-vum)
Placenta (pla-**sen**-tuh)

Preimplantation period of prenatal
  development (pre-im-plan-ta-shin)
Prenatal development (pre-nay-tal)
Primitive streak
Primordium (pry-more-de-um)
Proliferation (pro-lif-er-ay-shin)
Rubella virus (roo-bell-ah)

Somites (so-mites)
Sperm
Spina bifida (spi-nah bif-ah-dah)
Syphilis spirochete (sif-i-lis
  spi-ro-keet)
Teratogens (ter-ah-to-jens)
Tetracycline staining

(tet-rah-si-kleen)
Trilaminar embryonic disc
  (try-lam-i-nar)
Trophoblast layer (trof-oh-blast)
Yolk sac
Zygote (zy-gote)

PRENATAL DEVELOPMENT

In humans, **prenatal development** begins at the start of pregnancy and continues until the birth of the child. **Embryology** is the study of prenatal development and is introduced in this beginning of *Unit II.* Prenatal development consists of three distinct periods: the preimplantation period, the embryonic period, and the fetal period (Table 3-1). The preimplantation period and the embryonic period make up the first trimester of the pregnancy, and the fetal period comprises the last two trimesters.

TABLE 3-1

Periods of Prenatal Development

	PREIMPLANTATION PERIOD	EMBRYONIC PERIOD	FETAL PERIOD
Time span	First week	Second week to eighth week	Third to ninth month
Structure(s)*	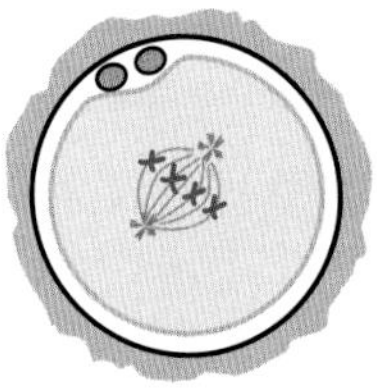 Zygote 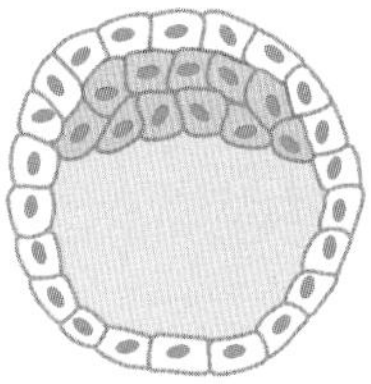 / Blastocyst	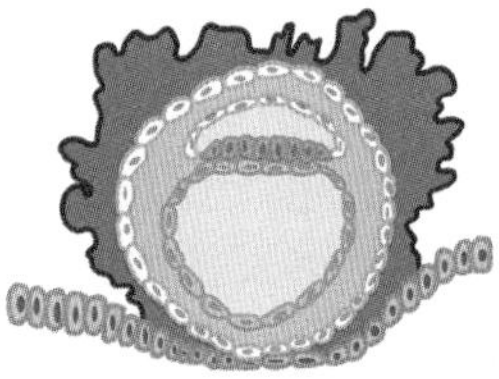 Blastocyst to Disc 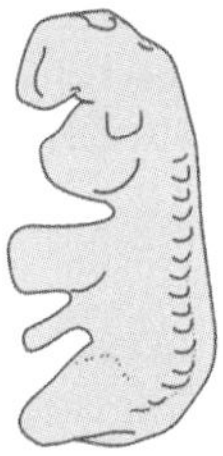 / Disc to Embryo 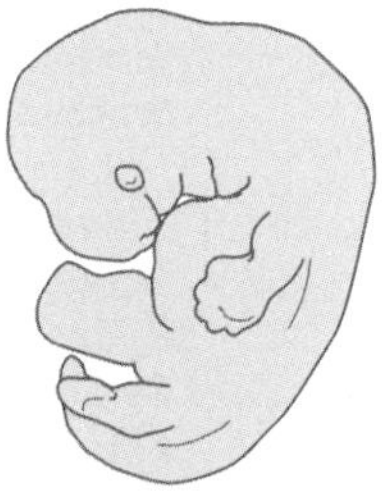 / Embryo	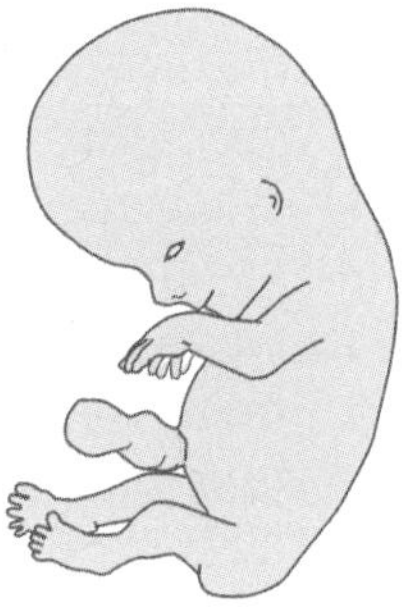 Embryo 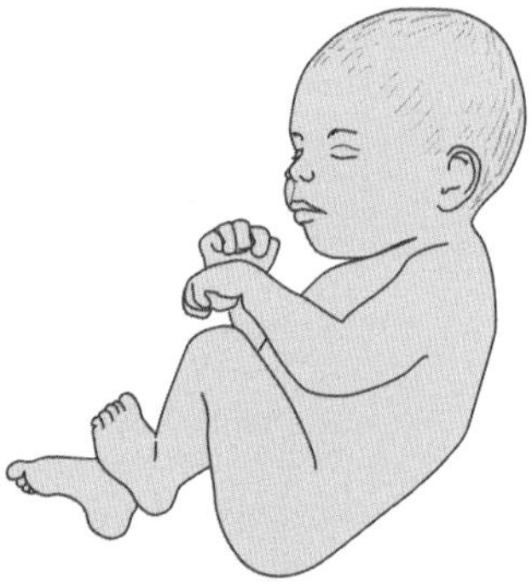 / Fetus
Structure(s) present	Zygote to blastocyst	Blastocyst to disc to embryo	Embryo to fetus
Description of period	Fertilization and implantation	Induction, proliferation, differentiation, morphogenesis, and maturation to form structures	Maturation of existing structures

*Note that structure size is not accurate or comparative.

Developmental Disturbances During
Prenatal Development

These developmental problems can include **congenital malformations,** or birth defects, which are developmental problems evident at birth. Most of these occur during both the preimplantation period and the embryonic period and thus the first trimester of the pregnancy (discussed later). Statistics show that such malformations occur with an incidence of 1 in 700 live births. This does not include anatomical variants, which are common, such as variation in the lesser details of a bone's shape.

Malformations can be due to genetic factors such as chromosome abnormalities or environmental agents or factors. These environmental agents or factors can include infections, drugs, and radiation and are called **teratogens** (Table 3-2). Women of reproductive age should avoid teratogens at the time of their first missed menstrual period and thereafter to protect the developing human (discussed later).

Malformations in the face, neck, and oral cavity range from serious clefts in the face or palate region to small deficiencies of the soft palate or cysts underneath an otherwise intact oral mucosa. It is important for dental professionals to remember that any orofacial congenital malformations discovered when examining a patient are understandable and traceable to a specific time in the embryological development of the individual. Thus one must understand the development of an individual's orofacial region, including its sequential process.

It is important for dental professionals to understand the major events of prenatal development to understand better the development of the structures of the face, neck, and oral tissue and the underlying relationships among these structures. Each of these structures has a **primordium,** the earliest indication of a part

TABLE 3-2

Known Teratogens Involved in Congenital Malformations

Drugs	Ethanol, tetracycline, phenytoin sodium, lithium, methotrexate, aminopterin, diethylstilbestrol, warfarin, thalidomide, isotretinoin (retinoic acid), androgens, progesterone
Chemicals	Methylmercury, polychlorinated biphenyls
Infections	Rubella virus, herpes simplex virus, human immunodeficiency virus, syphilis microbe
Radiation	High levels of ionizing type*

*Note that diagnostic levels of radiation should be avoided but have not been directly linked to congenital malformations.

or an organ during prenatal development. This information also helps in the appreciation of any developmental problems that may occur in these structures.

PREIMPLANTATION PERIOD OF PRENATAL DEVELOPMENT

The first period, the **preimplantation period of prenatal development,** or period of the unattached conceptus, takes place during the first week. At the beginning of the first week, a woman's **ovum** is penetrated by and united with a man's **sperm** during **fertilization** (Figure 3-1). This union of the ovum and sperm subsequently forms a fertilized egg, or **zygote.**

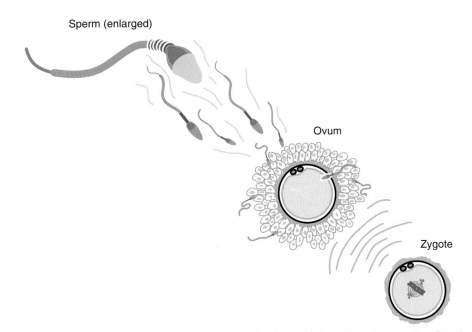

Sperm (enlarged)

Ovum

Zygote

FIGURE 3-1 The sperm fertilizes the ovum and unites with it to form the zygote, after the process of meiosis and during the first week of prenatal development. The ovum's and sperm's chromosomes join to form a zygote, a new individual.

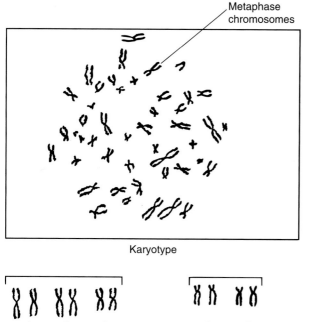

Karyotype

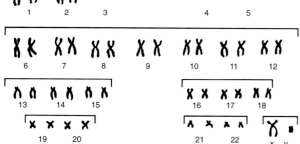

FIGURE 3-2 Example of a human karyotype, a photographic analysis of a person's chromosomes, which is done by orderly arrangement of the pairs.

During fertilization, the final stages of **meiosis** occur in the ovum. The result of this process is the joining of the ovum's chromosomes with those of the sperm. This joining of chromosomes from both biological parents forms a new individual with "shuffled" chromosomes. To allow this formation of a new individual, the sperm and ovum when joined have the proper number of chromosomes (diploid number of 46). If both these cells, sperm and ovum, carried the full complement of chromosomes, fertilization would result in a zygote with two times the proper number, resulting in severe congenital malformations and prenatal death.

This situation of excess chromosomes is avoided with meiosis, because during their development in the gonads, this process enables the ovum and sperm to reduce by one half the normal number of chromosomes (to a haploid number of 23). Thus the zygote has received half its chromosomes from the female and half from the male, with the resultant genetic material a reflection of both biological parents. The photographic analysis of a person's chromosomes is done by orderly arrangement of the pairs in a **karyotype** (Figure 3-2).

After fertilization, the zygote then undergoes **mitosis,** or individual cell division or **cleavage.** After initial cleavage, the solid ball of cells is known as a *morula.* Because of the ongoing process of mitosis and secretion of fluid by the cells within the morula, the zygote becomes a vesicle known as a **blastocyst,** or blastula (Figure 3-3). The rest of the first week is characterized by further mitotic cleavage, in which the blastocyst splits into smaller and more numerous cells as it undergoes successive cell divisions by mitosis.

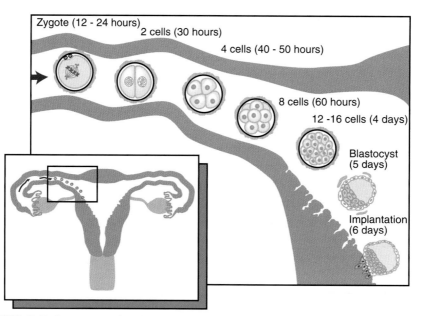

FIGURE 3-3 A zygote undergoing mitotic cleavage to form a blastocyst. After traveling, the blastocyst becomes implanted in the endometrium of the uterus.

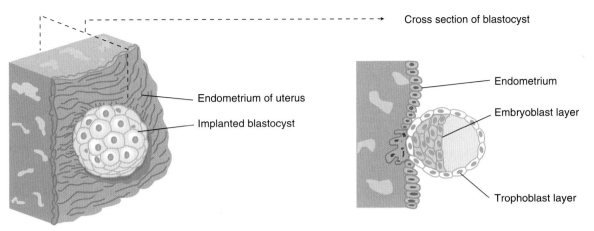

FIGURE 3-4 A blastocyst consists of a trophoblast layer and an embryoblast layer.

Mitosis takes place during growth or repair and is different from meiosis, which takes place during reproduction (mitosis is discussed further with cell structure in Chapter 7). Mitosis that occurs during cell division is the self-duplication of the chromosomes of the parent cell and their equal distribution to daughter cells. Thus the result is that the daughter cells have the same chromosome number and hereditary potential as the parent cells. As it grows by cleavage, the blastocyst travels from the site where fertilization took place to the uterus.

By the end of the first week, the blastocyst stops traveling and undergoes **implantation** and thus becomes embedded in the prepared endometrium, the innermost lining of the uterus. The ideal implantation site is the back wall of the body of the uterus toward the mother's spine. After 7 days of cleavage, the blastocyst consists of a layer of peripheral cells, the **trophoblast layer,** and a small inner mass of embryonic cells, or **embryoblast layer** (Figure 3-4). The trophoblast layer gives rise to important prenatal support tissues. The embryoblast layer gives rise to the embryo during the next prenatal period.

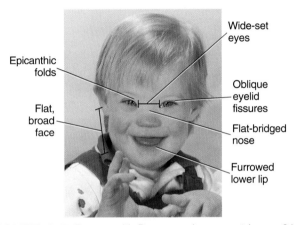

FIGURE 3-5 Person with Down syndrome, or trisomy 21, in which an extra chromosome number 21 is present after meiotic division. It is marked by certain oral and facial features. An affected child can have various levels of mental retardation. (From Zitelli BJ and Davis HW: *Atlas of Pediatric Physical Diagnosis*, ed 4, St. Louis, 2002, Mosby.)

Developmental Disturbances During Meiosis

If any disturbances occur in meiosis during fertilization, major congenital malformations result from the chromosomal abnormality. In **Down syndrome,** or trisomy 21, an extra chromosome number 21 is present after meiotic division (Figure 3-5). A child with this syndrome has a flat, broad face with wide-set eyes; a flat-bridged nose; epicanthic folds; oblique eyelid fissures; a furrowed lower lip; fissures of the tongue; hypertrophy of the lingual papillae; and other defects. An affected child can have various levels of mental retardation.

Children with Down syndrome may have increased levels of periodontal disease and fewer and abnormally shaped teeth, presenting challenges to oral hygiene care. The arched palate and poor use of tongue muscles lead to an open mouth position and protrusion of the normal-sized tongue. Therefore articulate speech is often difficult.

Implantation may occur outside the uterus, a condition called **ectopic pregnancy,** at this time and sometimes continue for up to 16 weeks of pregnancy before being noticed. Most ectopic pregnancies occur in the fallopian tube. This disturbance has several causes but is usually related to factors that delay or prevent transport of the dividing zygote to the uterus, such as scarred uterine tubes due to pelvic inflammatory disease. Ectopic pregnancies can rupture, causing loss of the embryo and threatening the life of the pregnant woman. Diagnosed quickly, ectopic pregnancies can be treated pharmacologically without surgery, reducing danger to the mother and preserving the site of the ectopic pregnancy.

EMBRYONIC PERIOD OF PRENATAL DEVELOPMENT

The second period, the **embryonic period of prenatal development,** extends from the beginning of the second week to the end of the eighth week. Certain physiological processes occur during this period (Table 3-3). These physiological processes include induction, proliferation, differentiation, morphogenesis, and maturation (discussed next). These processes cause the structure of the implanted blastocyst to become an **embryo.** These physiological processes also allow the teeth and associated structures, as well as other organ structures, to develop in the embryo (see Table 6-1).

The first physiological process involved in the beginning of most embryological development is the process of **induction,** which is the action of one group of cells on another that leads to the establishment of the developmental pathway in the responding tissue. Just what triggers cells to develop into structures from cellular interactions is poorly understood, but many problems can result from a failure of induction, leading to failure of initiation of certain embryological structures. Induction can also occur in the later stages of development.

Another type of physiological process that follows induction as well as the other processes is the dramatic process of **proliferation,** which is controlled levels of cellular growth present during most of embryological

TABLE 3-3

Developmental Processes in the Embryo

PROCESS	Description
Induction	Action of one group of cells on another that leads to the establishment of the developmental pathway in the responding tissue
Proliferation	Controlled cellular growth and accumulation of byproducts
Differentiation	Change in identical embryonic cells to become distinct structurally and functionally
Morphogenesis	Development of specific tissue structure or differing form due to embryonic cell migration and inductive interactions.
Maturation	Attainment of adult function and size due to proliferation, differentiation, and morphogenesis.

development. Finally, growth also occurs as a result of an accumulation of cellular byproducts.

Growth may be **interstitial,** which occurs from deep within a tissue or organ. In contrast, growth may be **appositional,** in which a tissue enlarges its size by the addition of layers on the outside of a structure. Soft tissue growth is usually interstitial, whereas hard tissues such as mature bone or dental tissues increase by apposition. Some tissues, such as cartilage and growing bone tissue, use both types of growth to attain their natural size.

It is important to note that growth is not just an increase in overall size, like a balloon being blown up, but involves differential rates for different tissues and organs. An example of this varied rate of growth is tooth eruption in a child, which occurs over many years, allowing for the associated growth of the jaw bones.

In the process of **differentiation,** a change occurs in the embryonic cells, which are identical genetically but become quite distinct structurally and functionally. Thus cells that perform specialized functions are formed by differentiation during the embryonic period. Although these functions are minimal at this time, the beginnings of all major tissues, organs, and organ systems are formed during this period from these specialized cells.

Differentiation occurs at various rates in the embryo. Many portions of the embryo are affected: cells, tissues, organs, and systems. Various terms describe each one of these types of differentiation, and it is important to note the specific delineation between each of them. **Cytodifferentiation** is the development of different cell types. **Histodifferentiation** is the development of different tissues within a structure. **Morphodifferentiation** is the development of the differing structure, or **morphology,** for each organ or system.

During the embryonic period, the complexity of the structure and function of these cells increases. This is accomplished by **morphogenesis,** the process of development of specific tissue structure or shape. Morphogenesis is from the migration of embryonic cells and inductive interactions of those cells. As previously mentioned, induction continues to occur during the embryonic period as a result of the new varieties of cells interacting with each other, producing an increasingly complex organism.

Finally, the physiological process of **maturation** of the tissues and organs begins during the embryological period and continues during the later fetal period. It is important to note that the physiological process of maturation of the individual tissues and organs also involves proliferation, differentiation, and morphogenesis. Thus maturation is not the attainment of just the correct adult size but also the correct adult form and function of tissues and organs.

An embryo is recognizably human at the end of the embryonic period, or the end of the eighth week, of prenatal development. This chapter discusses only the

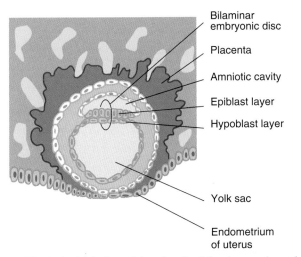

Bilaminar
embryonic disc

Placenta

Amniotic cavity

Epiblast layer

Hypoblast layer

Yolk sac

Endometrium
of uterus

FIGURE 3-6 A blastocyst forming the bilaminar embryonic disc, which consists of the epiblast layer and hypoblast layer and is surrounded by the amniotic cavity and yolk sac.

major events of the second, third, and fourth weeks of the embryonic period. The remaining weeks of prenatal development pertinent to dental practice are addressed in Chapters 4 and 5, which describe the ways in which the face, neck, and oral structures develop in the embryo.

Second Week of Prenatal Development

During the second week of prenatal development, within the embryonic period, the implanted blastocyst grows by increased proliferation of the embryonic cells, as well as cellular morphogenesis and differentiation. Every ridge, bump, and recess now indicate cellular differentiation. The increased number of embryonic cells creates the **embryonic cell layers,** or germ layers within the blastocyst. A **bilaminar embryonic disc** is eventually developed from the blastocyst (Figure 3-6). The bilaminar embryonic disc appears as a flattened, essentially circular plate of bilayered cells.

This bilaminar disc has a superior epiblast layer and an inferior **hypoblast layer.** The **epiblast layer** is composed of high columnar cells, and the hypoblast layer is composed of small cuboidal cells. The bilaminar disc develops into the embryo as prenatal development continues.

After its creation, the bilaminar disc is suspended in the uterus's endometrium between two fluid-filled cavities, the **amniotic cavity,** which faces the epiblast layer, and the **yolk sac,** which faces the hypoblast layer. The yolk sac serves as initial nourishment for the embryonic disc.

Later, the **placenta,** a prenatal organ that joins the pregnant woman and developing embryo, develops from the interactions of the trophoblast layer and endometrial tissues. The formation of the placenta and the developing umbilical circulation permit selective exchange of soluble bloodborne substances between the woman and the embryo.

Third Week of Prenatal Development

During the beginning of the third week of prenatal development, within the embryonic period, the **primitive streak** forms within the bilaminar disc (Figure 3-7). This furrowed, rod-shaped thickening in the middle of the disc results from an increased proliferation of cells in the midline area. The primitive streak causes the disc to have **bilateral symmetry,** with a right half and left half. Most of the further development of each half mirrors the other half of the embryo. If you could look at the embryo from a top view, it would resemble the sole of a shoe with the head end wider than the tail end and a slightly narrowed middle.

During the start of this third week, some cells from the epiblast layer move or migrate toward the hypoblast layer in the area of the primitive streak (Figure 3-8). These migratory cells locate in the middle between the epiblast and hypoblast layers, becoming **mesenchyme,** an embryonic connective tissue. Mesenchymal cells have the potential to proliferate and differentiate into diverse types of connective tissue–forming cells (e.g., fibroblasts, chondroblasts, and osteoblasts). Some of this tissue creates a new embryonic layer, called the **mesoderm.**

With three layers present, the bilaminar disc has become thickened into a **trilaminar embryonic disc** (Figure 3-9). Thus the trilaminar disc has three embryonic layers, or germ layers. With the creation of this new embryonic layer, the epiblast layer is now considered **ectoderm,** and the hypoblast layer is **endoderm.**

Within the trilaminar disc, each embryonic layer is distinct from the others and thus gives rise to specific tissues (Table 3-4). The ectoderm gives rise to the epidermis of the skin, the nervous system, and other structures. The mesoderm gives rise to muscle coats, connective tissues, vessels supplying tissues and organs, and other tissues. The endoderm gives rise to the epithelial linings of the respiratory passages and digestive tract, including some glandular organ cells.

Mesoderm and its related tissues are found in all areas of the future embryo except at certain embryonic membranes and the pharyngeal pouches (discussed later). In these areas without mesoderm, the ectoderm and endoderm fuse together, thereby preventing the migration of mesoderm between them.

The trilaminar disc has undergone so much growth during the past 3 weeks that certain anatomical structures of the disc become apparent. The disc now has a **cephalic end,** or head end. At the cephalic end, the **oropharyngeal membrane,** or buccopharyngeal membrane, forms. This membrane consists of only ectoderm externally and endoderm internally. This membrane is the location of the future primitive mouth of the embryo and thus the beginning of the digestive tract.

The disc also has a **caudal end,** or tail end (Figure 3-10). At the caudal end, the **cloacal membrane** forms.

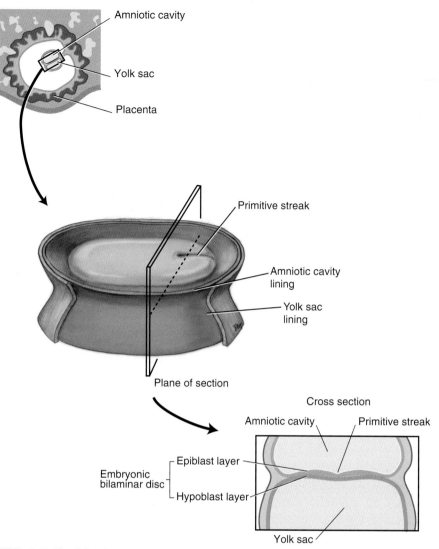

FIGURE 3-7 The bilaminar embryonic disc and formation of the primitive streak, with the resulting bilateral symmetry.

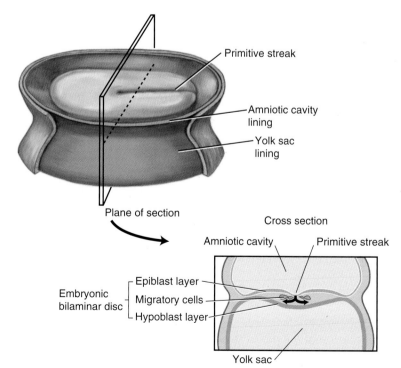

FIGURE 3-8 The bilaminar embryonic disc and migration of the epiblast layer cells toward the hypoblast layer to form a new layer, mesoderm.

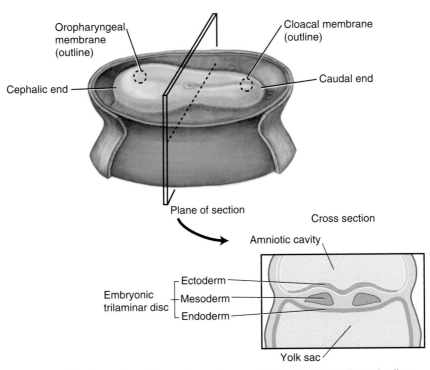

FIGURE 3-9 After formation of mesoderm, the resulting trilaminar embryonic disc consists of the ectoderm, mesoderm, and endoderm. Note the cephalic and caudal ends and also the oropharyngeal and cloacal membranes on the disc.

TABLE 3-4

Development of Embryonic Layers

	Ectoderm	Mesoderm	Endoderm	Neural Crest Cells*
Origin	Epiblast layer	Migrating cells from epiblast layer	Hypoblast layer	Migrating neuroectoderm
Morphology of the structure	Columnar	Varies	Cuboidal	Varies
Future systemic tissues	Epidermis; sensory epithelium of the eyes, ears, nose, nervous system, and neural crest cells; mammary and cutaneous glands	Dermis, muscle, bone, lymphatics, blood cells and bone marrow, cartilage, reproductive and excretory organs	Respiratory and digestive system linings, liver and pancreatic cells	Portions of the nervous system pigment cells, connective tissue proper, cartilage, bone, and certain dental tissues

*Note that the neural crest cells are included, but they are not present in the embryonic disc until the later portion of the third week. Many embryologists consider these cells from the neuroectoderm to be a fourth embryonic layer.

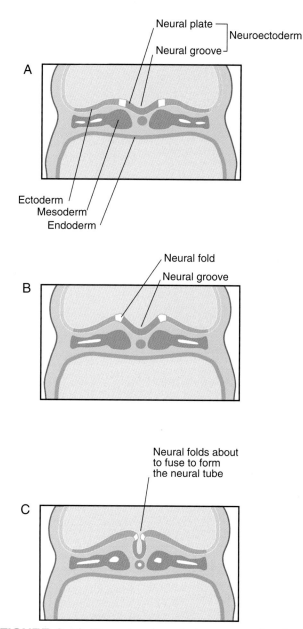

FIGURE 3-10 The embryo's central nervous system is beginning to form. This process includes several steps. **A:** Formation of the neuroectoderm from the ectoderm and its location at the neural plate. **B:** The neural plate then thickens to form the neural groove, surrounded by the neural folds. **C:** Then these folds meet and fuse, forming the neural tube.

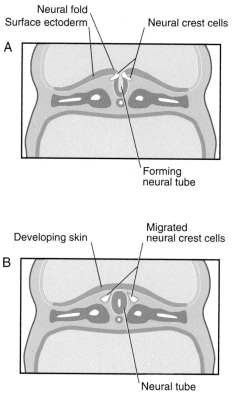

FIGURE 3-11 Neural crest cells from the neural folds **(A)** will migrate and disperse within the mesenchyme **(B)**.

This is the location of the future anus, the terminal end of the digestive tract. Similar to the oropharyngeal membrane, the cloacal membrane consists of only two embryonic layers, without any mesoderm.

During the later part of the third week of prenatal development, the **central nervous system (CNS)** begins to develop in the embryo. Many steps occur during this week to form the beginnings of the spinal cord and brain (the CNS is discussed further in Chapter 8). First, a specialized group of cells differentiates from the ectoderm. These cells are the **neuroectoderm**, and they are localized to the neural plate of

the embryo. The **neural plate** is a band of cells that extends the length of the embryo, from the cephalic end to the caudal end. This plate undergoes further growth and thickening, which cause it to deepen and invaginate centrally, forming the **neural groove.**

Near the end of the third week, the neural groove deepens further and is surrounded by the **neural folds.** As further growth of the neuroectoderm occurs, the neural folds meet superior to the neural groove, and a **neural tube** is formed during the fourth week. The neural tube undergoes **fusion** at its most superior portion and forms the future spinal cord as well as other neural tissues (see Table 3-4).

Other areas of the embryo also undergo fusion during the third week of prenatal development and in subsequent weeks, as the embryo develops. Unlike the process that the name *fusion* implies, this is usually not the joining of two separate surfaces on the embryo, as with the neural tube or later with the palate. In the case of facial fusion, the process of fusion is mainly the elimination of a groove between two adjacent swellings of tissues or processes on the surface of the embryo caused by merging of underlying tissues and migration into the groove. (The fusion of facial tissues is discussed in Chapter 4.)

In addition, during the third week, another specialized group of cells, the **neural crest cells,** develop from neuroectoderm (Figure 3-11). These cells migrate from the crests of the neural folds and disperse within the mesenchyme. These migrated cells are involved in the development of many face and neck structures, such as the branchial arches.

On reaching their predetermined destinations, the neural crest cells undergo differentiation into diverse cell types that are in part specified by local environmental influences. Many embryologists consider the neural crest cells to be a fourth embryonic layer (see Table 3-4). In the future, these cells are involved in the formation of portions of the nervous system, pigment cells, connective tissue proper, cartilage, bone, and certain dental tissues (by influencing ectomesenchyme), such as the pulp, dentin, cementum, and periodontal ligament. Thus neural crest cells are essential in the development of the face, neck, and oral tissues and are discussed further in Chapters 4 to 6.

By the end of the third week, the mesoderm additionally differentiates and begins to divide into paired cuboidal aggregates of cells called **somites** (Figure 3-12). These 38 paired blocks of mesoderm are located on each side of the developing midline portion of the central nervous system in the embryonic disc. The somites later appear as distinct elevations on the surface of the embryo. They continue to develop in the following weeks of prenatal development. The somites give rise to most of the skeletal structures of the head, neck, and trunk as well as the associated muscles and dermis of the skin.

Fourth Week of Prenatal Development

During the fourth week of prenatal development, the disc undergoes **embryonic folding** into an embryo, establishing for the first time the human axis and placing the tissues in their proper positions for further

Developmental Disturbance with Ectoderm

The syndrome of **ectodermal dysplasia** involves the abnormal development of one or more ectodermal structures (Figure 3-13). This syndrome has a hereditary etiology, and affected persons may have abnormalities of the teeth, skin, hair, nails, eyes, facial structure, and glands, because these are derived from ectoderm or associated embryological tissues. Children with all the features of this syndrome resemble "little old men." Persons with ectodermal dysplasia may suffer from partial or complete anodontia, the absence of some or all teeth in each dentition (see Chapter 6 for more discussion). The teeth present for both dentitions have frequent malformations. Partial or full dentures are used for both functional and cosmetic purposes and need to be reconstructed periodically as the jaws continue to grow. Implants may be considered after growth halts, if enough alveolar bone is present.

embryonic development. The folding of the flat embryonic disc also results in a somewhat tubular embryo (Figure 3-14). This folding results from extensive proliferation of the ectoderm and differentiation of basic tissues. This occurs mainly at the cephalic end, where the brain will form. This tissue grows beyond the oropharyngeal membrane and overhangs the developing heart.

Folding due to increased growth occurs not only at the cephalic end but also at the caudal end and at the sides of the embryo simultaneously. As a result of this folding, the positions of the embryonic layers take on a more recognizable placement for the further development of the embryo.

After folding of the disc, the endoderm lies inside the ectoderm, with mesoderm filling in the areas

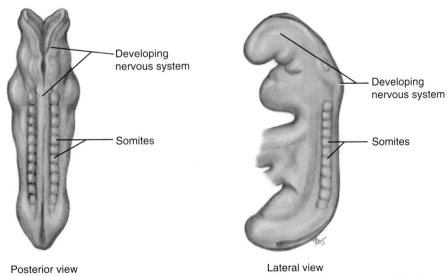

Posterior view   Lateral view

FIGURE 3-12 Differentiated mesoderm gives rise to the somites that are located on the sides of the developing nervous system.

between these two layers. This forms one long, hollow tube lined by endoderm from the cephalic end to the caudal end of the embryo—specifically, from the oropharyngeal membrane to the cloacal membrane. This tube is the future digestive tract and is separated into three major regions: the foregut, the midgut, and the hindgut.

The anterior portion of this tube is the **foregut,** which forms the primitive pharynx, or throat, and includes a portion of the primitive yolk sac as it becomes enclosed with folding. The other more posterior portions, the **midgut** and **hindgut,** form the rest

of the pharynx as well as the remainder of the digestive tract. During development of the digestive tract, four pairs of pouches form from evaginations on the lateral walls lining the pharynx. These are called the pharyngeal pouches (see Chapter 4).

Finally, during the fourth week, the face and neck begin to develop, with the primitive eyes, ears, nose, oral cavity, and jaw areas. The development of the face and neck is discussed in Chapter 4, and the development of the associated oral structures is described in Chapters 5 and 6.

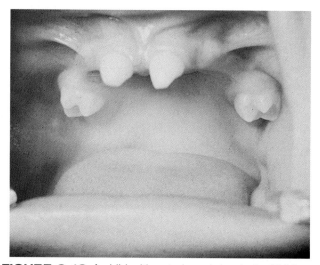

FIGURE 3-13 A child with ectodermal dysplasia. Children with this syndrome have abnormal development of ectodermal structures, resulting in certain facial features and an absence of teeth, or anodontia (partial in this case).

FETAL PERIOD OF PRENATAL DEVELOPMENT

The **fetal period of prenatal development** follows the embryonic period. The fetal period encompasses the beginning of the ninth week, or third month, to the ninth month. This is a period of time of maturation of existing structures as the embryo enlarges to become a **fetus.** This process involves not only the physiological process of maturation of the individual tissues and organs but also proliferation, differentiation, and morphogenesis.

Although developmental changes are not as dramatic as those that occur during the embryonic period, they are important because they allow the newly formed tissues and organs to function. Even though the embryo has been breathing since the third week, by the end of the fourth month, the fetal heartbeat can be detected. By the end of the 4-month mark, fetal movements can be felt by the pregnant woman.

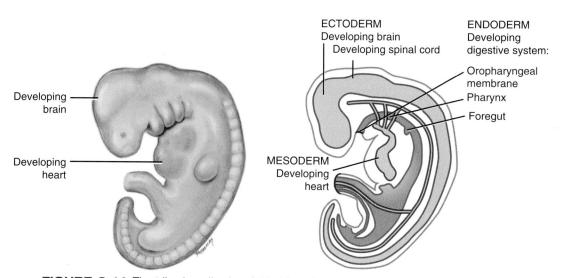

FIGURE 3-14 The trilaminar disc has folded into the embryo as a result of extensive growth of the ectoderm. The endoderm is thus inside the ectoderm, with the mesoderm filling in the areas between these two tissues, except at the two embryonic membranes. Note the developing brain, heart, and digestive tract.

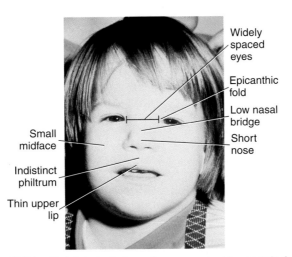

Widely spaced eyes

Epicanthic fold

Low nasal bridge

Short nose

Small midface

Indistinct philtrum

Thin upper lip

FIGURE 3-15 Child with fetal alcohol syndrome, marked by certain facial features and various levels of mental retardation. This syndrome is caused by the pregnant woman's use of ethanol during the embryonic period. (From Streissguth, Dwyer, Martin, and Smith: Teratogenic effects of alcohol in humans and laboratory animals. *Science* 209:18, 1990. Copyright 1990 American Association for the Advancement of Science.)

Developmental Disturbances During the Embryonic Period

Because the beginnings of all essential external and internal structures are formed during the embryonic period, this is considered the most critical period of development. Developmental disturbances during this period may give rise to major congenital malformations of the embryo (as discussed earlier in this chapter). Any teratogens can cross by way of the placenta. Thus teratogens can be present during the active differentiation of an organ or tissue, possibly raising the incidence of these malformations.

An example of an infective teratogen is the rubella virus. Rubella can be transmitted by way of the placenta to the embryo from the pregnant woman. This infection of the embryo can result in cataracts, cardiac defects, and deafness in the child. Another infective teratogen for the embryo is the **syphilis spirochete,** *Treponema pallidum,* because it produces defects in the incisors and molars as well as blindness, deafness, and paralysis. (Defects of the teeth are discussed in Chapters 16 and 17, respectively.)

An example of the result of a teratogenic drug effect during the embryonic period is **fetal alcohol syndrome.** Ethanol ingested by a pregnant woman easily crosses the placenta and can result in prenatal and postnatal growth deficiency, mental retardation, and other anomalies. An affected child may have a cluster of facial changes, such as small head circumference, a low nasal bridge, a short nose, a small midface, widely spaced eyes with epicanthic folds and eyelid fissures, an indistinct philtrum, and a thin upper lip (Figure 3-15). Oral changes such as anterior open bite and crowding of the dentition, mouth breathing, and

related gingivitis may occur, possibly on account of an increase in the habit of finger sucking.

Direct exposure to high levels of radiation can act as an environmental teratogen during the embryonic period. Radiation may injure embryonic cells, resulting in cell death, chromosome injury, and retardation of mental development and physical growth. The severity of embryonic damage is related to the absorbed dose, the dose rate, and the state of embryonic or fetal development at the time of exposure.

Human congenital abnormalities have not been proved to be caused by a diagnostic level of radiation such as that used in dentistry. Scattered radiation from a radiographic examination of the oral cavity administers a dose of only a few millirads to a pregnant woman. This amount is not teratogenic to an embryo. Nevertheless, even this small dose should be avoided unless an emergency situation requires it. Proper protective precautions should be used with all patients and, as always, with health-care personnel.

Failure of fusion of the neural tube results in neural tube defects of the tissue overlying the spinal cord, such as the meninges, vertebral arches, muscles, and skin. One type of neural tube defect is **spina bifida,** characterized by defects in the vertebral arches and various degrees of disability. Nutritional and environmental factors have an important role as teratogens that cause neural tube defects. Folic acid supplements are now being recommended during pregnancy to help prevent this defect as well as to prevent cleft lip and palate.

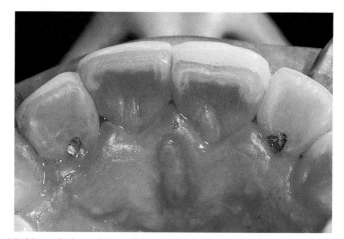

FIGURE 3-16 Lingual view of the permanent maxillary anterior teeth showing tetracycline staining. This staining was caused by the child's ingestion of the drug. Note the presence of prosthetic veneer crowns on the facial surface of the two central incisors. Similar staining can be seen in the primary dentition if the pregnant woman ingested the drug during the fetal period.

Developmental Disturbances During the Fetal Period

Congenital malformations can also occur during the fetal period. In **amniocentesis,** the most common invasive prenatal diagnostic procedure, amniotic fluid is sampled during the fourteenth to sixteenth weeks after the last missed menstrual period. It is performed in women of older age groups, when one or both parents have a chromosomal abnormality or neural tube defect, when a previous child was affected, or when the parents are carriers of inborn errors of metabolism or X-linked disorders such as hemophilia.

Systemic tetracycline antibiotic therapy of the pregnant woman can act as a teratogenic drug during the fetal period. This therapy of the woman can result in permanent tetracycline staining of the child's teeth or primary teeth that are developing at that time. This intrinsic yellow to yellow-brown **tetracycline staining** of the teeth can occur in slight, moderate, or severe degrees. The antibiotic becomes chemically bound to the dentin for the life of the tooth, and because of the transparency of enamel, this stain is visible (see Chapter 13 for more discussion).

The adult teeth, or permanent teeth, may also be affected if the drug is given during their development (Figure 3-16). If the permanent teeth are involved, treatment may require full-coverage crowns or veneers to alter the appearance of the teeth, although in some cases, vital tooth whitening may even out the coloration. Thus this type of antibiotic therapy should be avoided in pregnant women and children. Studies are now showing that overuse of amoxicillin in children with ear, nose, and throat infections may be involved in changes in enamel.

CHAPTER 4

Development of the Face and Neck

This chapter discusses the following topics:

- Development of the face

  - Stomodeum and oral cavity formation

  - Mandibular arch and lower face formation

  - Frontonasal process and upper face formation

  - Maxillary process and midface formation

- Development of the neck

  - Primitive pharynx formation

  - Branchial apparatus formation

After studying this chapter, the reader should be able to:

1. Define and pronounce the key terms in this chapter.
2. Discuss the events that occur during the development of the face and neck.
3. Integrate the knowledge of the development of the face and neck into understanding the observed structures and any developmental disturbances of these structures.

Key Terms

Branchial apparatus (brang-ke-al ap-pah-**ra**-tis), arches, grooves
Cervical cysts (ser-vi-kal)
Cleft lip (kleft)
Foregut (fore-gut)
Frontonasal process (frun-to-**nay**-zill)
Fusion (fu-zhin)
Hyoid arch (hi-oid)
Intermaxillary segment (in-ter-mak-si-lare-ee)
Lateral nasal processes

Mandibular arch, processes (man-dib-you-lar), symphysis (sim-fi-sis)
Maxillary process (mak-si-lare-ee)
Meckel's cartilage (mek-els)
Medial nasal processes
Nasal pits
Nasolacrimal groove (nay-zo-lak-ri-mal)
Neural crest cells
Oral epithelium (ep-ee-thee-lee-um)

Oropharyngeal membrane (or-oh-fah-**rin**-je-al)
Oronasal membrane (or-oh-**nay**-zil)
Pharyngeal pouches (fah-rin-je-il)
Placodes (plak-odes), lens, nasal (nay-zil), otic (o-tik)
Primitive pharynx (fare-inks)
Reichert's cartilage (rike-erts)
Stomodeum (sto-mo-**de**-um)

DEVELOPMENT OF THE FACE

The face and its related tissues begin to form during the fourth week of prenatal development, within the embryonic period. During this time, the rapidly growing brain of the embryo bulges over the oropharyngeal membrane and developing heart (Figures 4-1 and 4-2). The area of the future face is now squeezed between the developing brain and heart (see Chapter 3). Dental professionals must obtain knowledge about the development of the face to understand its underlying structural relationships and any developmental disturbances that may be present.

All three embryonic layers are involved in facial development (Table 4-1 and Box 4-1) (detailed information on the layers is discussed in Chapter 3). This development includes the formation of the primitive mouth, mandibular arch, maxillary process, frontonasal process, and nose. Facial development depends on the five facial processes (also called *prominences*) that form during the fourth week and surround the embryo's primitive mouth: the single frontonasal process and the paired maxillary and mandibular processes (Figure 4-3). These facial processes are then the centers of growth for the face. If the adult face is divided into thirds—upper, middle, and lower portions—these portions roughly correspond to the centers of facial growth. The upper portion of the face is derived from the frontonasal process, the middle from the maxillary processes, and the lower from the mandibular processes.

This facial development that starts in the fourth week will be completed later in the twelfth week, within the fetal period. The face changes shape considerably as it grows. Thus facial proportions develop during the fetal period. The development of the related oral structures is occurring at the same time and is discussed next in Chapter 5.

Most of the facial tissues develop by **fusion** of swellings or tissues on the *same* surface of the embryo (as discussed in Chapter 3). A cleft or groove is initially located between these adjacent swellings as they are created by growth, morphogenesis, and differentiation. During this type of fusion, these grooves are usually eliminated by underlying mesenchymal tissues migrating into the groove, making the embryonic surface smooth (Figure 4-4). This migration takes place because adjacent mesenchyme grows and merges beneath the external ectoderm. A slight groove or line is sometimes left on the facial surface, showing where the fusion of the swellings took place (see Chapter 2 for a discussion of facial lines). An exception to this type of facial fusion is what occurs during palatal development (see Chapter 5). In contrast to facial fusion, palatal fusion allows the fusion of swellings or tissue from *different* surfaces of the embryo.

The overall growth of the face is in an inferior and anterior direction in relation to the cranial base. The growth of the upper face is initially the most rapid, in keeping with its association with the developing brain. The forehead then ceases to grow significantly after age 12. In contrast, the middle and lower portions of the face grow more slowly over a prolonged period of

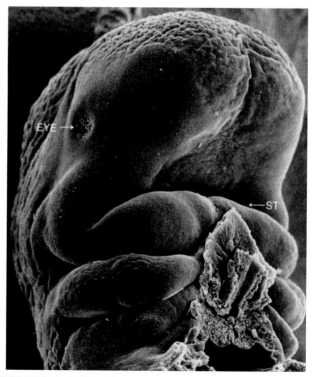

FIGURE 4-2 Scanning electron micrograph from a landmark article of the head and neck of an embryo at 4 weeks, showing the developing brain, face, and heart. Note the stomodeum (ST) and developing eye. (From Hinrichsen K: The early development of morphology and patterns of the face in the human embryo. *Advanced Anatomy of the Embryological Cell Biology* 98:1-79, 1985.)

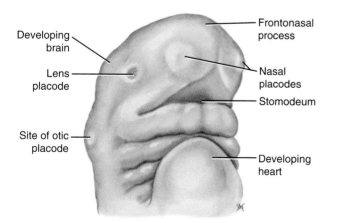

FIGURE 4-1 The embryo at the fourth week of prenatal development. The developing brain, face, and heart are noted.

TABLE 4-1

Embryonic Development of the Face

Embryonic Structures	Origin	Future Tissues
Stomodeum	Ectodermal depression enlarged by disintegration of oropharyngeal membrane	Oral cavity proper
Mandibular arch (first branchial arch)	Fused mandibular processes and neural crest cells	Lower lip, lower face, mandible with associated tissues (other arch derivatives in Table 4-2)
Maxillary process(es)	Superior and anterior swelling(s) from mandibular arch and neural crest cells	Midface, upper lip sides, cheeks, secondary palate, posterior portion of maxilla with associated tissues, zygomatic bones, portion of temporal bones
Frontonasal process	Ectodermal tissue and neural crest cells	Medial and lateral nasal processes
Nasal pits	Nasal placodes	Nasal cavities
Medial nasal process(es)	Frontonasal process medial to nasal pits	Middle of nose, philtrum region, intermaxillary segment
Intermaxillary segment	Fused medial nasal processes	Anterior portion of maxilla with associated tissues, primary palate, nasal septum
Lateral nasal process(es)	Frontonasal process lateral to nasal pits	Nasal alae
Nasolacrimal cord	Nasolacrimal groove	Lacrimal sac, nasolacrimal duct

---

BOX 4-1

Facial Development within the Fourth Week of Prenatal Development

Developmental Events
- Disintegration of the oropharyngeal membrane of the stomodeum enlarges the primitive mouth, allowing access to the primitive pharynx.
- Mandibular processes fuse to form the mandibular arch.
- Frontonasal process forms and gives rise to the nasal placodes, nasal pits, medial and lateral nasal processes, and intermaxillary segment.
- Maxillary process forms from mandibular arch.
- Maxillary process fuses with each medial nasal process to form the upper lip and with each mandibular arch to form the labial commissures.

time and finally cease to grow late in puberty. The eruption of the permanent third molars at approximately 17 to 21 years of age marks the end of the major growth of the lower two thirds of the face. The underlying facial bones developing also at this time depend on centers of bone formation by intramembranous ossification. (Bone development is discussed in Chapter 8.)

Stomodeum and Oral Cavity Formation

The primitive mouth, or **stomodeum**, initially appears as a shallow depression in the embryonic surface ectoderm at the cephalic end before the fourth week (see Figures 4-1 and 4-2). At this time, the stomodeum is limited in depth by the **oropharyngeal membrane.** This temporary membrane, consisting of external ectoderm overlying endoderm, was formed during the third week of prenatal development. The membrane also separates the stomodeum from the **primitive pharynx.** The primitive pharynx is the cranial portion of the foregut, the beginning of the future digestive tract.

The first event in the development of the face, during the fourth week of prenatal development, is disintegration of the oropharyngeal membrane (Figure 4-5). With this disintegration of the membrane, the primitive mouth is increased in depth, enlarging it. Access now occurs by way of the stomodeum from the internal primitive pharynx to the outside fluids of the amniotic cavity that surround the embryo. In the future, the stomodeum will give rise to the oral cavity,

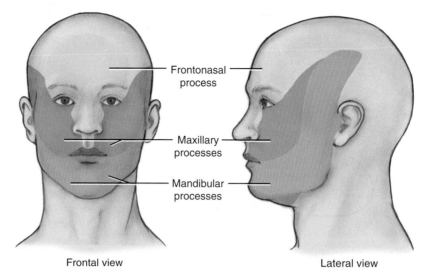

FIGURE 4-3 The adult face and its embryonic derivatives of five facial processes: the single frontonasal process and the paired maxillary and mandibular processes.

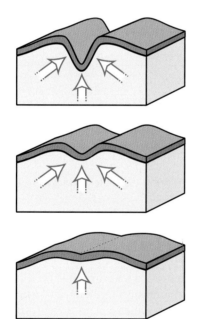

FIGURE 4-4 Facial fusion. This type of fusion involves elimination of a groove between two adjacent swellings of tissue on the *same* surface of the embryo, unlike palatal fusion, which is the fusion of two separate structures from two *different* surfaces.

which will be lined by **oral epithelium,** derived from ectoderm as a result of embryonic folding. The oral epithelium and underlying tissues will give rise to the teeth and associated tissues (see Chapter 6 for more discussion).

Mandibular Arch and Lower Face Formation

After formation of the stomodeum but still within the fourth week, two bulges of tissue appear inferior to the

primitive mouth, the two **mandibular processes** (see Figure 4-5). These processes consist of a core of mesenchyme formed in part by neural crest cells that migrate to the facial region, covered externally by ectoderm and internally by endoderm.

These paired mandibular processes then fuse at the midline to form the **mandibular arch.** After fusion, the mandibular arch then extends as a band of tissue inferior to the stomodeum and between the developing brain and heart. In the midline on the surface of the bony mandible is a faint ridge, an indication of the **mandibular symphysis,** where the mandible is formed by fusion of right and left processes (see Chapter 5). The mandibular arch and its related tissues are the first portions of the face to form after the creation of the stomodeum.

The mandibular arch is also considered the first branchial arch (discussed later). Thus this tissue depends on neural crest cells for its formation, as do all branchial arches. During the growth of the mandibular arch, cartilage forms within each side of the arch, and each cartilage is known as **Meckel's cartilage** (Table 4-2). Most of this cartilage disappears as the bony mandible forms by intramembranous ossification lateral to and in close association with it, yet only some of Meckel's cartilage makes a contribution to it (see Chapter 5). A portion of the cartilage participates in the formation of the middle ear bones.

In the future, the mandibular arch directly gives rise to the lower face, including the lower lip. The mandibular arch will also give rise to the mandible, with its mandibular teeth and associated tissues. The embryo's mandible initially appears underdeveloped, but it achieves its characteristic form as it develops further during the fetal period (see Chapter 5).

A part of the perichondrium surrounding Meckel's cartilage becomes ligaments of the jaws and middle

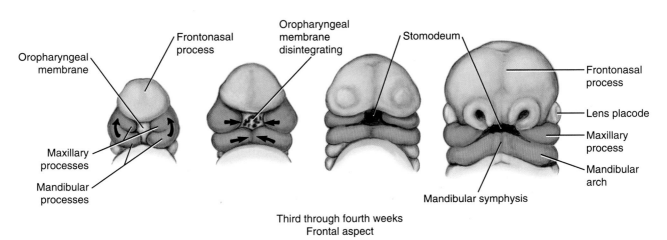

Third through fourth weeks
Frontal aspect

FIGURE 4-5 Disintegration of the oropharyngeal membrane enlarges the stomodeum of the embryo and allows access between the primitive mouth and the primitive pharynx. The mandibular processes also fuse, forming the mandibular arch inferior to the enlarged stomodeum.

TABLE 4-2

Branchial Arches and Derivative Structures

Arches	Future Nerves and Muscles	Future Skeletal Structures and Ligaments
First arches (mandibular)	Trigeminal nerve, muscles of mastication, mylohyoid and anterior belly of digastric, tensor tympani, tensor veli palatini muscles	Malleus and incus of middle ear, including anterior ligament of the malleus, sphenomandibular ligament, and portions of sphenoid bone (see also Table 4-1)
Second arches (hyoid)	Facial nerve, stapedius muscle, muscles of facial expression, posterior belly of the digastric muscle, stylohyoid muscle	Stapes and portions of malleus and incus of middle ear, stylohyoid ligament, styloid process of the temporal bone, lesser cornu of hyoid bone, upper portion of body of hyoid bone
Third arches	Glossopharyngeal nerve, stylopharyngeal muscle	Greater cornu of hyoid bone, lower portion of body of hyoid bone
Fourth through sixth arches	Superior laryngeal branch and recurrent laryngeal branch of vagus nerve, levator veli palatini muscles, pharyngeal constrictors, intrinsic muscles of the larynx	Laryngeal cartilages

ear. The mesoderm of the mandibular arch forms the muscles of mastication, as well as some palatal muscles and suprahyoid muscles. Thus because these muscles are derived from the mandibular arch, they are innervated by the nerve of the first arch, the fifth cranial nerve, the trigeminal nerve. The mandibular arch is also involved in the formation of the tongue (see Chapter 5).

During the fifth and sixth weeks, primitive muscle cells from the mesoderm in the mandibular arch begin to differentiate. These primitive muscle cells become oriented to the site of origin and insertion of the masticatory muscles that they will form. By the seventh week, the mandibular muscle mass has enlarged, and

the cells have begun to migrate into the areas where they will begin to differentiate into the four muscles of mastication: the masseter, medial and lateral pterygoids, and temporalis muscles. Muscle cell migration occurs before bone formation in the facial area.

By the tenth week, the mandibular muscle masses have become well organized bilaterally into the four muscles of mastication. Nerve branches from the trigeminal cranial nerve are incorporated early in these muscle masses. The muscle cells of the masseter and medial pterygoid muscles have formed a vertical sling that inserts into the site that will form the angle of the mandible. The temporalis muscle has differentiated in the temporal fossa and is inserting into the developing coronoid process. The lateral pterygoid muscle cells, which arise from the infratemporal fossa, extend horizontally into the condylar neck and the articular disc.

Frontonasal Process and Upper Face Formation

During this fourth week, the **frontonasal process** (see Figure 4-1) also forms. The frontonasal process is a bulge of tissue in the upper facial area, at the most cephalic end of the embryo, and is the cranial boundary of the stomodeum. In the future, the frontonasal process gives rise to the upper face, which includes the forehead, bridge of the nose, primary palate, nasal septum, and all structures related to the medial nasal processes.

PLACODE DEVELOPMENT

On the outer surface of the embryo are placodes, which are rounded areas of specialized, thickened ectoderm found at the location of developing special sense organs. Note that the facial area of the embryo has two **lens placodes,** which are on each side of the frontonasal process (see Figures 4-1 and 4-2). Later in development, these lens placodes migrate medially from their lateral positions and form the future eyes and related tissues.

The **otic placodes** are even more laterally and posteriorly placed and form pits that create the future internal ear and related tissues as they appear to rise to their mature position as a result of their relative growth. Portions of the nearby branchial apparatus of the embryonic neck later form the external and middle ear (discussed later).

In addition to the lens and otic placodes, the **nasal placodes** form in the anterior portion of the frontonasal process, just superior to the stomodeum, during the fourth week (see Figure 4-1). These two buttonlike structures form as bilateral ectodermal thickenings that later develop into olfactory cells for the sensation of smell, located in the mature nose.

NOSE AND PARANASAL SINUS FORMATION

During the fourth week, the tissue around the nasal placodes on the frontonasal process undergoes growth, thus starting the development of the nose. The placodes then become submerged, forming a depression in the center of each placode, the **nasal pits** or olfactory pits (Figure 4-6). These nasal pits later develop into the nasal cavities. Deepening of the nasal pits produces a nasal sac that grows internally toward the developing brain. At first the nasal sacs are separated from the stomodeum by the **oronasal membrane.** This temporary membrane disintegrates, bringing the nasal and oral cavities into communication in the area of the primitive choanae, posterior to the developing primary palate. At the same time, the superior, middle, and inferior conchae are developing on the lateral walls of the developing nasal cavities.

Some of the paranasal sinuses develop later during the fetal period, and others develop after birth. All form as outgrowths of the walls of the nasal cavities and become air-filled extensions of the nasal cavities in the adjacent bones, such as in the maxillae and the frontal bone. The development of the paranasal sinuses with their histology is discussed further in Chapter 11.

The middle portion of the tissue growing around the nasal placodes appears as two crescent-shaped swellings located between the nasal pits. These are named the **medial nasal processes** (see Figure 4-6). In the future, the medial nasal processes will fuse together externally to form the middle portion of the nose from the root to the apex and the center portion of the upper lip and also the philtrum region.

The paired medial nasal processes also fuse internally and grow inferiorly on the inside of the stomodeum, forming the **intermaxillary segment,** or premaxillary segment (Figure 4-7; see also Figure 5-1). The intermaxillary segment is involved in the formation of the maxillary incisor teeth and associated tissues, primary palate, and nasal septum. (The latter two items are discussed in Chapter 5.)

On the outer portion of the nasal pits are two other crescent-shaped swellings, the **lateral nasal processes** (see Figure 4-6). In the future, the lateral nasal processes form the alae, or sides of the nose. Fusion of the lateral nasal, maxillary, and medial nasal processes forms the nares, or nostrils. The embryonic nose remains visually flat, however, until the fetal period, when facial development is completed.

Maxillary Process and Midface Formation

During the fourth week of prenatal development, within the embryonic period, an adjacent swelling forms from increased growth of the mandibular arch. This swelling, the **maxillary process,** grows superiorly and anteriorly on each side of the stomodeum (see Figure 4-5). Because it is formed from the mandibular arch, the maxillary process is also formed from mesenchyme provided by neural crest cells.

In the future, the maxillary processes will form the midface. This includes the sides of the upper lip, the cheeks, the secondary palate, and the posterior portion of the maxilla, with the maxillary canines and posterior teeth and associated tissues. This tissue also forms the zygomatic bones and portions of the temporal bones.

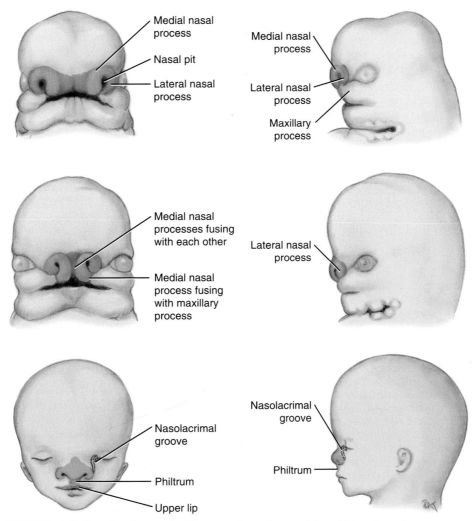

FIGURE 4-6 The development of the nose from the medial and lateral nasal processes.

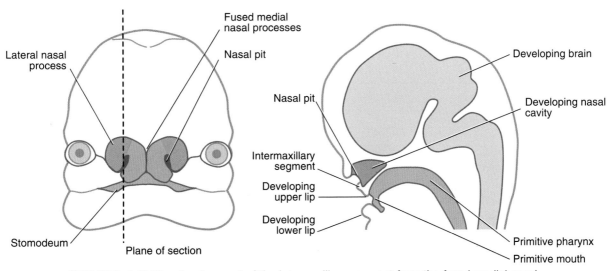

FIGURE 4-7 The development of the intermaxillary segment from the fused medial nasal processes on the inside of the stomodeum.

UPPER LIP AND LABIAL COMMISSURE FORMATION

During the fourth week, the upper lip is formed when each maxillary process fuses with each medial nasal process as a result of the underlying growth of the mesenchyme (see Figure 4-6). Thus the maxillary processes contribute to the sides of the upper lip, and the two medial nasal processes contribute to the middle of the upper lip. Fusion of these processes to form the upper lip is completed during the sixth week of prenatal development, when the grooves between the processes are obliterated. The maxillary processes on each side of the developing face partially fuse with the mandibular arch to form the labial commissures, or corners, of the mouth.

Developmental Disturbances with the Lips and Related Tissues

Failure of fusion of the maxillary processes with the medial nasal process can result in **cleft lip,** with varying degrees of disfigurement and disability (Figures 4-8 and 4-9). This disturbance may be hereditary or associated with environmental factors. It may be isolated or associated with other developmental abnormalities, such as cleft palate. Cleft lip, with or without cleft palate, occurs in about one in 1000 live births. These cleft lips result from a failure of the mesenchyme to grow beneath the ectoderm to obliterate any grooves between these processes or even a deficiency or absence of mesenchyme in the area.

These clefts of the lip are located at one side or both sides of the upper lip. The cleft lip may be unilateral or bilateral. It may vary from a notch in the vermilion border of the upper lip (incomplete cleft) to more severe cases (complete cleft) that extend into the floor of the nostril and through the alveolar process of the maxilla.

Cleft lip is more common and more severe in males, and more commonly unilateral, occuring on the left side. It can complicate nursing and feeding of the child as well as speech development, appearance, and oronasal infection levels. Cleft lip is treated by oral and plastic surgery, with dental intervention. Speech and hearing therapy may be needed also.

LACRIMAL TISSUE FORMATION

The maxillary process also fuses with the lateral nasal process along the line of the **nasolacrimal groove,** which extends from the medial corner of the eye to the nasal cavity (see Figure 4-6). This establishes a continuity between the side of the nose, formed by the lateral nasal process, and the cheek region, formed by the maxillary process. This fusion also forms the nasolacrimal cord, a rodlike ectodermal thickening in the floor of the nasolacrimal groove. Its cranial portion expands to form the lacrimal sac of the eye. The cord later canalizes as a result of cell degeneration to become the nasolacrimal duct, draining the tears of the eye (lacrimal fluid) through its inferior meatus in the lateral wall of the nasal cavity after birth.

DEVELOPMENT OF THE NECK

The development of the neck parallels the development of the face in time span. It begins during the fourth week of prenatal development, within the embryonic period, and is completed during the fetal period. The neck and its associated tissues develop from the primitive pharynx and the branchial apparatus. Dental professionals must obtain knowledge about the development of the neck to understand its underlying structural relationships and any developmental disturbances that may be present.

Primitive Pharynx Formation

The beginnings of the embryo's hollow tube are derived from the anterior portion of the foregut and will form the primitive pharynx, the future oral portion of the throat, or oropharynx (Figure 4-10; see also Figure 2-17). The foregut is originally derived from the embryonic endoderm layer (see Chapter 3). The primitive pharynx widens cranially where it joins the primitive mouth of the stomodeum and narrows

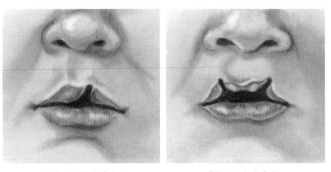

Unilateral cleft lip   Bilateral cleft lip

FIGURE 4-8 Two cleft lip deformities.

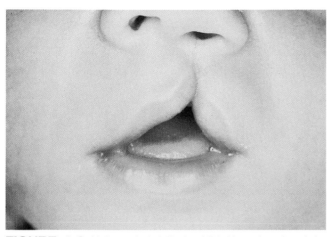

FIGURE 4-9 Unilateral cleft lip in child. Note that the cleft is to the side of the midline of the oral cavity, where the facial processes failed to fuse.

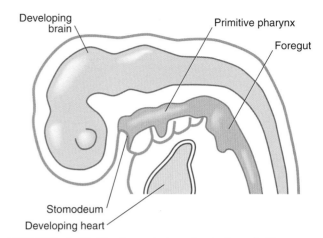

FIGURE 4-10 The foregut gives rise to the primitive pharynx, which will form the oropharynx.

caudally as it joins the esophagus. The endoderm of the pharynx lines the internal portions of the branchial arches and passes into balloonlike areas called the **pharyngeal pouches** (both structures are discussed later). This same endoderm, however, does not come to line the oral cavity proper or nasal cavity. Instead, the oral cavity proper and nasal cavity are lined by ectoderm as a result of embryonic folding.

The caudal part of the primitive pharynx forms the esophagus, which leads to the stomach. A ventral outgrowth forms the laryngopharynx, larynx, and trachea and ends in the superior portion of the developing lungs. The thyroid gland is also an anterior outpocketing from the ventral wall of the pharynx. Development of the thyroid gland is discussed with its histology in Chapter 11.

Branchial Apparatus Formation

The **branchial apparatus** consists of the branchial arches, branchial grooves and membranes, and pharyngeal pouches. The name *branchial* is used because it refers to gill formation in the neck area for respiratory function in lower life forms. No gills form in human embryos; thus the term *pharyngeal* is often used instead of *branchial* in discussions of these embryonic structures.

BRANCHIAL ARCH FORMATION

During the fourth week of prenatal development, stacked bilateral swellings of tissue appear inferior to the stomodeum and include the mandibular arch. These are the **branchial arches,** or pharyngeal arches, with the mandibular arch being the first branchial arch and the others numbered in craniocaudal sequence (Figure 4-11). These branchial arches are six pairs of

U-shaped bars with a core of mesenchyme formed by **neural crest cells** that migrate to the neck region. The branchial arches are covered externally by ectoderm and lined internally by endoderm. These arches support the lateral walls of the primitive pharynx.

The branchial arches are located bilaterally, oriented in an anterior-posterior direction on the embryo, bending to surround and support the developing pharynx. It is important to note that the **fifth branchial arches** are so rudimentary that they are absent in humans or are included with the fourth branchial arches. The branchial arches give rise to important structures of the face and neck (see Table 4-2).

Each paired branchial arch has its own developing cartilage, nerve, vascular, and muscular components within each mesodermal core. The first two pairs of arches become developed to the greatest extent of all the arches and are also the only ones named. In general, the first pair of arches form the middle and lower face, and the lower four pairs of arches are involved in the formation of the structures of the neck. The mandibular arch, or **first branchial arch,** and its associated tissues were described earlier.

Forming within the **second branchial arch,** or **hyoid arch**, is cartilage similar to the cartilage in the mandibular arch. This cartilage in the second branchial arch is called **Reichert's cartilage**, and most of it disappears; however, parts of it are responsible for a middle ear bone, a process of the temporal bone, and portions of the hyoid bone.

Additionally, the perichondrium surrounding Reichert's cartilage gives rise to the ligament of the hyoid bone. The mesoderm of the hyoid arches helps form the muscles of facial expression, the middle ear muscles, and a suprahyoid muscle. Because these muscles are derived from the hyoid arches, they are all innervated by the nerve of the second arches, the

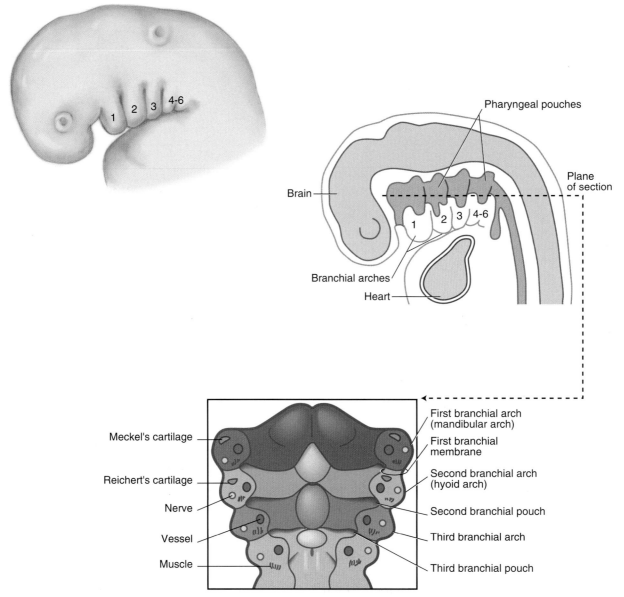

FIGURE 4-11 The embryo during the fourth week of prenatal development. The branchial arches are highlighted.

seventh cranial nerve, and the facial nerve. The hyoid arches, along with the third and fourth branchial arches, are also involved in formation of the tongue (see Chapter 5).

During the seventh week, the muscle cells from the mesoderm of the hyoid arches have begun to differentiate. These muscle cells then begin to migrate over the mandibular muscle masses. By the tenth week, the muscle cells have migrated superiorly all over the face, forming a thin sheet of muscle masses. Both superficial and deep groups of muscle fibers eventually develop from these muscle masses and become attached to the newly differentiating bones of the facial skeleton as the muscles of facial expression. The nerve from the seventh cranial nerve is incorporated early in these muscle masses.

The **third branchial arch** has an unnamed cartilage associated with it. This cartilage will be responsible for the formation of portions of the hyoid bone. The only muscle to be derived from the mesoderm of each third arch is a pharyngeal muscle. Each pair of arches is innervated by the ninth cranial nerve, the glossopharyngeal nerve.

Both the **fourth branchial arch** and the **sixth branchial arch** also have unnamed cartilage associated with them. These arches fuse and participate in the formation of most of the laryngeal cartilages. The mesoderm of these arches is associated with the muscles of the larynx and pharynx. These tissues are innervated by the ninth and tenth cranial nerves, although the nerves of these arches are branches of the tenth cranial nerve, the vagus.

BRANCHIAL GROOVE AND MEMBRANE FORMATION

Between neighboring branchial arches, external grooves are noted on each side of the embryo. These are the **branchial grooves,** or pharyngeal grooves (see Figure 4-11). Only the first branchial groove, which is located between the first and second branchial arches at approximately the same level as the first pharyngeal pouches (discussed later), gives rise to a definitive mature structure of the head and neck.

The first branchial groove becomes deeper to the extent that the ectoderm of the branchial groove contacts the endoderm of the pharyngeal pouches. Thus only a thin, double-layered membrane, the first branchial membrane or pharyngeal membrane, separates the groove from the pouches, although mesenchyme later separates these two layers. This membrane, with its three layers, develops into the tympanic membrane (eardrum). Thus the first groove forms the external auditory meatus. Other branchial membranes appear in the bottom of each of the four branchial grooves, although they are only temporary structures in the human embryo.

By the end of the seventh week, the last four branchial grooves are obliterated as a result of a sudden spurt of growth experienced by the pair of hyoid arches, which grow in an inferior direction and eventually form the neck. This obliteration of grooves gives the mature neck a smooth contour.

PHARYNGEAL POUCH FORMATION

Four well-defined pairs of **pharyngeal pouches** develop as endodermal evaginations from the lateral walls lining the pharynx (see Figure 4-11). The pouches develop as balloonlike structures in a craniocaudal sequence between the branchial arches. The fifth pharyngeal pouches are absent or rudimentary. Many tissues of the face and neck are developed from the pharyngeal pouches (Table 4-3).

The first pharyngeal pouches form between the first and second branchial arches and become the auditory tubes. Palatine tonsillar tissue is derived from the lining of the second pharyngeal pouches and also from the pharyngeal walls. The thymus gland and parathyroid glands appear to be derived from the lining of the

TABLE 4-3

Pharyngeal Pouches and Derivative Structures

Pouches	Future Tissues
First pouches	Tympanic membrane (with first branchial groove), tympanic cavity, mastoid antrum, auditory tube
Second pouches	Crypts and lymphatic nodules of the palatine tonsils
Third and fourth pouches	Parathyroid and thymus glands

third and fourth pharyngeal pouches. Additionally, a portion of the thymus gland may be of ectodermal origin.

The thymus's growth and development are not complete at birth. The thymus is a relatively large lymphatic organ during the perinatal period and then later starts to diminish in relative size during puberty. By adulthood, the thymus is often scarcely recognizable; however, it still is functioning by secreting thymic hormones and by maturing lymphocytes (T-cells).

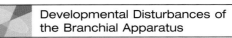 Developmental Disturbances of the Branchial Apparatus

Most congenital malformations in the neck originate during transformation of the branchial apparatus into its mature derivatives (see Chapter 3 for a general discussion of congenital malformations). Some of these are a result of the persistence of parts of the branchial apparatus that normally disappear during development of the neck and its associated tissues.

The branchial grooves occasionally do not become obliterated, and thus portions remain as cervical sinuses or **cervical cysts.** These cysts may drain through sinuses along the neck but may also remain free in the neck tissue just inferior to the angle of the mandible and anywhere along the anterior border of the sternocleidomastoid muscle. These cysts do not become apparent until they produce a slowly enlarging, painless swelling.

CHAPTER 5

Development of Orofacial Structures

■ ■ ■

This chapter discusses the following topics:

- Orofacial development
- Palatal development
  - Primary palate formation
  - Secondary palate formation
  - Completion of palate
- Nasal cavity and septum development
- Tongue development
  - Body of tongue formation
  - Base of tongue formation
  - Completion of tongue formation

■ ■ ■

After studying this chapter, the reader should be able to:

1. Define and pronounce the key terms in this chapter.
2. Discuss the events that occur during the development of the orofacial structures.
3. Integrate the knowledge of the development of the orofacial structures into understanding the present structure of the tissues and any developmental disturbances involved in these structures.

■ ■ ■

Key Terms

Ankyloglossia
 (ang-ke-lo-gloss-ee-ah)
Branchial arches (brang-ke-al)
Cleft palate (kleft), uvula
Copula (kop-u-lah)
Epiglottic swelling (ep-ee-glot-ik)

Foramen cecum (for-ay-men se-kum)
Fusion (fu-zhin)
Intermaxillary segment (in-ter-mak-si-lare-ee)
Lateral lingual swellings
Palatal shelves

Primary palate
Secondary palate
Sulcus terminalis
 (sul-kus ter-mi-nal-is)
Tuberculum impar (too-ber-ku-lum im-par)

OROFACIAL DEVELOPMENT

The orofacial structures discussed in this chapter develop during the fourth week to the twelfth week of prenatal development, spanning the later embryonic and early fetal periods. The development of the stomodeum was discussed in Chapter 4. This chapter continues with embryonic development, starting from where the sequence left off in the previous chapter on the development of the face and neck, and discusses the development of the vastly differing oral structures: the palate, nasal septum and cavity, and tongue. The development of other oral structures, such as the jaw bones, temporomandibular joint, and salivary glands, is discussed with their histology in later chapters.

Dental professionals must obtain knowledge about the development of the oral structures to understand

TABLE 5-1

Development of the Palate

Time Period	Palatal Portions Involved
Fifth to sixth weeks	Primary palate: intermaxillary segment from fused medial nasal processes
Sixth to twelfth weeks	Secondary palate: fused palatal shelves from maxillary processes
Twelfth week	Final palate: fusion of all three processes

their underlying structural relationships and any developmental disturbances that may be present.

PALATAL DEVELOPMENT

The formation of the palate in the embryo and later in the fetus takes place during several weeks of prenatal development (Table 5-1). It is formed from two separate embryonic structures: the primary palate and the secondary palate. Thus the palate, both hard and soft, begins formation in the fifth week of prenatal development, within the embryonic period. The palate is then completed during the twelfth week, within the fetal period. Thus the palate is developed in three consecutive stages: the formation of the primary palate, the formation of the secondary palate, and the completion of the palate.

Most of the tissues of the orofacial region develop by fusion of swellings or tissues of the embryo (as discussed in Chapter 3 and then in more detail in Chapter 4). In contrast with facial fusion, which allows the fusion of swellings or tissue on the *same* surface of the embryo, palatal fusion allows the fusion of swellings or tissue from *different* surfaces of the embryo (Figure 5-1).

Primary Palate Formation

During the fifth week of prenatal development, still within the embryonic period, the **intermaxillary segment** forms (Figure 5-2). The intermaxillary segment arises as a result of fusion of the two medial nasal processes within the embryo. The intermaxillary segment is an internal wedge-shaped mass that extends inferiorly and deep to the nasal pits, on the inside of the stomodeum or primitive mouth, and develops into the floor of the nasal pits and the nasal septum. Thus it is located between the internal surfaces of the maxillary processes of the developing maxilla.

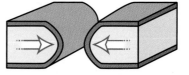
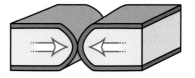
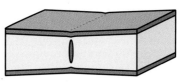

FIGURE 5-1 Palatal fusion. In contrast with facial fusion, which allows the fusion of swellings or tissue on the *same* surface of the embryo, palatal fusion allows the fusion of swellings or tissue from *different* surfaces of the embryo.

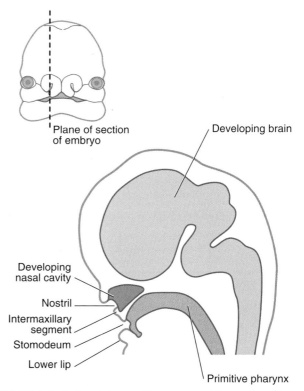

FIGURE 5-2 The intermaxillary segment forms from the fusion of the two medial nasal processes on the inside of the stomodeum of the embryo.

The intermaxillary segment gives rise to the **primary palate,** or primitive palate, a triangular mass. At this time, the primary palate serves only as a partial separation between the developing nasal and oral cavities (Figure 5-3). In the future, the primary palate will form the premaxillary portion of the maxilla, the anterior one third of the final, or definitive, palate. This small portion of the hard palate is anterior to the inci-

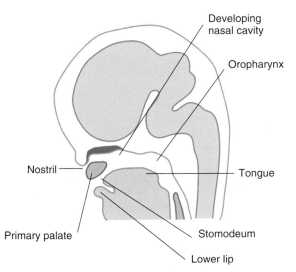

FIGURE 5-3 The primary palate forms from the intermaxillary segment, which serves as a partial separation between the developing nasal and oral cavities.

sive foramen and will contain the maxillary incisor teeth. The formation of the primary palate completes the first stage of palate development.

Secondary Palate Formation

During the sixth week of prenatal development, within the embryonic period, the bilateral maxillary processes give rise to two **palatal shelves,** or lateral palatine processes (Figures 5-4 and 5-5). These shelves grow inferiorly and deep on the inside of the stomodeum in a vertical direction, along both sides of the developing tongue. The tongue is forming on the floor of the pharynx at this time, and as it grows, it fills the common nasal and oral cavity (discussed later).

As the developing tongue muscles begin to function, the tongue contracts and moves out of the way of these developing palatal shelves. The tongue avoids being an obstacle by moving anteriorly and inferiorly. This process is aided by the growth of the lower jaw primordium. This movement of the tongue so that it is now confined solely to the oral cavity proper occurs around the eighth week of prenatal development.

Because of unknown shelf-elevating forces, the palatal shelves, after growing in a vertical direction, "flip" in a superior direction within a few hours. Thus the shelves move into a horizontal position, now superior to the developing tongue. Next, the two palatal shelves elongate and move medially toward each other, fusing to form the **secondary palate.**

The secondary palate will give rise to the posterior two thirds of the hard palate, which will contain the maxillary canines and posterior teeth, posterior to the incisive foramen (Figure 5-6). It also gives rise to the soft palate and its uvula. The median palatine raphe on the surface of the mucosa and underneath,

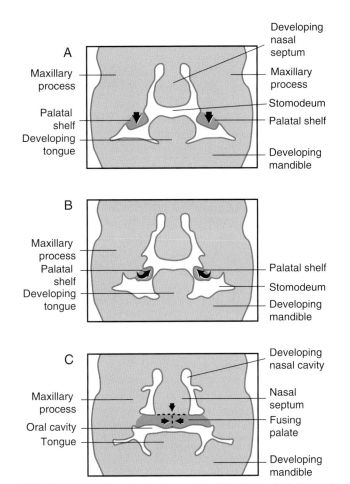

FIGURE 5-4 The developing palate (highlighted). **A:** Palatal shelves form from the maxillary process deep on the inside of the stomodeum. Note the indication of the vertical movement of the growing shelves and the position of the developing tongue. **B:** Palatal shelves grow in a horizontal direction toward each other, after "flipping" in a superior direction, to form the secondary palate. **C:** Fusion of the three processes, the primary palate and two palatal shelves, to form the final palate in the fetus.

the median palatine suture on the adult bone, indicate the line of fusion of the palatal shelves (see Chapter 2 for description of these features). The formation of the secondary palate completes the second stage of palate development.

Completion of Palate

To complete the palate, the secondary palate meets the posterior portion of the primary palate, and fuses together (see Figures 5-4 and 5-5). These three processes are completely fused, forming the final palate, both hard and soft portions, during the twelfth week of prenatal development. The oral cavity thus becomes separated from the nasal cavity, which has begun to undergo development of its nasal septum (discussed next).

Bone formation, or ossification, has already begun in the anterior hard palate by the time palatal fusion is

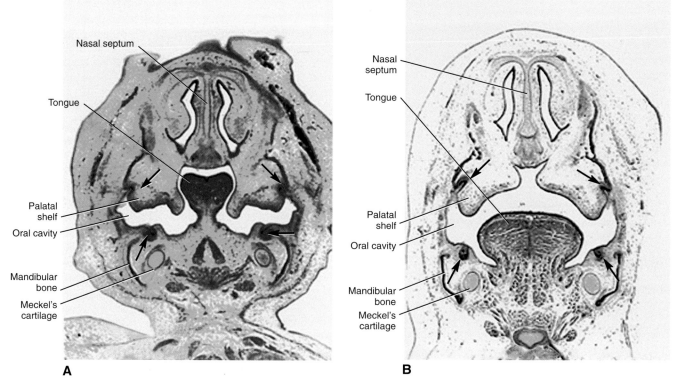

A   **B**

FIGURE 5-5 Photomicrographs of the palatal shelves during the formation of the palate. Note the position of the tongue, oral cavity, nasal septum with its nasal cavity, developing Meckel's cartilage and mandibular bone over time between the two time periods. The arrows point to the developing teeth in each set of the developing jaws. (From Nanci A. *Ten Cate's Oral Histology*, ed 6. Mosby, St. Louis, 2003.)

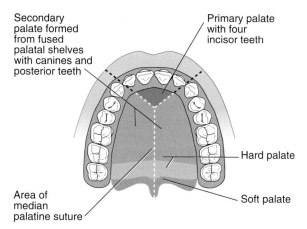

FIGURE 5-6 The adult palate and its developmental portions.

completed. (Histology is discussed in Chapter 8.) In contrast, in the posteriorly placed soft palate, mesenchyme from the first and second branchial arches migrates into the area to form the palatal muscles (discussed later).

A small paired nasopalatine canal persists near the median plane of the mature palate at the site of the junction of the primary palate and the secondary palate (see Figure 5-6). This canal is represented in the mature hard palate by the incisive foramen, the common opening for the bilateral incisive canals. An irregular suture extends from the incisive foramen to the alveolar process of the maxilla, between the lateral incisor and canine teeth on each side. It demarcates where the primary and secondary palates fused. This bony fusion is completed within the first year postnatally, and the overlying epithelium has already fused by that time.

Developmental Disturbances with the Palate and Related Tissues

Failure of fusion of the palatal shelves with the primary palate or with each other results in **cleft palate**, with varying degrees of disability (Figure 5-7). This disturbance may be hereditary or related to environmental factors. It may also be isolated or associated with other abnormalities, such as cleft lip (Figure 5-8). It may involve only the soft palate or may extend through to the hard palate. **Cleft uvula** is the mildest form of cleft palate. Cleft palate, with or without cleft lip, occurs once in 2500 live births. Isolated forms of cleft palate are less common than cleft lip and are more common in female subjects, unlike cleft lip, which is more common in male subjects.

Complications can include difficulty with nursing or feeding the child, oronasal infections, and problems in speech and appearance. Treatment includes oral and plastic surgery, with dental intervention. Speech and hearing therapy may also be necessary.

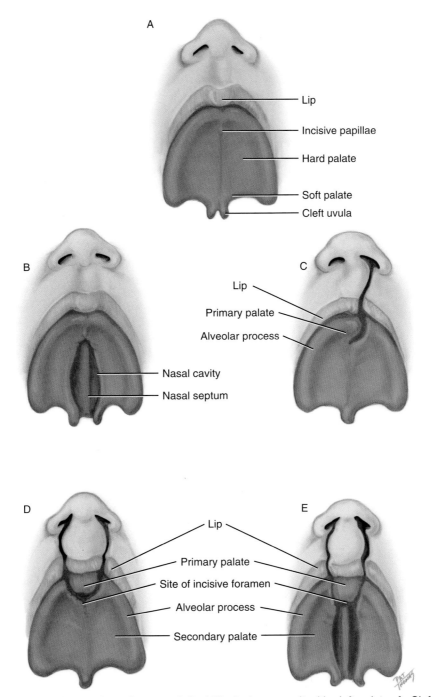

FIGURE 5-7 The various degrees of disability that can result with cleft palate. **A:** Cleft uvula. **B:** Bilateral cleft of the posterior palate. **C:** Complete unilateral cleft of the lip and alveolar process of the maxilla with a unilateral cleft of the primary palate. **D:** Complete bilateral cleft of the lip and alveolar process with bilateral cleft of the primary palate. **E:** Complete bilateral cleft of the lip and alveolar process with complete bilateral cleft of the primary and secondary palatal portions.

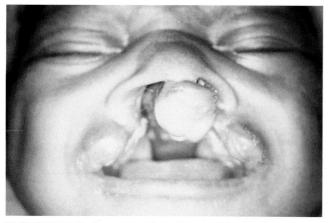

FIGURE 5-8 Complete bilateral cleft of the lip and alveolar process with complete bilateral cleft of the primary and secondary palatal portions.

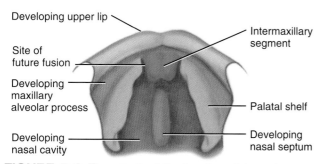

FIGURE 5-9 The growth of the fused medial nasal processes and the early stages in the formation of the nasal septum.

NASAL CAVITY AND SEPTUM DEVELOPMENT

The nasal cavity forms at the same time as the palate. It will serve as part of the respiratory system. The future nasal septum of the nasal cavity is also developing when the palate is forming. The structure of the nasal septum, similar to the primary palate, is a growth from the fused medial nasal processes (Figure 5-9). The tissues that form the nasal septum will grow inferiorly and deep to the medial nasal processes and superior to the stomodeum.

The vertical nasal septum then fuses with the horizontally oriented final palate after it forms (Figure 5-10 and see Figure 5-5). This fusion begins in the ninth week and is completed by the twelfth week. With the formation of the nasal septum and final palate, the paired nasal cavity and the single oral cavity in the fetus become completely separate. The nasal cavity and oral cavity also undergo development of different types of mucosa, such as lining, respiratory, and oral mucosa, respectively (see Chapters 9 and 11).

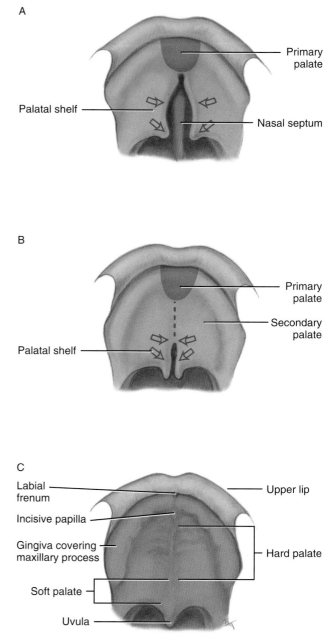

FIGURE 5-10 The later stages of nasal septum development **(A, B)** and fusion with the final palate to separate the nasal and oral cavities completely **(C)**.

The nasal septum has considerable influence on determining orofacial form. It transmits septal growth "pull and thrust" to facial bones such as the maxilla, as it expands its vertical length a dramatic sevenfold between the tenth week of prenatal development and birth.

TONGUE DEVELOPMENT

The tongue develops during the fourth to eighth weeks of prenatal development (Table 5-2). It develops from independent swellings located internally on the

TABLE 5-2

Development of the Tongue

Time Period	Tongue Portions Involved
Fourth to eighth weeks	Body: tuberculum impar and lateral lingual swellings Base: Copula overgrowing second branchial arches
Eighth week	Tongue: Merging of anterior swellings of the body and copula of the base

floor of the primitive pharynx, formed by the first four **branchial arches.**

Specifically, the body of the tongue develops from the first branchial arches, and the base originates later from the second, third, and fourth branchial arches. The grooves between these swellings are eliminated by fusion similar to that on the external face, with growth, migration, and merging of the mesenchyme inferior to the ectoderm into the grooves.

Body of Tongue Formation

During the fourth week of prenatal development, within the embryonic period, the tongue begins its development (see Chapter 2 for a description of the tongue and its features). This tongue development begins as a triangular median swelling, the **tuberculum impar,** or median tongue bud (Figure 5-11). The single tuberculum impar is located in the midline, on the floor of the primitive pharynx, in the embryo's conjoined nasal and oral cavities.

Later, two oval **lateral lingual swellings,** or distal tongue buds, develop on each side of the tuberculum impar. All these anterior swellings are from the growth of mesenchyme of the first branchial arches, or mandibular arches. The paired lateral lingual swellings grow in size and merge with each other (see Figure 5-11, A). Then the two fused swellings overgrow and encompass the disappearing tuberculum impar to form the anterior two thirds, or body, of the tongue, which lies within the oral cavity proper. The median lingual sulcus is a superficial demarcation of the line of fusion of the two lateral lingual swellings (as well as of a deeper fibrous structure). The tuberculum impar does not form any recognizable portion of the mature tongue. Around the lingual swellings, the cells degenerate, forming a sulcus, which frees the body of the tongue from the floor of the mouth, except for the midline lingual frenum.

Base of Tongue Formation

Immediately posterior to these fused anterior swellings, a pair of swellings, the **copula,** becomes evident (see Figure 5-11, B). The copula is formed from the fusion of mesenchyme of mainly the third and parts of the fourth branchial arches. The copula gradually overgrows the second branchial arches, or hyoid arches, to form the base of the tongue, or posterior one third.

Even farther posterior to the copula is the projection of a third median swelling, the **epiglottic swelling,** which develops from the mesenchyme of the posterior parts of the fourth branchial arches (see Figure 5-11, C). This swelling marks the development of the most posterior region of the tongue and of the future epiglottis.

Completion of Tongue Formation

As the tongue develops still further, the copula of the tongue base, after overgrowing the second branchial arches, merges with the anterior swellings of the first branchial arches of the tongue body during the eighth week of prenatal development (see Figure 5-11). This fusion is superficially demarcated by the **sulcus terminalis** in the mature tongue, an inverted V-shaped groove marking the border between the base of the tongue and its body.

The sulcus terminalis points backward toward the oropharynx at a small pitlike depression called the **foramen cecum,** which is the beginning of the thyroglossal duct. This duct is the origin of and pathway showing the thyroid gland's migration into the neck region. This duct later becomes obliterated (discussed with the histology of the thyroid gland in Chapter 11). No similar anatomical landmark is found between the base of the tongue and the epiglottic region.

By the end of the eighth week, the tongue has completed the fusion of these swellings. The tongue then contracts and moves anteriorly and inferiorly to avoid becoming an obstacle to the developing palatal shelves. Thus the tongue moves out of the pharynx into the oral cavity proper. The entire tongue is in the oral cavity proper at birth; its base and epiglottic region descend into the oropharynx by 4 years of age, while the body remains in the oral cavity proper. The tongue normally doubles in length, breadth, and thickness between birth and puberty, when it reaches its maximum size in most persons.

The intrinsic muscles of the tongue are believed to originate from the mesoderm of the occipital somites, not from the branchial arches. Primitive muscle cells from these somites migrate into the developing tongue, taking their motor nerve supply, the twelfth cranial, or hypoglossal, nerve. This explains how the

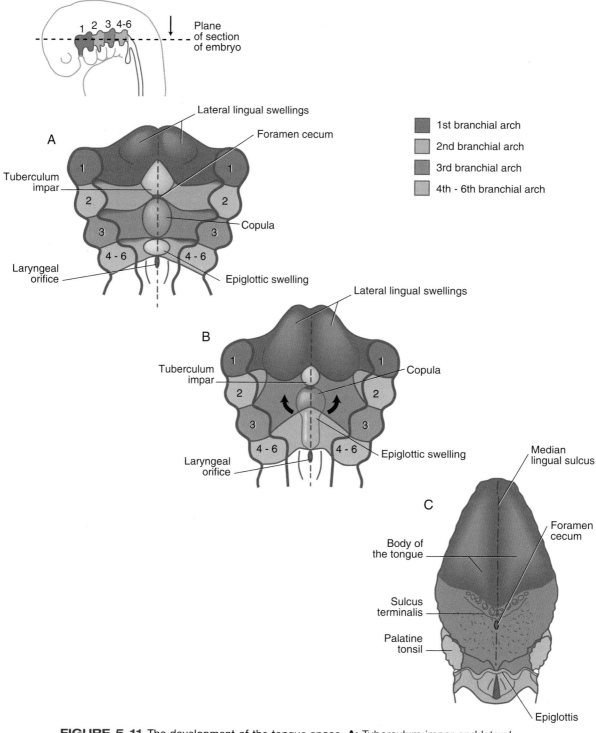

FIGURE 5-11 The development of the tongue space. **A:** Tuberculum impar and lateral lingual swellings and their involvement in the formation of the body of the tongue. **B:** Copula and its involvement in the formation of the base of the tongue. **C:** Fusion of the anterior swellings and the posterior swellings to form the tongue.

single structure of the tongue is innervated by various cranial nerves: It develops from the first four pairs of branchial arches (each with its own cranial nerve) and the occipital somites.

The lingual papillae, small elevated structures of specialized mucosa, appear toward the end of the eighth week. The circumvallate papillae and foliate papillae appear first, close to the terminal branches of the glossopharyngeal nerve. The fungiform papillae appear later, near the terminations of the chorda tympani branches of the facial nerve. The final lingual papillae to form, the filiform papillae, develop during the early fetal period, which comprises the tenth to eleventh weeks.

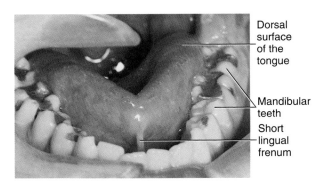

Dorsal surface of the tongue

Mandibular teeth

Short lingual frenum

FIGURE 5-12 Ankyloglossia, resulting from a short lingual frenum.

The taste buds that are associated with some lingual papillae develop during the eleventh to thirteenth weeks by inductive interaction between the epithelial cells of the tongue and invading nerve cells from the chorda tympani of the facial nerve and the glossopharyngeal nerve.

Developmental Disturbances of the Tongue

Abnormalities of the tongue are uncommon. One type that is more common than others is **ankyloglossia**, described as "tongue-tied," which results in a short lingual frenum that extends to the tongue apex (Figure 5-12). This restricts the movement of the tongue to varying degrees. The lingual frenum usually stretches with time; thus surgical correction may not be necessary. This disturbance may be associated with other craniofacial abnormalities.

CHAPTER 6

Tooth Development and Eruption

■ ■ ■

This chapter discusses the following topics:

- Tooth development
  - Initiation stage
  - Bud stage
  - Cap stage
  - Bell stage
  - Apposition and maturation stages
- Root development
  - Root dentin formation

- Cementum and pulp formation
- Periodontal ligament and alveolar bone development
- Multirooted teeth
- Primary tooth eruption and shedding
- Permanent tooth eruption

■ ■ ■

After studying this chapter, the reader should be able to:

1. Define and pronounce the key terms in this chapter.
2. Discuss the events that occur during the development of the teeth and associated structures and during tooth eruption.
3. Integrate the knowledge of the development of the teeth and associated structures and tooth eruption into understanding the present anatomy of these structures and any developmental disturbances.

■ ■ ■

Key Terms

Accessory roots
Active eruption
Alveolar bone
Ameloblasts (ah-**mel**-oh-blasts)
Amelogenesis (ah-mel-oh-**jen**-i-sis), imperfecta (im-per-**fek**-tah)
Anodontia (an-ah-**don**-she-ah)
Apposition (ap-oh-**zish**-in)
Basement membrane
Bell stage
Bud stage
Cap stage
Cells of the dental papilla: inner, central, outer (pah-**pil**-ah)

Cementoblasts (see-men-tah-blasts)
Cementocytes (see-**men**-toe-sites)
Cementogenesis (see-men-toe-**jen**-i-sis)
Cementoid (see-**men**-toyd)
Cementum (see-**men**-tum)
Cervical loop (**ser**-vi-kal)
Concrescence (kahn-**kres**-ens)
Dens in dente (denz in **den**-tay)
Dental lamina (**lam**-i-nah), papilla (pah-**pil**-ah), sac
Dentigerous cyst (den-**ti**-jer-os)
Dentin dysplasia (dis-**play**-ze-ah)

Dentinal tubule
Dentinocemental junction
Dentinoenamel junction
Dentinogenesis (den-tin-oh-**jen**-i-sis), imperfecta (im-per-**fek**-tah)
Dentition (den-**tish**-in): permanent, period, primary, mixed
Differentiation (dif-er-en-she-**ay**-shin)
Dilaceration (di-las-er-**ay**-shun)
Ectoderm (**ek**-toe-derm)
Ectodermal dysplasia (ek-toe-derm-al dis-**play**-ze-ah)
Ectomesenchyme (ek-toe-mes-eng-kime)

Enamel epithelium: inner, outer
Enamel organ, dysplasia
  (dis-**play**-ze-ah), pearls
Epithelial rests of Malassez
  (mal-ah-**say**)
Fusion (fu-**zhin**)
Gemination (jem-i-**nay**-shin)
Hertwig's epithelial root sheath
  (hirt-**wigz**)
Induction
Initiation stage
Macrodontia (mak-roe-**don**-she-ah)
Matrix (**may**-triks): enamel
Microdontia (mi-kro-**don**-she-ah)
Morphogenesis (mor-fo-**jen**-is-is)
Nasmyth's membrane (**nas**-miths)

Neural crest cells
Nonsuccedaneous (non-
  suk-seh-**dane**-ee-us)
Odontoblasts (oh-**don**-toe-blasts)
Odontoblastic process
  (oh-**don**-toe-blast-ik)
Odontoclasts (oh-**don**-toe-klasts)
Odontogenesis (oh-**don**-to-jen-eh-sis)
Oral epithelium
Passive eruption
Periodontal ligament
Preameloblasts
  (pre-ah-**mel**-oh-blasts)
Predentin
Proliferation (pro-lif-er-**ay**-shin)
Reduced enamel epithelium

Repolarization (re-po-ler-i-**za**-shun)
Resorption (re-**sorp**-shun)
Root trunk
Stellate reticulum
  (**stel**-ate reh-**tik**-u-lum)
Stratum intermedium (**stra**-tum
  in-ter-**mede**-ee-um)
Succedaneous
  (suk-seh-**dane**-ee-us)
Successional dental lamina
  (suk-**sesh**-shun-al)
Supernumerary teeth
  (soo-per-**nu**-mer-air-ee)
Tomes' process (tomes)
Tooth fairy, germ
Tubercles (**tu**-ber-kls)

TOOTH DEVELOPMENT

The term **dentition** is used to describe the natural teeth in the jaw bones. There are two dentitions: primary dentition and permanent dentition. A child's **primary dentition** develops during the prenatal period and consists of 20 teeth, which erupt and are later shed or lost (see Chapter 18 for more discussion). As the primary teeth are shed and the jaws grow and mature, the **permanent dentition,** consisting of as many as 32 teeth, gradually erupts and replaces the primary dentition.

An overlapping period between the primary and permanent dentition during the preteen years is referred to as the **mixed dentition period,** when an individual has some teeth from both dentitions. This chapter initially focuses on the development of the primary dentition and then its eruption and shedding. The final discussion in this chapter centers on the eruption of the permanent dentition. The process of development for both dentitions is similar; only the time frames are different. The dental anatomy associated with both these dentitions is discussed further in Chapter 15.

Tooth development, or **odontogenesis,** takes place in many stages, which occur in a stepwise fashion for both dentitions (Table 6-1). Odontogenesis is a continuous process, and there is no clear-cut beginning or end point between these stages. These stages are used to help students focus on the different events in odontogenesis and are based on the appearance of the developing structures. After initiation of odontogenesis, identifiable stages in tooth development include the bud stage, the cap stage, and the bell stage. Odontogenesis then progresses to the apposition stage with the formation and maturation of the hard dental structures, such as enamel, dentin, and cementum (Table 6-2).

During these stages of odontogenesis, many physiological processes occur. These in many ways parallel the processes that occur in the formation of other embryonic structures, such as the face (see Chapter 3 for a description of these processes in embryonic development; see also Table 3-3). These physiological processes include initiation, proliferation, differentiation, morphogenesis, and maturation. Except for the initiation process, many of these processes overlap and are somewhat continuous during odontogenesis. However, one individual process does tend to be predominant in any given stage of odontogenesis.

In the past, the study of odontogenesis included a discussion of developmental lobes that were thought to be growth centers during tooth development. These are portions of the crown of the tooth that are clinically and microscopically visible on account of their depressions. Whether there is any justification for including them in a discussion of tooth formation remains controversial; developmental lobes may simply be evidence of the tooth form only. They are included in this text for completeness.

Not all the teeth in each dentition begin to develop at the same time. The initial teeth for both dentitions develop in the anterior mandibular region, followed later by the anterior maxillary region, and then development progresses posteriorly in both jaws. This posterior progression of odontogenesis allows time for the jaws to grow to accommodate the increased number of primary teeth, the larger primary molars, and then finally the overall larger permanent teeth.

The primary dentition develops during both the embryonic and fetal periods. Most of the permanent dentition is formed during the fetal period. Tooth development continues for years after birth, however, especially considering the formation of the permanent second and third molars (see Unit IV and Appendix D for timelines for the development of each tooth and each dentition). Thus teeth have the longest developmental period of any set of organs in the body.

TABLE 6-1

Stages of Tooth Development

Stage/Time Span*	Microscopic Appearance	Main Processes Involved	Description
Initiation stage/sixth to seventh weeks		Induction	Ectoderm lining stomodeum gives rise to oral epithelium and then to dental lamina, adjacent to deeper ectomesenchyme, which is influenced by the neural crest cells. Both tissues are separated by a basement membrane.
Bud stage/eighth week		Proliferation	Growth of dental lamina into bud that penetrates growing ectomesenchyme.
Cap stage/ninth to tenth weeks		Proliferation, differentiation, morphogenesis	Enamel organ forms into cap, surrounding mass of dental papilla from the ectomesenchyme and surrounded by mass of dental sac also from the ectomesenchyme. Formation of the tooth germ.
Bell stage/eleventh to twelfth weeks		Proliferation, differentiation, morphogenesis	Differentiation of enamel organ into bell with four cell types and dental papilla into two cell types.
Apposition stage/varies per tooth		Induction, proliferation	Dental tissues secreted as matrix in successive layers.
Maturation stage/varies per tooth		Maturation	Dental tissues fully mineralize to their mature levels.

*Note that these are approximate prenatal time spans for the development of the primary dentition.

TABLE 6-2

Comparison of the Dental Hard Tissues

	Enamel	Dentin	Cementum	Alveolar Bone
Embryological background	Enamel organ	Dental papilla	Dental papilla	Mesoderm
Type of tissue	Epithelial	Connective tissue	Connective tissue	Connective tissue
Formative cells	Ameloblasts	Odontoblasts	Cementoblasts	Osteoblasts
Incremental lines	Lines of Retzius	Imbrication lines of von Ebner	Arrest and reversal lines	Arrest and reversal lines
Mature cells	None (lost with eruption)	Only dentinal tubules with processes	Cementocytes	Osteocytes
Resorptive cells	Odontoclasts	Odontoclasts	Odontoclasts	Osteoclasts
Mineral levels	96%	70%	65%	60%
Organic and water levels	1% organic and 3% water	20% organic and 10% water	23% organic and 12% water	25% organic and 15% water
Tissue formation after eruption	None	Possible	Possible	Possible
Vascularity	None	None	None	Present
Innervation	None	Present	None	Present

Dental professionals must have a clear understanding of the stages of odontogenesis and their physiological basis. Developmental disturbances can occur within each stage of odontogenesis, affecting the physiological process or processeses taking place (Table 6-3). These developmental disturbances can have ramifications that may affect the clinical treatment of a patient.

Initiation Stage of Tooth Development

Odontogenesis of the primary dentition begins between the sixth and seventh week of prenatal development, during the embryonic period (Figure 6-1). This first stage of tooth development, known as the **initiation stage,** involves the physiological process of **induction,** which is an interaction between the embryological tissues. Studies show that mesenchymal tissues must influence the ectodermal tissues in order for initiation of odontogenesis to occur, but the mechanisms are unknown at this time.

At the beginning of the sixth week, the embryo's stomodeum, or primitive mouth, is lined by **ectoderm,**

as was discussed in Chapter 4. The outer portion of the ectoderm gives rise to **oral epithelium.** The oral epithelium consists of two horseshoe-shaped bands of tissue at the surface of the stomodeum, one for each future jaw or arch. At the same time, deep to the forming oral epithelium, there is a type of mesenchyme originally from the ectoderm, **ectomesenchyme,** which is influenced by **neural crest cells** that have migrated to the area (see Figure 6-1).

An important acellular structure separates the oral epithelium and the ectomesenchyme in the stomodeum, the **basement membrane.** This basement membrane is similar to the one separating all epithelial and connective tissues (see Chapter 8 for further discussion of the basement membrane).

During the later portion of the seventh week, the oral epithelium grows deeper into the ectomesenchyme and is induced to produce a layer called the **dental lamina** (Figure 6-2). This growth occurs in the developing jaw areas where the two future curved dental arches of the primary dentition will form. The dental lamina begins initially to form in the midline for both arches and progresses posteriorly.

Text continued on p. 70.

TABLE 6-3

Common Dental Developmental Disturbances

Disturbance	Stage	Description	Etiological Factors	Clinical Ramifications
Anodontia	Initiation stage	Absence of single or multiple teeth	Hereditary, endocrine dysfunction, systemic disease, excess radiation exposure	May cause disruption of occlusion and aesthetic problems. May need partial or full dentures, bridges, and/or implants to replace teeth.
Supernumerary teeth	Initiation stage	Development of one or more extra teeth	Hereditary	Occurs commonly between the maxillary centrals, distal to third molars and premolar region. May cause crowding, failure of normal eruption, and disruption of occlusion.

Continued

TABLE 6-3

Common Dental Developmental Disturbances—cont'd

Disturbance	Stage	Description	Etiological Factors	Clinical Ramifications
Macrodontia/ microdontia	Bud stage	Abnormally large or small teeth	Hereditary in localized form. Endocrine dysfunction is complete	Commonly involves permanent maxillary lateral incisor and third molars.
Dens in dente	Cap stage	Enamel organ invaginates into the dental papilla	Hereditary	Commonly affects the permanent maxillary lateral incisor. Tooth may have deep lingual pit and need endodontic therapy.

TABLE 6-3

Common Dental Developmental Disturbances—cont'd

Disturbance	Stage	Description	Etiological Factors	Clinical Ramifications
Gemination	Cap stage	Tooth germ tries to divide	Hereditary	Large single-rooted tooth with one pulp cavity and exhibits "twinning" in crown area. Normal number of teeth in dentition. May cause problems in appearance and spacing.
Fusion	Cap stage	Union of two adjacent tooth germs	Pressure on area	Large tooth with two pulp cavities. One fewer tooth in dentition. May cause problems in appearance and spacing.

Continued

TABLE 6-3

Common Dental Developmental Disturbances—cont'd

Disturbance	Stage	Description	Etiological Factors	Clinical Ramifications
Tubercle	Cap stage	Extra cusp due to effects on enamel organ	Trauma, pressure or metabolic disease	Common on permanent molars or cingulum of anterior teeth.
Enamel pearl	Apposition and maturation stages	Sphere of enamel on root	Displacement of ameloblasts to root surface	May be confused as calculus deposit on root.

TABLE 6-3

Common Dental Developmental Disturbances—cont'd

Disturbance	Stage	Description	Etiological Factors	Clinical Ramifications
Enamel dysplasia	Apposition and maturation stages	Faulty development of enamel from interference involving ameloblasts	Local or systemic or hereditary	Pitting and intrinsic color changes in enamel. Changes in thickness of enamel possible. Problems in function and aesthetics.
Concrescence	Apposition and maturation stages	Union of root structure of two or more teeth by cementum	Traumatic injury or crowding of teeth	Common with permanent maxillary molars.

(All courtesy of Fehrenbach and Associates, Seattle, WA).

Developmental Disturbances During the Initiation Stage

Lack of initiation results in the absence of a single tooth (partial) or multiple teeth (complete), which is called **anodontia**. Partial anodontia is more common and most commonly occurs (listed in order of occurrence) with the permanent maxillary lateral incisors, third molars, and mandibular second premolars (see Table 6-3). Anodontia can be associated with the syndrome of **ectodermal dysplasia** because many portions of the tooth are indirectly or directly of ectodermal origin. (This syndrome is discussed in Chapter 3.) Anodontia can also result from endocrine dysfunction, systemic disease, and exposure to excess radiation, such as that in radiation therapy. It may cause disruption of occlusion and aesthetic problems. Patients may need partial or full dentures, bridges, or implants to replace the missing teeth.

In contrast, abnormal initiation may result in the development of one or more extra teeth, or **supernumerary teeth** (see Table 6-3). These extra teeth are initiated from the dental lamina and have a hereditary etiology. Certain areas of both dentitions commonly have supernumerary teeth, such as (listed in order of occurrence) between the maxillary central incisors (mesiodens, as discussed in Chapter 16), distal to the maxillary third molars (distomolar), and in the premolar region (perimolar) of both dental arches. Supernumerary teeth are smaller than normal, and most are accidentally discovered on radiographic examination. These extra teeth may be erupted or nonerupted and in both cases may cause crowding, noneruption of normal teeth, and disruption of occlusion. Thus removal is often necessary.

Bud Stage of Tooth Development

The second stage of odontogenesis is called the **bud stage** and occurs at the beginning of the eighth week of prenatal development for the primary dentition (Figures 6-3 and 6-4). This stage is named for an extensive proliferation, or growth, of the dental lamina into buds or oval masses penetrating into the ectomesenchyme. At the end of the proliferation process involving the primary dentition's dental lamina, both the future maxillary arch and the future mandibular arch will each have 10 buds. The underlying ectomesenchyme also undergoes proliferation. A basement membrane remains between the bud and the growing ectomesenchyme.

Each of these buds from the dental lamina, together with the surrounding ectomesenchyme, will develop into a tooth germ and its associated supporting tissues. Thus all the teeth and their associated tissues develop from both ectoderm and the mesenchymal tissue, ectomesenchyme, which is influenced by neural crest cells.

Only proliferation of the two tissues occurs during this stage; no structural change occurs in the cells of

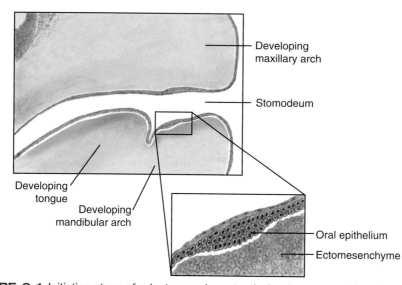

FIGURE 6-1 Initiation stage of odontogenesis, or tooth development, of the primary teeth highlighting the developing mandibular arch. It is now lined by oral epithelium, with the deeper ectomesenchyme influenced by neural crest cells. A similar situation is also occuring in the maxillary arch.

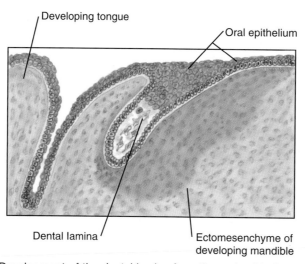

FIGURE 6-2 Development of the dental lamina from the oral epithelium in the mandibular arch, where primary teeth will later form during the initiation stage of tooth development. A similar situation is also occuring in the maxillary arch.

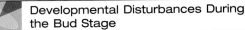
Developmental Disturbances During the Bud Stage

Abnormal proliferation can cause a single tooth (partial) or a complete dentition to be larger or smaller than normal. Abnormally large teeth result in **macrodontia**; abnormally small teeth result in **microdontia** (see Table 6-3). Individual teeth can sometimes appear larger than normal as a result of splitting of the enamel organ or fusion of two adjacent tooth germs, but this is not true of partial macrodontia (these other disturbances are discussed later). Hereditary factors are involved, and teeth commonly affected with true partial microdontia are the permanent maxillary lateral incisor (peg lateral) and permanent third molars (peg molars). Both of these teeth are discussed individually in Chapters 16 and 17, respectively. Complete macrodontia or microdontia rarely occurs and can be due to dysfunction of the pituitary gland.

the dental lamina or ectomesenchyme as later occurs with differentiation and morphogenesis. In areas where teeth will not be developing, the dental lamina only remains thickened; it lines the stomodeum but does not produce buds. Later, this non–tooth-producing portion of the dental lamina disintegrates as the developing oral mucosa comes to line the oral cavity.

Cap Stage of Tooth Development

The third stage of odontogenesis is called the **cap stage** and occurs for the primary dentition between the ninth and tenth week of prenatal development, during the

fetal period (Figures 6-5 and 6-6). The physiological process of proliferation continues during this stage, but the tooth bud of the dental lamina does *not* grow into a large sphere surrounded by ectomesenchyme. Instead, there is unequal growth in different parts of the tooth bud, leading to formation of a cap shape attached to the dental lamina.

Thus not only does proliferation characterize this stage, but various levels of **differentiation** (cytodifferentiation, histodifferentiation, and morphodifferentiation) are also active during the cap stage. Additionally during this stage, a primordium of the tooth (or tooth

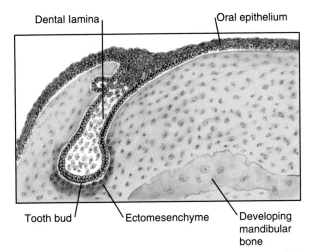
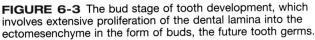

FIGURE 6-3 The bud stage of tooth development, which involves extensive proliferation of the dental lamina into the ectomesenchyme in the form of buds, the future tooth germs.

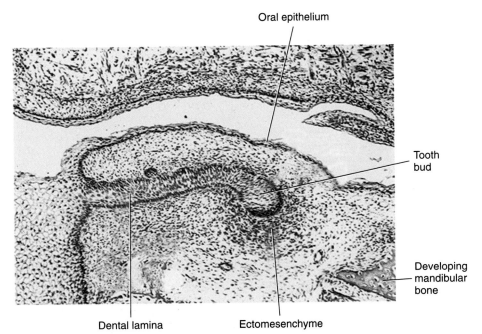

FIGURE 6-4 Photomicrograph of the bud stage of tooth development, which involves extensive proliferation of the dental lamina into the ectomesenchyme in the form of buds, the future tooth germs. (From Nanci A. *Ten Cate's Oral Histology*, ed 6. Mosby, St. Louis, 2003.)

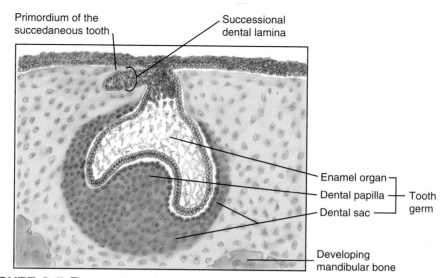

Primordium of the
succedaneous tooth

Successional
dental lamina

Enamel organ ┐
Dental papilla ┤ Tooth
Dental sac ┘ germ

Developing
mandibular bone

FIGURE 6-5 The cap stage of tooth development, which involves proliferation and differentiation, forming the tooth germ, the primordium of a primary tooth. Note the components of the tooth germ: the enamel organ, dental papilla, and dental sac. Also note that the developing primordium of the permanent succedaneous tooth lingual to the primary tooth germ is in the bud stage.

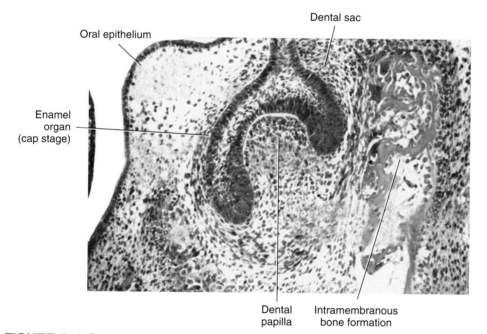

Dental sac

Oral epithelium

Enamel
organ
(cap stage)

Dental   Intramembranous
papilla   bone formation

FIGURE 6-6 Photomicrograph of the cap stage of tooth development, showing the tooth germ and its components from the dental lamina as well as the adjacent ectomesenchyme. The dental lamina is derived from the oral epithelium lining the developing oral cavity (*arrow*). (From Nanci A. *Ten Cate's Oral Histology,* ed 6. Mosby, St. Louis, 2003.)

germ) develops with a specific form. Therefore the predominant physiological process during the cap stage is one of **morphogenesis.**

From these combined physiological processes, a depression results in the deepest part of each tooth bud of dental lamina and forms a cap, or **enamel organ.** The innermost margin of the cap shape of the enamel organ signals the tooth's future crown form. In the future, the enamel organ will produce enamel for the outer surface of the tooth. Note that the enamel organ was originally derived from ectoderm, making enamel an ectodermal product.

A portion of the ectomesenchyme deep to the buds has now condensed into a mass within the concavity of the cap of the enamel organ. This inner mass of ectomesenchyme is now called the **dental papilla.** The dental papilla will produce the future dentin and pulp tissue for the inner portion of the tooth. Note that the dental papilla is originally derived from ectomesenchyme, which is influenced by neural crest cells. Thus dentin and pulp tissues are of mesenchymal origin. A basement membrane still exists between the enamel organ and the dental papilla and is the site of the future dentinoenamel junction.

TABLE 6-4

Components of Tooth Germ During Cap Stage

Component	Description of Component	Future Dental Tissue Produced
Enamel organ	Formation of tooth bud in a cap shape with deep central depression	Enamel
Dental papilla	Condensed mass of ectomesenchyme within the concavity of the enamel organ	Dentin and pulp
Dental sac	Condensed mass of ectomesenchyme surrounding the enamel organ	Cementum, periodontal ligament, alveolar bone

The remaining ectomesenchyme surrounding the outside of the cap or enamel organ condenses into the **dental sac,** or dental follicle. In the future, the capsulelike dental sac will produce the periodontium, the supporting tissues of the tooth: cementum, periodontal ligament, and alveolar bone. Note that the dental sac is originally derived from ectomesenchyme; thus the supporting dental tissues are of mesenchymal origin. A basement membrane still separates the enamel organ and dental sac.

At the end of the cap stage, these three embryological structures—the enamel organ, dental papilla, and dental sac—are now considered together to be the **tooth germ,** the primordium of the tooth (Table 6-4). These initial tooth germs housed within each developing dental arch will develop into the primary dentition.

Already at the tenth week of prenatal development, during the cap stage for each primary tooth, initiation is occurring for the anterior teeth of the permanent dentition. Each primordium for these initially formed permanent teeth appears as an extension of the dental lamina into the ectomesenchyme lingual to the developing primary tooth germs. Its site of origin is called the **successional dental lamina** (see also Figure 6-26).

Permanent teeth formed with primary predecessors are called **succedaneous** and include the anterior teeth and premolars, which replace the primary anterior teeth and molars, respectively. The permanent succedaneous tooth's crown will erupt lingual to its primary predecessor's root (or roots) if the primary tooth has not been fully shed or lost.

The permanent molars are **nonsuccedaneous** and have no primary predecessors. These six permanent molars per dental arch develop from a posterior exten-

Developmental Disturbances During the Cap Stage

During the cap stage, the enamel organ may abnormally invaginate into the dental papilla, resulting in **dens in dente** (see Table 6-3). The teeth most commonly affected are the permanent maxillary incisors, especially the lateral incisor (see Chapter 16 for more discussion). Dens in dente usually leaves the tooth with a deep lingual pit in the area where the invagination occurs and may appear as a "tooth within a tooth" on radiographic examination. This lingual pit may lead to pulpal exposure and pathology and subsequent endodontic therapy. Therefore early detection is important. Hereditary factors may be involved in dens in dente.

Another disturbance that can occur during the cap stage is **gemination** (see Table 6-3). This disturbance occurs as the single tooth germ tries unsuccessfully to divide into two tooth germs. This results in a large single-rooted tooth with a common pulp cavity. The tooth exhibits "twinning" in the crown area, with false macrodontia. The appearance of splitting can be detected as a cleft with varying depths in the incisal surface, or it may manifest as two crowns. The number of teeth in either dentition with this disturbance is usually normal. Gemination usually occurs in the anterior teeth in either dentition and may be due to hereditary factors. This can create problems in appearance, spacing, and thus periodontal health and is verified by radiographic examination.

Another disturbance that can occur during the cap stage is **fusion** (see Table 6-3). This results from the union of two adjacent tooth germs, possibly resulting from pressure in the area. This leads to a large, falsely macrodontic tooth and is verified by radiographic examination. Radiographs show two distinct pulp cavities, but the enamel, dentin, and pulp are united. The arch of the dentition with this disturbance has one less tooth. The fusion usually occurs only in the crown area of the tooth, but it can involve both the crown and root. This disturbance occurs more commonly with the anterior teeth of the primary dentition and can present problems in appearance and spacing.

Teeth may also have extra cusps, or **tubercles** (see Table 6-3) that appear as small, round enamel extensions. They are noted mainly on the permanent molars, especially the third molars, but can be found on any tooth in both dentitions. Tubercles may also be present as a lingual extension on the cingulum on permanent maxillary anterior teeth, especially lateral incisors and canines. This disturbance may be due to trauma, pressure, or metabolic disease that affects the enamel organ that forms the crown area.

sion of the dental lamina distal to the primary second molar's dental lamina and its associated ectomesenchyme for each quadrant.

Bell Stage of Tooth Development

The fourth stage of odontogenesis is the **bell stage** (Figures 6-7 and 6-8), which occurs for the primary dentition between the eleventh and twelfth week of prenatal development. It is characterized by continuation of the ongoing processes of proliferation, differentiation, and morphogenesis. However, differentiation on all levels occurs to its furthest extent, and

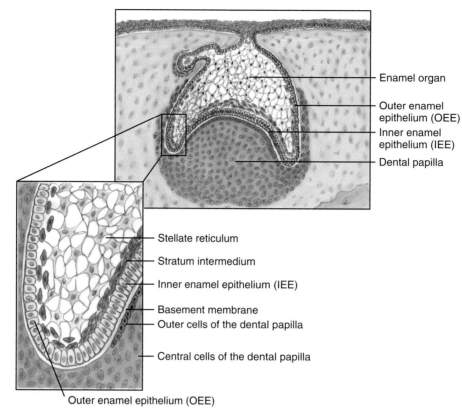

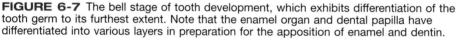

FIGURE 6-7 The bell stage of tooth development, which exhibits differentiation of the tooth germ to its furthest extent. Note that the enamel organ and dental papilla have differentiated into various layers in preparation for the apposition of enamel and dentin.

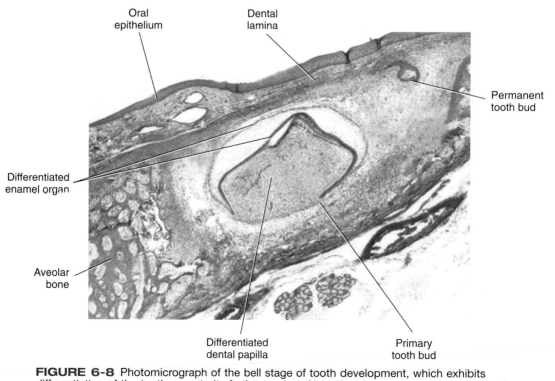

FIGURE 6-8 Photomicrograph of the bell stage of tooth development, which exhibits differentiation of the tooth germ to its furthest extent. Note that the enamel organ and dental papilla have differentiated into various layers in preparation for the apposition of enamel and dentin. (From Nanci A. *Ten Cate's Oral Histology,* ed 6. Mosby, St. Louis, 2003.)

TABLE 6-5

Cell Layers of the Tooth During the Bell Stage (from Outer to Inner)

Cell Layers	Description of Layer	Role in Tooth Formation
Dental sac	Increasing amount of collagen fibers forming around the enamel organ	Will differentiate into cementum, periodontal ligament, and alveolar bone
Outer enamel epithelium (OEE)	Outer cuboidal cells of enamel organ	Serves as protective barrier for enamel organ
Stellate reticulum	More outer star-shaped cells in many layers, forming a network within the enamel organ	Supports the production of enamel matrix
Stratum intermedium	More inner compressed layer of flat to cuboidal cells	Supports the production of enamel matrix
Inner enamel epithelium (IEE)	Innermost tall, columnar cells of enamel organ	Will differentiate into ameloblasts that form enamel matrix
Outer cells of dental papilla	Outer layer of cells of the dental papilla nearest the inner enamel epithelium of the enamel organ (note the presence of basement membrane between this outer layer and the IEE)	Will differentiate into odontoblasts that form dentin matrix
Inner cells of dental papilla	Inner cell mass of the dental papilla	Will differentiate into pulp tissue

as a result, four different types of cells are now found within the enamel organ (Table 6-5). These cell types form layers and include the inner enamel epithelium, the outer enamel epithelium, the stellate reticulum, and the stratum intermedium. Thus the cap shape of the enamel organ evident during the last stage assumes a bell shape.

The outer cuboidal cells of the enamel organ are the **outer enamel epithelium (OEE)**. The OEE will serve as a protective barrier for the rest of the enamel organ during enamel production. The innermost tall columnar cells of the enamel organ are the **inner enamel epithelium (IEE)**. In the future, the IEE will differentiate into enamel-secreting cells (ameloblasts). A basement membrane remains between the IEE and the adjacent dental papilla.

Between the outer and inner enamel epithelium are two layers, the **stellate reticulum** and **stratum intermedium**. The more outer stellate reticulum consists of star-shaped cells in many layers, forming a network. The more inner stratum intermedium is made up of a compressed layer of flat to cuboidal cells. Both of these two intermediately placed layers of the enamel organ help support the production of enamel.

At the same time, the dental papilla within the concavity of the enamel organ is also undergoing extensive differentiation so that it now consists of two types of tissues or layers: the **outer cells of the dental papilla** and the **central cells of the dental papilla** (see Table 6-5). In the future, the outer cells of the dental papilla (or peripheral cells) will differentiate into dentin-secreting cells (odontoblasts), whereas the inner cells are the primordium of the pulp. The outer dental sac increases in the amount of collagen fibers but undergoes differentiation into its dental tissues later than the enamel organ and dental papilla do.

Apposition and Maturation Stages of Tooth Development

The final stages of odontogenesis include **apposition,** during which the enamel, dentin, and cementum are secreted in successive layers. These tissues are initially secreted as a **matrix,** which is an extracellular substance that is partially calcified yet serves as a framework for later calcification. The other final stage, maturation, is reached when the dental tissues subsequently fully mineralize. The time period of these two final stages varies according to the tooth involved but overall involves the same chronology as the initiation of odontogenesis. The results of the maturation of each hard dental tissue are noted in Table 6-2 and should be consulted as the study of dental histology begins.

During the stage of apposition, many inductions occur between the ectodermal tissue of the enamel organ and mesenchymal tissues of the dental papilla and dental sac. Studies show that these interactions are necessary for the production of enamel, dentin, and cementum by the proliferation or growth of cellular

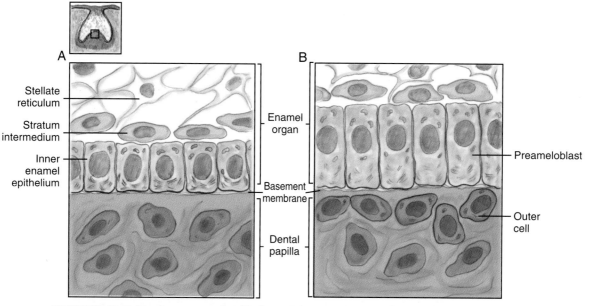

FIGURE 6-9 The inner enamel epithelium of the enamel organ differentiating into the preameloblasts, the future cells that will secrete enamel matrix. **A:** Inner enamel epithelial cells with central nuclei lined up along the basement membrane. **B:** Inner enamel epithelial cells that have elongated and repolarized their nuclei to become preameloblasts. Also note the location of the outer cells of the dental papilla.

byproducts. Acting not only as a boundary between the two tissues, the basement membrane conveys communications between the cells of the enamel organ, the dental papilla, and the dental sac, allowing these tissue interactions.

This portion of the chapter mainly focuses on the production of enamel and coronal dentin, and the maturation and histology of these tissues are discussed in Chapters 12 and 13. The development of the crown of the tooth is discussed first. This follows the same timeline as tooth development, given that development begins in the crown and then proceeds to the root (evident on most periapical radiographs of a mixed dentition). Root development with root dentin and cementum formation is discussed later in this chapter. The events in the production of enamel and coronal dentin include the formation of preameloblasts, odontoblasts and dentin matrix, ameloblasts, dentinoenamel junction, and enamel matrix (see Table 6-5).

FORMATION OF PREAMELOBLASTS

After the formation of the IEE in the bell-shaped enamel organ, these innermost cells grow even more columnar or elongate as they differentiate into **preameloblasts** (Figure 6-9). During this differentiation, the nucleus in each cell moves away from the center of the cell to the position farthest away from the basement membrane. This movement of all the nuclei in the IEE cells occurs during cellular **repolarization,** and studies show its importance in the change of the IEE cells into preameloblasts. In the future, the preameloblasts will induce dental papilla cells to differ-

entiate and will themselves differentiate into cells that secrete enamel matrix.

FORMATION OF ODONTOBLASTS AND DENTIN MATRIX

After the IEE differentiates into preameloblasts, the outer cells of the dental papilla are induced by the preameloblasts to differentiate into **odontoblasts** (Figures 6-10 and 6-11). These cells also undergo repolarization, which results in their nuclei moving from the center to a position in the cell farthest from the basement membrane. These repolarized cells are also lined up adjacent to the basement membrane but in a mirror-image orientation compared with the preameloblasts. The odontoblasts now begin **dentinogenesis,** which is the apposition of dentin matrix, or **predentin,** on their side of the basement membrane. Thus the odontoblasts start their secretory activity some time before enamel matrix production begins. This explains why the dentin layer in any location in a developing tooth is slightly thicker than the corresponding layer of enamel matrix.

FORMATION OF AMELOBLASTS, DENTINOENAMEL JUNCTION, AND ENAMEL MATRIX

After the differentiation of odontoblasts from the outer cells of the dental papilla and their formation of predentin, the basement membrane between the preameloblasts and the odontoblasts disintegrates. This disintegration of the basement membrane allows the

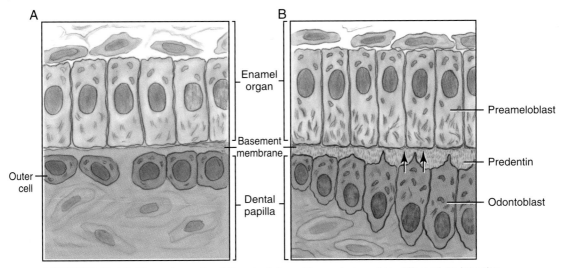

FIGURE 6-10 The outer cells of the dental papilla are induced to differentiate into the odontoblasts and form predentin. **A:** Outer cells of the dental papilla lining up along the basement membrane, with repolarization of their nuclei, becoming odontoblasts. **B:** The odontoblasts start dentinogenesis, the apposition of predentin on their side of the basement membrane.

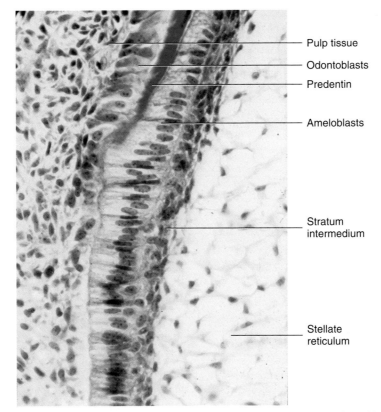

FIGURE 6-11 Photomicrograph of the formation of predentin from the odontoblasts. The predentin is enclosing the forming pulp tissue. Note the stellate reticulum, stratum intermedium, and ameloblasts from the inner enamel epithelium. (From Nanci A. *Ten Cate's Oral Histology,* ed 6. Mosby, St. Louis, 2003.)

preameloblasts to come into contact with the newly formed predentin. This induces the preameloblasts to differentiate into **ameloblasts**.

Ameloblasts begin **amelogenesis**, or the apposition of **enamel matrix,** laying it down on their side of the now disintegrating basement membrane (Figures 6-12,

6-13, 6-14, and 6-15). The enamel matrix is secreted from **Tomes' process,** a tapered portion of each ameloblast that faces the disintegrating basement membrane.

With the enamel matrix in contact with the predentin, mineralization of the disintegrating basement

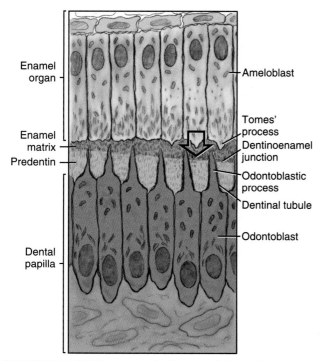

Enamel organ

Enamel matrix

Predentin

Dental papilla

Ameloblast

Tomes' process

Dentinoenamel junction

Odontoblastic process

Dentinal tubule

Odontoblast

FIGURE 6-12 The preameloblasts are induced to differentiate into ameloblasts. The ameloblasts begin amelogenesis, the apposition of enamel matrix on their side of the basement membrane. Note that the predentin layer is thicker than the enamel matrix layer because the odontoblasts differentiate and start matrix production earlier than the ameloblasts. Also note the formation of the dentinoenamel junction from the mineralization of the disintegrating basement membrane.

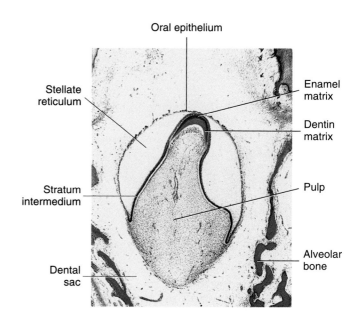

Oral epithelium

Stellate reticulum

Enamel matrix

Dentin matrix

Stratum intermedium

Pulp

Dental sac

Alveolar bone

FIGURE 6-14 Photomicrograph during the apposition stage, showing enamel and dentin matrix formation. (From Nanci A. *Ten Cate's Oral Histology*, ed 6. Mosby, St. Louis, 2003.)

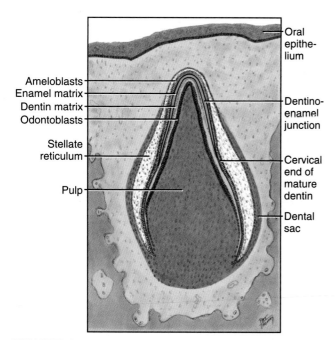

Ameloblasts
Enamel matrix
Dentin matrix
Odontoblasts

Stellate reticulum

Pulp

Oral epithelium

Dentino-enamel junction

Cervical end of mature dentin

Dental sac

FIGURE 6-13 Tooth development during the apposition stage, showing enamel and dentin matrix formation.

membrane now occurs, forming the **dentinoenamel junction (DEJ),** the inner junction between the dentin and enamel tissues. Apposition of both types of dental matrix becomes regular and rhythmic, as the cellular bodies of both the odontoblasts and ameloblasts retreat away from the DEJ.

The odontoblasts, unlike the ameloblasts, will leave attached cellular extensions in the length of the predentin called the **odontoblastic process.** Each odontoblastic process is contained in a mineralized cylinder, the **dentinal tubule.** The calcification or maturation of each type of matrix occurs later and is a different process for both enamel and dentin. The cell bodies of odontoblasts will remain within pulp tissue. The cell bodies of the ameloblasts will be involved in the eruption and mineralization process but will be lost after eruption.

ROOT DEVELOPMENT

The process of root development takes place after the crown is completely shaped and the tooth is starting to erupt into the oral cavity. Most nondental personnel find it remarkable that the tooth is formed starting with the crown and then moving to the apex of the root.

The structure responsible for root development is the **cervical loop** (Figure 6-18, A). The cervical loop is the most cervical portion of the enamel organ, a bilayer rim that consists of only IEE and OEE.

Developmental Disturbances During Apposition and Maturation Stages

Factors may interfere with the metabolic processes of the ameloblasts, resulting in **enamel dysplasia**, the faulty development of enamel (see Table 6-3). Many different types are possible, and they have either a local or a systemic etiology. Local enamel dysplasia may result from trauma or infection of a small group of ameloblasts. Systemic dysplasia involves larger numbers of ameloblasts and may result from traumatic birth, systemic infections, nutritional deficiencies, or dental fluorosis (excess systemic fluoride).

Any tooth in which amelogenesis is active during the metabolic interference may be affected, and changes in focal areas, the entire tooth, or the complete dentition may be noted. A type of enamel dysplasia, enamel hypoplasia, results from a reduction in the *quantity* of enamel matrix. As a result, the teeth appear with pitting and grooves in the enamel surface.

Enamel hypoplasia can be involved in Hutchinson's incisors and mulberry molars caused by the teratogenic potential of congenital syphilis (discussed in Chapters 3, 16, and 17). From the labial view, Hutchinson's incisors have a crown with a screwdriver shape that is wider cervically and narrow incisally, with a notched incisal edge. Mulberry molars have enamel tubercles on the occlusal surface.

Enamel dysplasia may also involve enamel hypocalcification. This disturbance results in reduction in the *quality* of the enamel maturation. The teeth appear more opaque, yellower, or even browner because of an intrinsic staining of enamel. Enamel hypoplasia and hypocalcification may occur together, a common finding in dental fluorosis (see Chapter 12 for more discussion).

A certain type of enamel dysplasia, **amelogenesis imperfecta**, has a hereditary etiology and can affect all teeth of both dentitions (Figure 6-16). With this disturbance, the teeth have very thin enamel portions that chip off or have no enamel at all. The crowns are yellow and are composed of dentin. They undergo extreme attrition, the mechanical loss of tooth material resulting from mastication. No treatment is required, unless full-coverage crowns are desired for cosmetic appearance and to prevent further attrition.

In addition, **dentin dysplasia**, or the faulty development of dentin, can result from an interference with the metabolic processes of the odontoblasts during dentinogenesis, but it is more rare than enamel dysplasias. This dysplastic condition can also be due to local or systemic factors, similar to enamel dysplasias, and can involve either dentin hypoplasia or hypocalcification or both types of dentin dysplasia.

One type of dentin dysplasia is **dentinogenesis imperfecta,** which has a hereditary basis (Figure 6-17). This disturbance results in blue-gray or brown teeth with an opalescent sheen. The enamel portion is normal but chips off because of a lack of support by the abnormal dentin, leaving dentinal crowns. The result is severe attrition because the dentin is less mineralized overall. This type of dentin has an irregular maturation quality (as discussed in Chapter 13 with regard to interglobular dentin). No treatment is required unless full-coverage crowns are desired for cosmetic appearance and prevention of further attrition.

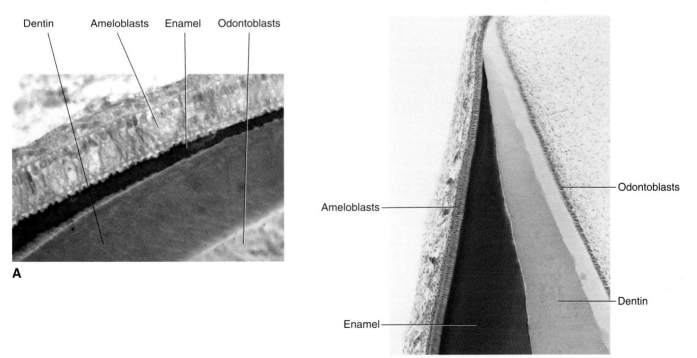

FIGURE 6-15 Photomicrographs of enamel formation from ameloblasts and dentin formation from odontoblasts. Note the stellate reticulum and stratum intermedium covering the ameloblasts. (**A:** From Nanci **A.** *Ten Cate's Oral Histology,* ed 6. Mosby, St. Louis, 2003. **B:** Courtesy of Dr. James McIntosh, PhD, Department of Biomedical Sciences, Baylor College of Dentistry, Dallas, TX.)

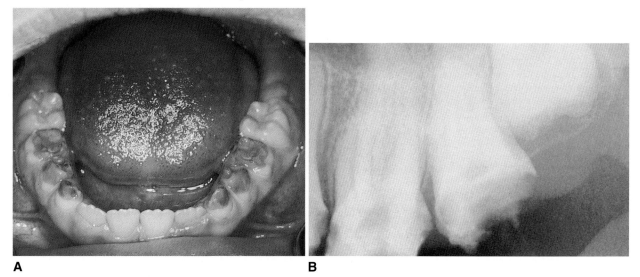

A   **B**

FIGURE 6-16 Amelogenesis imperfecta in the permanent dentition, a hereditary type of enamel dysplasia. The teeth have either no enamel or a very thin enamel portion that chips off, leaving the yellow crowns of dentin, which undergo extreme attrition. **A:** Clinical considerations. **B:** Radiographic presentation.

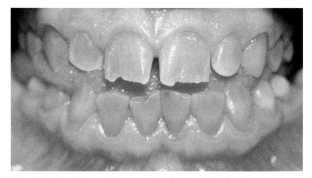

FIGURE 6-17 Dentinogenesis imperfecta in the permanent dentition, a hereditary type of dentin dysplasia that results in blue-gray teeth with an opalescent sheen and chipped-off enamel and dentin crowns with severe attrition.

The cervical loop begins to grow deeper into the surrounding ectomesenchyme of the dental sac, elongating and moving away from the newly completed crown area to enclose more of the dental papilla tissue and form **Hertwig's epithelial root sheath (HERS)** (Figures 6-18, B and C). The function of this sheath or membrane is to shape the root (or roots) and induce dentin formation in the root area so that it is continuous with coronal dentin. This chapter first discusses root development in a single-rooted tooth and then later in multirooted teeth.

Root Dentin Formation

Root dentin forms when the outer cells of the dental papilla in the root area are induced to undergo differentiation and become odontoblasts (Figure 6-19). This induction occurs similarly to the process that happens in the crown area to produce coronal dentin, under the influence of the IEE of HERS. Lacking the intermediate layers of the stellate reticulum and stratum intermedium, HERS may induce odontoblastic differentiation but fails to differentiate into enamel-forming ameloblasts. This accounts for the absence of enamel in the roots.

After the differentiation of odontoblasts in the root area, these cells undergo dentinogenesis and begin to secrete predentin. As in the crown area, a basement membrane is located between the inner enamel epithelium of the sheath and the odontoblasts in the root area.

When root dentin formation is completed, this portion of the basement membrane also disintegrates, as does the entire HERS. After this disintegration of the root sheath, its cells may become the **epithelial rests of Malassez.** These groups of epithelial cells become located in the mature periodontal ligament and can become cystic, presenting future problems (see Chapter 14).

Developmental Disturbances During Root Formation

Misplaced ameloblasts can migrate to the root area, causing enamel to be abnormally formed on the cemental root surface. These are called **enamel pearls** (see Table 6-3). They appear as small, spherical enamel projections on the root surface, especially at the cementoenamel junction (CEJ) or in the furcation area on molars where the roots divide. They may have a tiny dentin and pulp core and appear radiopaque on radiographs. Enamel pearls may be confused with a calculus deposit upon exploration of the root surface but cannot be removed.

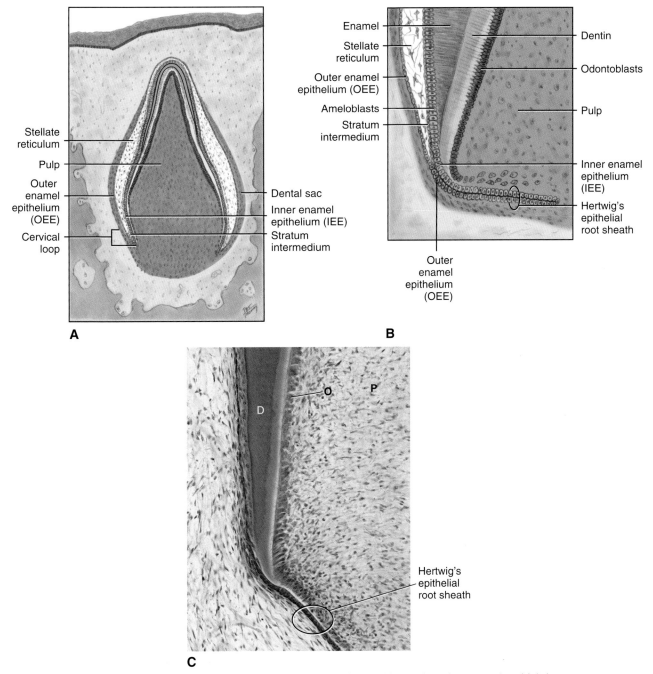

FIGURE 6-18 Stages in root development. **A:** Cervical loop of a primary tooth, which is composed of the most cervical portion of the enamel organ and is responsible for root development. Note that the cervical loop is composed of only the inner and outer enamel epithelium. **B:** Hertwig's epithelial root sheath is formed from elongation of the cervical loop, which is responsible for the shape of the root (or roots) and the induction of root dentin. **C:** Microscopic view of a portion of the root sheath (*circled*). Odontoblasts (*O*) are within the pulp tissue (*P*) after forming dentin (*D*). (Courtesy of Dr. James McIntosh, PhD, Department of Biomedical Sciences, Baylor College of Dentistry, Dallas, TX.)

Cementum and Pulp Formation

The apposition of cementum, or **cementogenesis,** in the root area also occurs when HERS disintegrates (Figure 6-20). This disintegration of the sheath allows the undifferentiated cells of the dental sac to come into contact with the newly formed surface of root dentin. This contact of the dental sac cells with the dentin surface induces these cells to become immature **cementoblasts.**

The cementoblasts move to cover the root dentin area and undergo cementogenesis, laying down

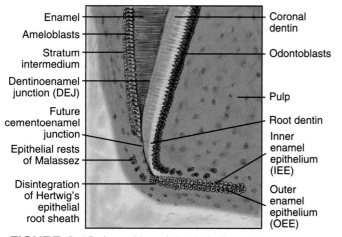

FIGURE 6-19 Apposition of dentin in the root area resulting from the induction of the outer cells of the dental papilla to differentiate into odontoblasts.

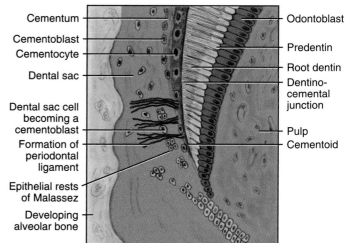

FIGURE 6-20 Apposition of cementum in the root area after Hertwig's epithelial root sheath disintegration and the induction of dental sac cells to differentiate into cementoblasts. The cementoblasts begin to produce cementum matrix, or cementoid, and some cells become entrapped during the later stages of apposition. Note the developing periodontal ligament and alveolar bone adjacent to the cementum.

cementum matrix, or **cementoid.** Unlike ameloblasts and odontoblasts, which leave no cellular bodies in their secreted products, many cementoblasts become entrapped by the cementum they produce and become mature **cementocytes** in the later stages of apposition. As the cementoid surrounding the cementocytes becomes calcified, or matured, it is then considered **cementum** (see Chapter 14). As a result of the apposition of cementum over the dentin, the **dentinocemental junction (DCJ)** is formed. Also at this time, the **central cells of the dental papilla** are forming into the **pulp.** The pulp tissue is surrounded by the newly formed dentin (see Chapter 13 for further discussion of the pulp and dentin).

Periodontal Ligament and Alveolar Bone Development

As the crown and root develop, the surrounding supporting tissues of the tooth are also developing (see Figure 6-20). The ectomesenchyme from the dental sac begins to form the **periodontal ligament (PDL)** adjacent to the newly formed cementum. This process involves forming collagen fibers that are immediately organized into the fiber bundles of the PDL. The ends of these fibers insert into the outer portion of the cementum and the surrounding alveolar bone to support the tooth.

The ectomesenchyme of the dental sac also begins to mineralize to form the tooth sockets or alveoli of the **alveolar bone** surrounding the PDL (see Chapter 14 for further discussion of periodontal ligament and alveolar bone development and histology).

 Developmental Disturbances with Cementum Formation

Excess cementum formation can occur with **concrescence** (see Table 6-3). This is the union of the root structure of two or more teeth through the cementum only, usually occurring with permanent maxillary molars (see Chapter 17). The teeth involved are originally separate but join as a result of the excessive cementum deposition on one or more teeth after eruption. Traumatic injury or crowding of the teeth in the area during the apposition and maturation stage of tooth development may be the cause. This may present problems during extraction and endodontic treatment, and thus preoperative radiographs are important in the detection of this disturbance.

Multirooted Teeth

Like anterior teeth, multirooted premolars and molars originate as a single root on the base of the crown. This portion on these posterior teeth is called the **root trunk.** The cervical cross section of the root trunk initially follows the form of the crown. However, the root of a posterior tooth divides from the root trunk into the correct number of root branches for its tooth type (see Chapter 17 for a discussion on roots of posterior teeth). Differential growth of HERS causes the root trunk of the multirooted teeth to divide into two or three roots (Figure 6-21). During the formation of the enamel

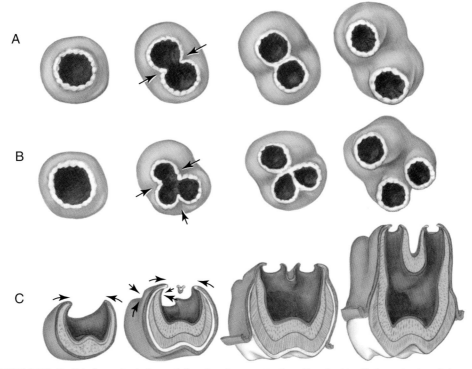

FIGURE 6-21 An apical view of the development of multirooted teeth from horizontal extensions of the cervical loop. **(A, B):** Process in a two-rooted tooth. **B:** Process in a three-rooted tooth. **C:** Section of a developing tooth with the roots still forming. The growing division of three roots is seen on this permanent maxillary molar.

organ on a multirooted tooth, elongation of its cervical loop occurs in such a way that long, tonguelike horizontal epithelial extensions or flaps develop within. Two or three such extensions can be present on multirooted teeth, depending on the similar number of roots on the mature tooth.

The usually single cervical opening of the coronal enamel organ is then divided into two or three openings by these horizontal extensions. On the pulpal surfaces of these holes, dentin formation starts after the induction of the odontoblasts and disintegration of HERS and the associated basement membrane. Only at the periphery of each opening are cementoblasts induced to form cementum on the newly formed dentin. Root development then proceeds in the same way as described for a single-rooted tooth.

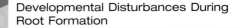
Developmental Disturbances During Root Formation

A disturbance that can occur during root development is **dilaceration**, distorted root (or roots) or crown angulation in a formed tooth (see Chapters 16 and 17 for more discussion, mainly in relation to permanent maxillary lateral incisors and canines, as well as molars). Dilaceration results from distortion of HERS caused by injury or pressure. This disturbance can occur in any tooth or group of teeth. Dilaceration can cause problems during extraction and endodontic therapy and underlines the importance of preoperative radiographic examination. This is contrast to flexion, which is a deviation or bend restricted just to the root portion of the tooth. Usually the bend is less than 90 degrees. It may also be a result of trauma to the developing tooth.

Teeth may also have extra roots, or **accessory roots** (supernumerary roots). This disturbance may be due to trauma, pressure, or metabolic disease that affects HERS. Any tooth may be affected, but it occurs mainly with the permanent third molars and is rare in incisors. Accessory roots can present problems in extraction and endodontic therapy. Preoperative radiographic examination is necessary to rule out this disturbance.

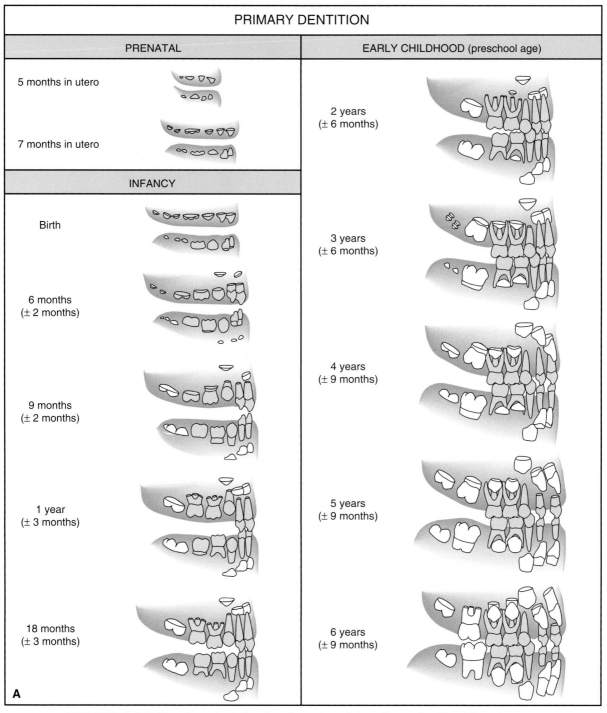

FIGURE 6-22 The chronological order of eruption of the primary dentition **(A)** and permanent dentition **(B)**. (Adapted with permission from Schour and Massler: The development of the human dentition. *Journal of the American Dental Association* 28:1153, 1941.)

PRIMARY TOOTH ERUPTION AND SHEDDING

Eruption of the primary dentition takes place in chronological order, as does the permanent dentition later (Figure 6-22). This process involves **active eruption,** which is the actual vertical movement of the tooth. This is not the **passive eruption** that occurs as

we age, when the gingiva recedes and no actual tooth movement takes place. Passive eruption is usually completed by age 24 ± 6.2 years. In studies, only 12% of patients exhibited delayed passive eruption. In a fully erupted tooth, the gingival margin is located on the enamel 0.5 to 2.0 mm coronal to the CEJ.

How tooth eruption occurs is understood, but *why* can only be theorized. No one can certify what forces "push" teeth through the soft tissues or can identify

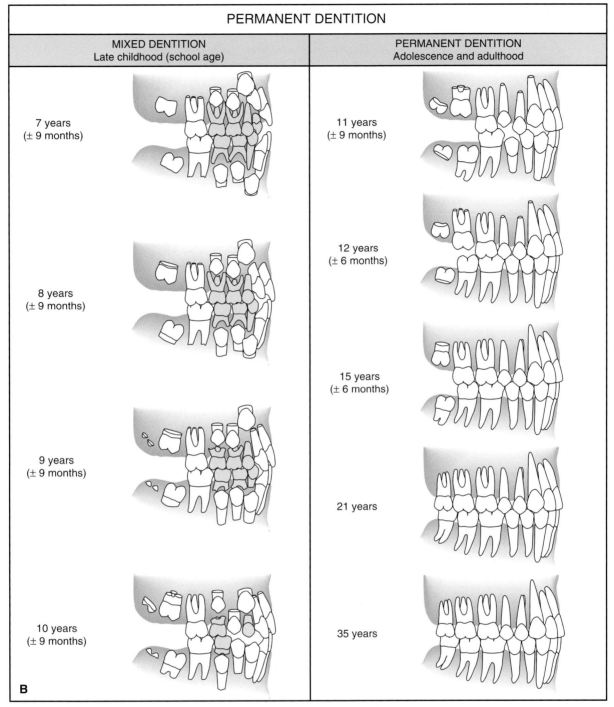

FIGURE 6-22, cont'd.

the timing mechanism that coincides with these eruptions. Each theory for eruption presents a problem in its conception. Root growth, existence of a temporary ligament, vascular pressure, contractile collagen, and hormonal signals to genetic targets all have been used to explain eruption. The timelines for eruption for both dentitions are included in Unit IV and actual eruption times for primary and permanent dentition in Chapter 18 and Appendix D.

Active eruption of a primary tooth has many stages in the movement of the tooth. After enamel apposition ceases in the crown area of each primary or permanent tooth, the ameloblasts place an acellular dental cuticle on the new enamel surface. In addition, the layers of the enamel organ are compressed, forming the **reduced enamel epithelium (REE)** (Figures 6-23 and 6-24). The REE appears as a few layers of flattened cells overlying the new enamel surface. As this formation of the REE occurs for a primary tooth, it can begin to erupt into the oral cavity.

To allow for the eruption process, the REE first fuses with the oral epithelium lining the oral cavity (Figure

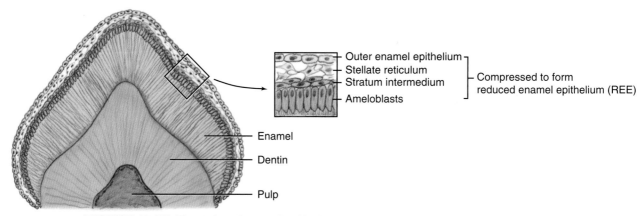

FIGURE 6-23 The reduced enamel epithelium is produced after the completion of enamel apposition when the enamel organ undergoes compression of its many layers on the enamel surface.

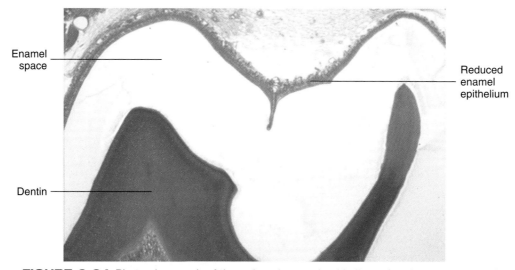

FIGURE 6-24 Photomicrograph of the reduced enamel epithelium after the completion of enamel apposition when the enamel organ undergoes compression of its many layers on the enamel surface (enamel space). (From Nanci A. *Ten Cate's Oral Histology*, ed 6. Mosby, St. Louis, 2003.)

6-25). Second, enzymes from the REE disintegrate the central portion of the fused tissue, leaving an epithelial tunnel for the tooth to erupt through into the surrounding oral epithelium of the oral cavity. This tissue disintegration causes an inflammatory response known as "teething," which may be accompanied by tenderness and edema of the local tissues. Proper oral hygiene can reduce the amount of inflammation and thus the discomfort associated with these oral changes.

As a primary tooth actively erupts, the coronal portion of the fused epithelial tissues peels back off the crown, leaving the cervical portion still attached to the neck of the tooth. This fused tissue that remains near the CEJ after the tooth erupts then serves as the initial junctional epithelium of the tooth and creates a seal between the tissue and the tooth surface. This tissue is later replaced by a definitive junctional epithelium as the root is formed (see Chapter 10).

The primary tooth is then lost, exfoliated or shed, as the succedaneous permanent tooth develops lingual to it. The process involving loss of the primary tooth consists of differentiation of osteoclasts, which absorb the alveolar bone between the two teeth, and **odonto-clasts**, which cause **resorption**, or removal of portions of the primary's root of dentin and cementum as well as small portions of the enamel crown.

The process of shedding of the primary tooth is intermittent ("on again/off again") because at the same time that osteoblasts differentiate to replace the resorbed bone, odontoblasts and cementoblasts also differentiate to replace the resorbed portions of the root. Thus a loose primary tooth may become tightened just when the supervising adults take a child to the dentist to have it removed because it is driving the child crazy as the child plays with it. When the primary tooth is lost, the **tooth fairy** is called to action, with rates now approaching very high levels.

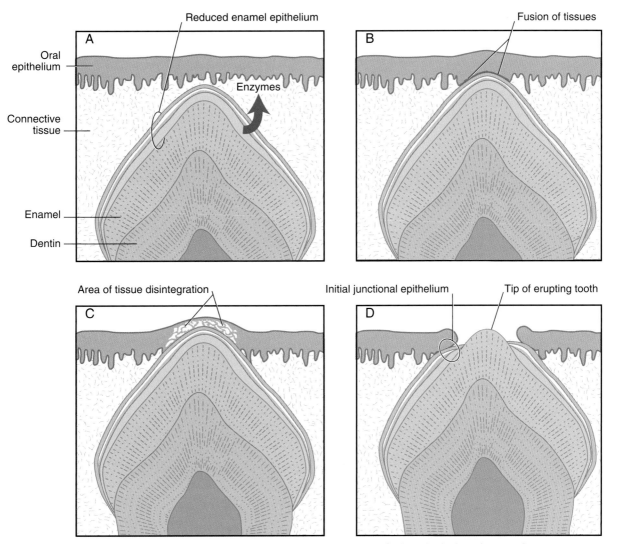

FIGURE 6-25 Stages in the process of tooth eruption. **A:** Oral cavity before the eruption process begins. Reduced enamel epithelium covers the newly formed enamel. **B:** Fusion of the reduced enamel epithelium with the oral epithelium. **C:** Disintegration of the central fused tissue, leaving a tunnel for tooth movement. **D:** Coronal fused tissues peel back from the crown during eruption, leaving the initial junctional epithelium near the cementoenamel junction.

Clinical Considerations with the Eruption Process

A residue may form on newly erupted teeth of both dentitions that may leave the teeth extrinsically stained. This residue, **Nasmyth's membrane,** consists of the fused tissue of the REE and oral epithelium as well as the dental cuticle placed by the ameloblasts on the new enamel surface (Figure 6-26). Nasmyth's membrane then easily picks up stain from food debris. It is hard to remove except by thorough but gently selective polishing. Caregivers may need to be reassured that it is only extrinsic stain on a child's newly erupted teeth.

PERMANENT TOOTH ERUPTION

The succedaneous permanent tooth erupts into the oral cavity in a position lingual to the roots of the shedding or shed primary tooth, just as it develops that way (Figure 6-27). The only exception to this is the permanent maxillary incisors, which move to a more facial position as they erupt into the oral cavity.

The process of eruption for a succedaneous tooth is the same as for the primary tooth: The REE fuses with the oral epithelium to create a tissue that degenerates, leaving an epithelial-lined eruption tunnel. The process of the nonsuccedaneous permanent tooth's eruption is similar also, but no primary tooth is shed. Both succedaneous and nonsuccedaneous permanent

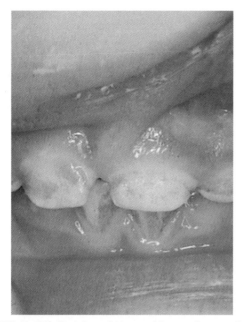

FIGURE 6-26 Staining of Nasmyth's membrane after eruption of the teeth. The entire crown area of the primary dentition is affected.

teeth erupt in chronological order (see Figure 6-22). A permanent tooth often starts to erupt before the primary tooth is fully shed, and problems in spacing can arise. Preventive orthodontic therapy can prevent some of these situations. Thus it is important for children with retained primary teeth to seek dental consultation early.

 Clinical Considerations with Eruption of the Permanent Dentition

The crown of a permanent tooth is formed initially as shown on a periapical radiograph of a mixed dentition or skull sections (Figures 6-28 and 6-29). After a permanent tooth erupts in the oral cavity, its root begins to form in the cervical area. Thus prevention of traumatic injury to the permanent teeth before they are fully anchored into the jaws is very important. Sport bite guards, which consist of individually formed plastic coverings for the teeth, are recommended for children active in all types of sports. Any injury to a child's dentition must be seen promptly by a dentist.

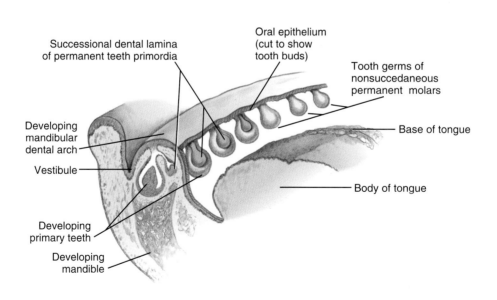

Section through fetal mandible

FIGURE 6-27 Development of the succedaneous permanent teeth lingual to the primary teeth on a section of a fetal mandible.

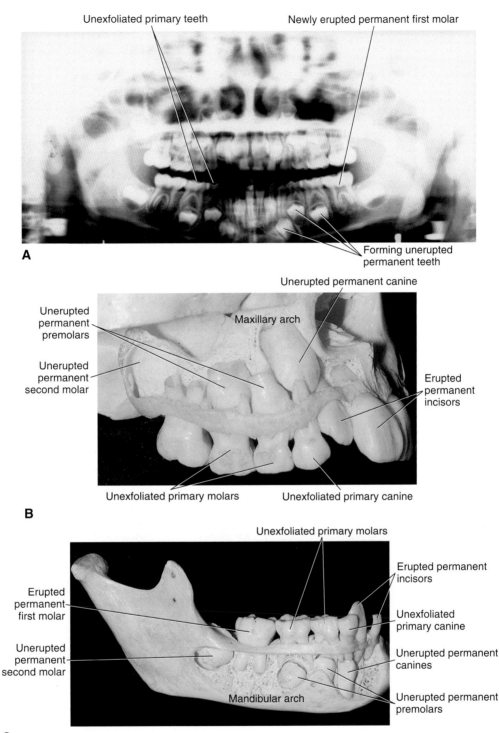

Unexfoliated primary teeth

Newly erupted permanent first molar

Forming unerupted permanent teeth

A

Unerupted permanent canine

Unerupted permanent premolars

Maxillary arch

Unerupted permanent second molar

Erupted permanent incisors

Unexfoliated primary molars

Unexfoliated primary canine

B

Unexfoliated primary molars

Erupted permanent incisors

Erupted permanent first molar

Unexfoliated primary canine

Unerupted permanent second molar

Unerupted permanent canines

Mandibular arch

Unerupted permanent premolars

C

FIGURE 6-28 Examples of a mixed dentition with primary teeth being shed and the permanent dentition erupting. **A:** Radiograph of a mixed dentition. Note the permanent teeth still forming within the jawbones of each arch. **B** and **C:** Maxilla and mandible of a skull, with a section of facial compact bone removed.

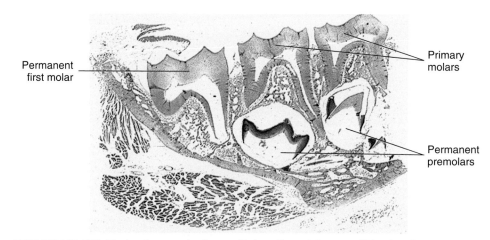

Permanent first molar

Primary molars

Permanent premolars

FIGURE 6-29 Photomicrograph of a sagittal section of the mandible showing a mixed dentition: two functioning primary mandibular molars and a partially erupted permanent mandibular first molar, as well as the developing permanent mandibular premolars. (From Nanci A. *Ten Cate's Oral Histology*, ed 6. Mosby, St. Louis, 2003.)

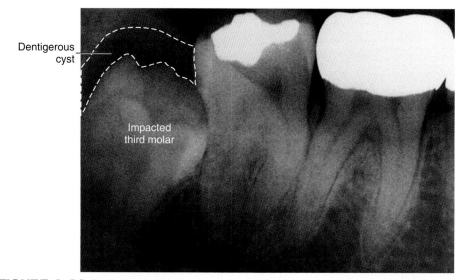

Dentigerous cyst

Impacted third molar

FIGURE 6-30 Radiograph of a dentigerous cyst (*outlined*) that is formed around the crown of an impacted and unerupted permanent mandibular third molar.

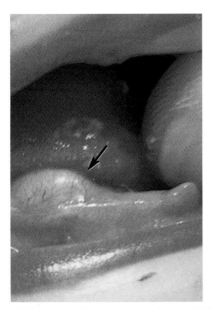

FIGURE 6-31 An eruption cyst (*arrow*) in a child. This less serious type of dentigerous cyst has formed over an erupting primary mandibular incisor.

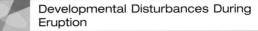

Developmental Disturbances During Eruption

An odontogenic cyst that forms from the REE after the crown has completely formed and matured is called a **dentigerous cyst,** or follicular cyst (Figure 6-30). This initially asymptomatic cyst forms around the crown of a nonerupted impacted or developing tooth, most commonly the permanent third molars. When the cyst of a nonerupted tooth becomes larger, it may cause displaced teeth, jaw fracture, and pain. This type of cyst must be completely removed surgically, because it may become neoplastic otherwise.

If a dentigerous cyst appears on a developing tooth, it is called an eruption cyst and appears as fluctuant, blue, vesicle-like gingival lesion on a partially erupted tooth (Figure 6-31). With eruption of the tooth, the cyst disintegrates, and no further treatment is needed. Because it appears to enlarge as the tooth erupts, caregivers may need to be reassured that this lesion is not serious.

UNIT III

DENTAL HISTOLOGY

CHAPTER 7

Overview of the Cell

This chapter discusses the following topics:

- The cell
  - Cell membrane and cytoplasm
  - Organelles
  - Inclusions
- Cell division
- Extracellular materials
- Intercellular junctions

After studying this chapter, the reader should be able to:

1. Define and pronounce the key terms in this chapter.
2. Discuss the components of the cell, the cell membrane, cytoplasm, organelles, and inclusions.
3. Describe cell division and the phases of mitosis that are involved.
4. Describe the extracellular materials surrounding the cell and its intercellular junctions.
5. Integrate the knowledge of a background of the cell into the histology of the orofacial tissues and the pathology that may occur within them.

Key Terms

Anaphase (an-ah-faz)
Cell
Cell membrane
Centrioles (sen-tree-ols)
Centromere (sen-tro-mere)
Centrosome (sen-tro-some)
Chromatids (kro-mah-tids)
Chromatin (kro-mah-tin)
Chromosomes (kro-mah-somes)
Cytoplasm (cy-to-plazm)
Cytoskeleton (site-oh-skel-it-on)
Desmosome (des-mo-som)
Endocytosis (en-do-sigh-toe-sis)
Endoplasmic reticulum
 (en-do-plas-mik rey-tik-u-lum)
Exocytosis (ek-so-sigh-toe-sis)

Golgi complex (gol-jee)
Hemidesmosome
 (hem-eye-des-mo-som)
Histology (his-tol-oh-jee)
Inclusions (in-kloo-zhins)
Intercellular substance
Intermediate filaments (fil-ah-ments)
Interphase (in-ter-faz)
Keratin (ker-ah-tin)
Lysosomes (li-sah-somes)
Metaphase (met-ah-faz)
Mitochondria (mite-ah-kon-dree-ah)
Microfilaments (my-kroh-fil-ah-ments)
Microtubules (my-kroh-too-bules)
Mitosis (my-toe-sis)
Nuclear envelope (noo-kle-er), pores

Nucleolus (noo-kle-oh-lis)
Nucleoplasm (noo-kle-ah-plazm)
Nucleus (noo-kle-is) (plural, nuclei,
 noo-kle-eye)
Organ
Organelles (or-gah-nels)
Phagocytosis (fag-oh-sigh-toe-sis)
Prophase (pro-faz)
Ribosomes (ry-bo-somes)
System
Telophase (tel-oh- faz)
Tissue, fluid
Tonofilaments (ton-oh-fil-ah-ments)
Vacuoles (vak-you-oles)

THE CELL

The organization of the body histologically is initially discussed in this beginning of *Unit III*. The smallest living unit of organization in the body is the **cell** (Figures 7-1 and 7-2 and Table 7-1). Each cell is capable of performing various functions. Each cell has a cell membrane, cytoplasm, organelles, and inclusions. Every cell is a world unto itself, like a small enclosed town, surrounded by a boundary, having "factories" and other "industries" that make it almost self-sufficient.

However, cells also interact with the extracellular environment in many ways. Cells can perform **exocytosis,** which is an active transport of material from a vesicle within the cell out into the extracellular environment. Exocytosis occurs when there is fusion of a vesicle membrane with the cell membrane and subsequent expulsion of the contained material.

The uptake of materials from the extracellular environment into the cell is called **endocytosis.** Endocytosis can take place as an invagination of the cell membrane. Endocytosis can also take place as **phagocytosis,** which is the engulfing and then digesting of solid waste and foreign material by the cell through enzymatic breakdown of the material (discussed later in regard to lysosomes).

Cells also interact with one another. Cells with similar characteristics of form and function are grouped together to form a **tissue** (see Table 7-1). Thus tissues are collections of similarly specialized cells, most often surrounded by extracellular materials. Tissues bond together to form an **organ,** a somewhat independent body part that performs a specific function or functions. Organs can function together as a **system.**

Cells in a tissue undergo cellular division to reproduce themselves and replace the dead tissue cells. As a result of the division process, two daughter cells that are identical to each other and to the original parent cell are formed. This process consists of different phases and is discussed with regard to different components of the cell. It will be described at the end of this chapter.

Histology is the study of the microscopic structure and function of cells and their tissues. Another term for histology is *microanatomy,* because the dimensions of the anatomical structures studied are on a microscopic scale. A dental professional must understand the basic unit, the cell, to then understand the larger concepts involved in the histology of tissues, such as those in the oral cavity. This chapter gives an overview of the cell and its various components, and then Chapter 8 presents a review of basic tissues in the body. A discussion of the histology of the tissues

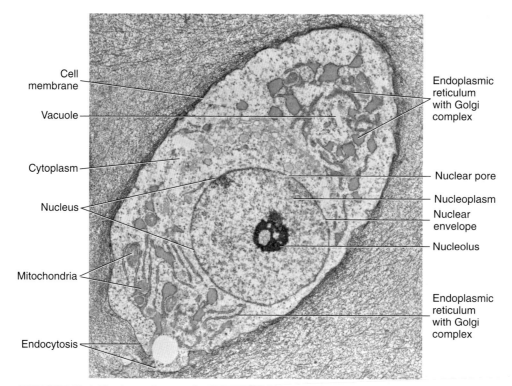

FIGURE 7-1 Electron micrograph of the cell and some of its most visible contents. Note the prominent nucleus and cell membrane. (Courtesy of the late Herbert K. Kashiwa, PhD, Associate Professor, Department of Biological Structure, University of Washington, Seattle, WA.)

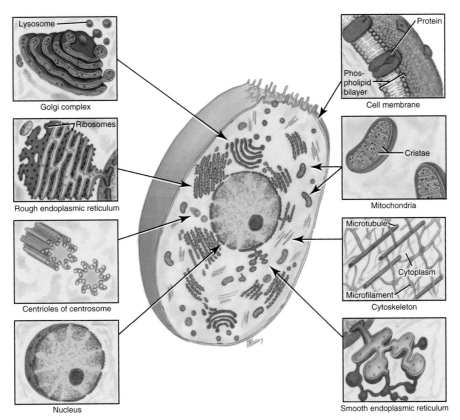

FIGURE 7-2 The cell and its cell membrane, cytoplasm, organelles, and inclusions.

TABLE 7-1

Components of the Human Body With Examples

Cell	Smallest living unit of organization: Epithelial cell, neuron, myofiber, chondrocyte, fibroblast, erythrocyte, macrophage, sperm
Tissue	Collection of similarly specialized cells: Epithelium, nervous tissue, muscle, cartilage, bone, blood
Organ	Independent body part formed from tissues: Skin, brain, heart, liver
System	Organs functioning together: Central nervous system, respiratory system, immune system, cardiovascular system

and organs of the oral cavity follows later in this unit.

Cell Membrane and Cytoplasm

The **cell membrane,** or plasma membrane, completely surrounds the cell (see Figures 7-1 and 7-2). Despite its fragile microscopic appearance, it is a tough and resourceful guardian, or "gatekeeper," of the cell's interior. The usual cell membrane is an intricate bilayer, consisting predominantly of phospholipids and proteins. The phospholipids serve largely as a diffusion regulator. The proteins of the cell membrane serve as structural reinforcements as well as receptors for specific hormones, neurotransmitters, and immunoglobulins (antibodies). The cell membrane is associated with many of the mechanisms of intercellular junctions and other functions of the cell.

The **cytoplasm** includes the semifluid portion contained within the cell membrane boundary as well as the skeletal system of support (or cytoskeleton, discussed later in this chapter). The cytoplasm contains not only a number of structures but also spaces or cavities, or **vacuoles.**

Organelles

The **organelles** are specialized, metabolically active structures within the cell (see Figures 7-1 and 7-2). The organelles allow each cell to function according to its genetic code. Organelles also subdivide the cell into compartments. The major organelles of the cell include the nucleus, mitochondria, ribosomes, endoplasmic reticulum, Golgi complex, lysosomes, and cytoskeleton.

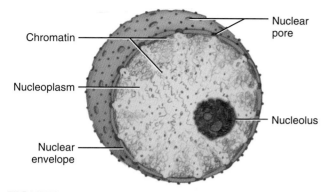

Chromatin

Nucleoplasm

Nuclear envelope

Nuclear pore

Nucleolus

FIGURE 7-3 The nucleus and its various components: the nucleoplasm, nuclear envelope, nuclear pores, chromatin, and nucleolus.

NUCLEUS

The **nucleus (plural, nuclei)** is the largest, densest, and most conspicuous organelle in the cell when it is viewed microscopically (see Figures 7-1 and 7-2 and Figure 7-3). A nucleus is found in all cells except mature red blood cells, and most cells have a single nucleus. Some cells are mulinucleated, such as skeletal muscle cells.

When stained with basic histological dyes, the chief nucleic acid in the nucleoplasm (DNA, in the form of **chromatin**) shows up well as diffuse stippling when the cell is viewed microscopically. In an actively dividing cell, the chromatin condenses into microscopically visible, discrete, rodlike **chromosomes.** Each chromosome has a **centromere,** a clear, constricted area near the middle. Chromosomes become two filamentous, or threadlike, **chromatids,** or daughter chromosomes, during cell division, joined by a centromere. After cell division, major segments of the chromosomes again become uncoiled and dispersed among the other components of the nucleoplasm.

The nucleus is the cell's "memory bank": It stores the genetic code. From its sequence of nucleotides in the chromatin, deoxyribonucleic acid (DNA) and ribonucleic acid (RNA) give directions for everything the cell is and will be. Thus they control all functions the cell performs. The nucleus is also the "command center" of the cell, controlling the other organelles in the cell. The nucleus is influenced by what occurs inside the cell as well as outside the cell. Only certain genes are "turned on" to participate in the production of specific proteins at any particular time.

The chemical messages that result in genes' switching on or off in the nucleus come from the cytoplasm, where, in turn, they are generated as a result of interaction between the surface membrane and the environment. Although genes contain the total range of the cell's possibilities, the cellular environment dictates which of these possibilities for differentiation, growth, development, and specialization will be expressed.

As would be expected, the nucleus is constantly active. Before cell division, new DNA must be synthesized and every single gene must be replicated. These genes, linked into chromosomes, are then separated into duplicate sets during cell division. In the nucleus, three very important types of RNA are produced: messenger RNA (mRNA) molecules, which are complementary copies of distinct segments of DNA; transfer RNA (tRNA) molecules, which are molecules capable of specifically binding to and transporting amino acid units for protein synthesis; and ribosomal RNA (rRNA), which will be discussed later.

In addition to all the hereditary activity associated with cell division, genes on the DNA selectively direct the synthesis of thousands of enzymes and other integral and cytoplasmic proteins, as well as any secretory products. This process involves transcription of information from various parts of the DNA molecules into new strands of mRNA, which carry the encoded instructions into the cytoplasm for processing through the process of translation involving tRNA, and rRNA, and amino acids.

The fluid portion within the nucleus is the **nucleoplasm,** which contains important molecules used in the construction of ribosomes, nucleic acids, and other nuclear materials. The nucleus is completely surrounded by the **nuclear envelope,** a membrane similar to the cell membrane, except that it is double-layered. The nuclear envelope is associated with many other organelles of the cell. The nuclear envelope may be pierced by **nuclear pores,** which act as avenues of communication between the inner nucleoplasm and the outer cytoplasm. The number and distribution of these nuclear pores vary with cell type, with level of cell activity, and in states of differentiation of the same cell type.

Contained in the nucleus is the **nucleolus,** a prominent, rounded nuclear organelle that is usually centrally placed in the nucleoplasm when the cell is viewed microscopically (see Figure 7-3). The nucleolus mainly produces rRNA and the nucleotides of the two other types of RNA. The roles of the nucleolus and ribosomes with rRNA in protein synthesis are discussed later. Without a nucleolus, no protein synthetic activity would occur within the cell.

MITOCHONDRIA

The **mitochondria** are the most numerous organelles in the cell. They are associated with energy conversion and are the "power plants" of the cell. They are a major source of adenosine triphosphate (ATP) and therefore are the site of many metabolic reactions (see Figures 7-1 and 7-2). Microscopically, mitochondria resemble small bags with a larger bag fitted inside because each bag is folded back on itself. These inner folds exist to increase the surface area for more dense packing of the particular protein and enzyme molecules involved in aerobic cellular respiration. Internal to the folds, mitochondrial DNA, calcium and magnesium granules, enzymes, electrolytes, and water are present in a matrix.

Most of a cell's energy comes from mitochondria and is produced by two of the pathways of aerobic cellular respiration. These involve both Krebs cycle, with its multienzyme system, and the hydrogen pathway, which uses the electron transport chain of enzymes. Besides supplying energy, mitochondria help balance the concentration of water, calcium, and other ions in the cytoplasm.

RIBOSOMES

The **ribosomes** are another organelle of the cell and are tiny spheres (see Figure 7-2). The ribosomes are made in the nucleolus from rRNA and protein molecules and are assembled in the cytoplasm. They function as "protein factories" for the cell. They can be free in the cytoplasm, bound to membranes, or within mitochondria. Their position changes depending on the type of protein being made. They can be bound either to the outer nuclear membrane or onto the surface of the rough endoplasmic reticulum (discussed next).

Ribosomes can also be found singly or in clusters within the cell. As many as 30 separate ribosomes may be attached sequentially to a single molecule of mRNA, with each ribosome making its own protein copy as it works its way along the length of the mRNA transcript. Within these ribosomes, free amino acids are being joined together in accordance with the particular order specified by the mRNA transcript to sequence the required protein chain.

ENDOPLASMIC RETICULUM

Endoplasmic reticulum (**ER**) is so called because it is arranged in a network and is more concentrated in the cell's inner or endoplasmic region than in the peripheral or ectoplasmic region (see Figures 7-1 and 7-2). The ER consists of parallel membrane-bound channels. All the membranes of the ER interconnect, forming a system of channels and folds microscopically. This system is continuous with the nuclear envelope.

The ER can be classified as either smooth or rough on the basis of the absence or presence of ribosomes, each giving a different microscopic appearance to the structure. The smooth ER (SER), which is free of ribosomes, appears microscopically smooth in surface texture. Rough ER (RER) is dotted with ribosomes on its outer surface, which makes it appear microscopically rough.

The outer layer of the nuclear envelope connects with all the ER in the cell, both smooth and rough. The ER's primary functions are modification, storage, segregation, and finally transport of proteins that the cell manufactures (on the ribosomes) for use in other sections of the cell or even outside the cell.

GOLGI COMPLEX

Once the newly created protein has been modified by the ER, it is transferred to the **Golgi complex** for subsequent segregation, packaging, and transport of protein compounds (see Figures 7-1 and 7-2). The Golgi complex is the second largest organelle after the nucleus and is composed of stacks of three to twenty flattened, smooth-membraned vesicular sacs arranged parallel to one another.

Vesicles of protein molecules from the RER fuse with the Golgi complex, transferring protein molecules to be further modified, concentrated, and packaged by the Golgi complex. After this modification and packaging, the Golgi complex wraps up large numbers of these molecules into a single membranous vesicle and then sends it on its way to the cell's surface to be released by the process of exocytosis. These protein molecules, which include hormones, enzymes, and other secretory products, are released into the extracellular space or into capillaries as these vesicles fuse with the cell membrane. These products put together in the Golgi complex can include such substances as mucus for the salivary glands or insulin for the pancreas.

The modifications by the Golgi complex to the protein molecules include adding carbohydrates, thus forming glycoproteins, as it does in the production of mucus. The Golgi complex also may remove part of a polypeptide chain, as it does in the case of insulin. The Golgi complex not only prepares proteins for export by exocytosis but also produces a separate organelle, lysosomes (discussed next).

LYSOSOMES

The **lysosomes** are organelles produced by the Golgi complex (see Figure 7-2). They function in both intracellular and extracellular digestion by the cell. This digestive function is due to their ability to lyse, or digest, waste and foreign material, which occurs during phagocytosis (Figure 7-4). Lysosomes break down many kinds of molecules by way of the powerful hydrolytic and digestive enzymes contained within them. The main hydrolytic enzyme in lysosomes is hyaluronidase. Lysosomes are membrane-bound vesicles that develop as a bud that pinches off of the end of one of the Golgi complex's flattened sacs. The enzymes of the lysosomes originally are produced on the RER and then transported for packing to the Golgi complex, where the lysosomes originate.

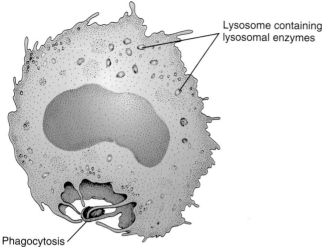

Lysosome containing
lysosomal enzymes

Phagocytosis
of bacterium

FIGURE 7-4 Phagocytosis. This is the engulfing and digesting of solid waste and foreign material (such as a bacterium, as seen here) by a white blood cell (monocyte) through enzymatic breakdown of the matter from its enclosed lysosomes. (From Fehrenbach MJ: Inflammation and repair. Ibsen OAC, Phelan JA, Editors: *Oral Pathology for Dental Hygienists*, ed 4. WB Saunders, Philadelphia, 2004.)

As the substances are broken down into sufficiently small and simple products, the usable material diffuses out of the lysosome into the cell's cytoplasm to be incorporated into new molecules being synthesized, a situation of cellular recycling. Indigestible material remains in the lysosome and becomes a residual body. It either migrates to the cell surface to be released by exocytosis or remains as a remnant in the lysosome and becomes an inclusion (discussed later). Although all cells except red blood cells are capable of some digestive activity, other cells, such as certain white blood cells, have differentiated to specialize in digestive processes, especially phagocytosis.

CENTROSOME

The **centrosome** is a dense, somewhat oval-shaped organelle. A pair of cylindrical structures are contained in it, called **centrioles.** The centrosome is always located near the nucleus. This location is important because the centrosome plays a significant role in forming the mitotic spindle apparatus during cell division. There are two centrioles within the centrosome, and each is composed of triplets of microtubules arranged in a cartwheel pattern. Without this self-replicating centriole-centrosome unit, an animal cell cannot reproduce (discussed later).

CYTOSKELETON

The interior of the cell is neither liquid nor gel in nature but somewhat between the two. It also has a three-dimensional system of support, the **cytoskeleton.** The components of the cytoskeleton include microfilaments, intermediate filaments, and microtubules. This design lends basic stability to the cell as a whole, functioning like reinforced girders. It also acts to compartmentalize the cytoplasm, creating preferred "freeways" for the movement of molecules formed by cellular processes.

Both **microfilaments** and **microtubules** consist of specialized proteins. Microfilaments are delicate, threadlike microscopic structures. Microtubules are slender, hollow, tubular microscopic structures that may appear individually, doubly, or as triplets. Microtubules assist microfilaments in the maintenance of overall cell shape and in the transport of intracellular materials. Additionally, microtubules form the internal framework of cilia and flagella, centrioles, and the mitotic spindle for cell division (discussed later).

Certain cells exhibit projections for the purpose of moving substances along the surface of the cell or for moving the entire cell in the extracellular environment. If the projections on the cell are shorter and more numerous, they are called *cilia.* If the projections are fewer and longer, they are called *flagella.*

Both cilia and flagella are useful in human reproduction. An egg is propelled within the fallopian tube by cilia, and sperm are propelled by their own flagella. Structurally, there is no major difference between cilia and flagella except for their relative lengths. Both consist of pairs of multiple microtubules that form a ring around two single microtubules. Cilia are also noted in the respiratory mucosa lining the nasal cavity and paranasal sinuses as they move the mucous coating of those tissues.

The **intermediate filaments** are of various types of thicker, threadlike microscopic structures within the cell. One type of intermediate filament, **tonofilaments,** has a major role in intercellular junctions. Another type of intermediate filament is one that forms **keratin,** which is found in calloused epithelial tissues.

Inclusions

The cell also contains **inclusions,** which are metabolically inert substances or structures that are transient (see Figure 7-2). These include masses of organic chemicals and often are recognizable microscopically. These inclusions are released from storage by the cell and used as demand dictates. Lipids and glycogen can be decomposed for energy from inclusions in the cell. Melanin, a pigment, is stored as inclusions in certain cells of the skin and oral mucosa (see Chapter 8). Inclusions also include residual bodies: spent lysosomes and their digested material.

TABLE 7-2

Process of Mitosis During Cell Division

Phases	Microscopic Appearance	

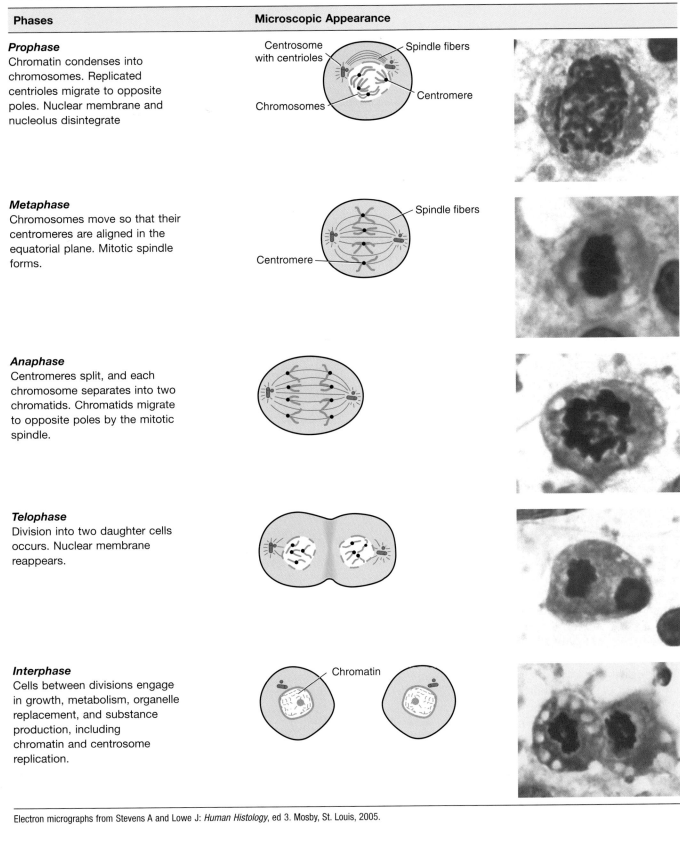

Prophase
Chromatin condenses into chromosomes. Replicated centrioles migrate to opposite poles. Nuclear membrane and nucleolus disintegrate

Centrosome with centrioles · Spindle fibers · Chromosomes · Centromere

Metaphase
Chromosomes move so that their centromeres are aligned in the equatorial plane. Mitotic spindle forms.

Spindle fibers · Centromere

Anaphase
Centromeres split, and each chromosome separates into two chromatids. Chromatids migrate to opposite poles by the mitotic spindle.

Telophase
Division into two daughter cells occurs. Nuclear membrane reappears.

Interphase
Cells between divisions engage in growth, metabolism, organelle replacement, and substance production, including chromatin and centrosome replication.

Chromatin

Electron micrographs from Stevens A and Lowe J: *Human Histology*, ed 3. Mosby, St. Louis, 2005.

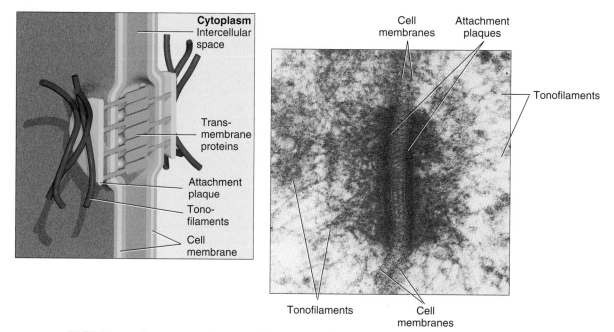

FIGURE 7-5 Desmosomal intercellular junctions between cells in a diagram and electron micrograph. Note the attachment plaque, which is the attachment device that involves the tonofilaments. Cell adhesion between cell membranes is mediated by transmembrane proteins. (From Stevens A, Lowe J: *Human Histology*, ed 3. Mosby, St. Louis, 2005.)

CELL DIVISION

Cell division is a complex process involving many of the organelles of the cell (Table 7-2). Before cell division, the nuclear material (DNA) is replicated; then, during the part of cell division known as **mitosis**, this material is divided so that the resulting two daughter cells are identical to the parent cell. Then, other cytoplasmic components of the cell also are divided. Mitosis during cell division comprises four phases: **prophase, metaphase, anaphase,** and **telophase.**

EXTRACELLULAR MATERIALS

The cells in tissues are surrounded by extracellular materials. These include both tissue fluid and intercellular substance. **Tissue fluid,** or interstitial fluid, provides a medium for dissolving, mixing, and transporting substances and for carrying out chemical reactions. Similar to blood plasma in its content of ions and diffusible substances, tissue fluid contains a small amount of plasma proteins.

Tissue fluid enters the tissue to surround the cells by diffusing through the capillary walls as a filtrate from the plasma of the blood. Tissue fluid then drains back into the blood as lymph through osmosis via the lymphatic system. The amount of tissue fluid varies from tissue to tissue, and variations can also occur within any tissue. An excess amount of tissue fluid, or edema, can accumulate when an injured tissue undergoes an inflammatory response, leading to tissue enlargement.

Intercellular substance, or ground substance, is shapeless, colorless, and transparent. It fills the spaces between cells in a tissue. It serves as a barrier to the penetration of foreign substances into the tissues. It also serves as a medium for the exchange of gases and metabolic substances. The cells produce the intercellular substance among them. One of the most common ingredients of intercellular substance is hyaluronic acid.

INTERCELLULAR JUNCTIONS

Some cells in tissues are joined by intercellular junctions. These are mechanical attachments between cells and possibly between cells and nearby noncellular surfaces. With these intercellular junctions, the cell membranes come close together but do not completely attach. Higher-power microscopes are needed to visualize these attachments, which appear as dense bodies. All intercellular junctions involve some sort of intricate attachment device. The attachment device includes an attachment plaque located within the cell and tonofilaments.

An intercellular junction between cells is a **desmosome,** such as that seen in the upper layers of the skin (Figure 7-5). The desmosome appears to be disc-shaped and can be likened to a "spot weld." Desmosomes cause an artifact when epithelial cells are fixed and dried for prolonged microscopic study. Desmosomes tend to cause the regularly plump cells to appear prickled or star-shaped in stratified squamous epithelium as the desmosomes maintain their junctional stronghold between the shrinking cells

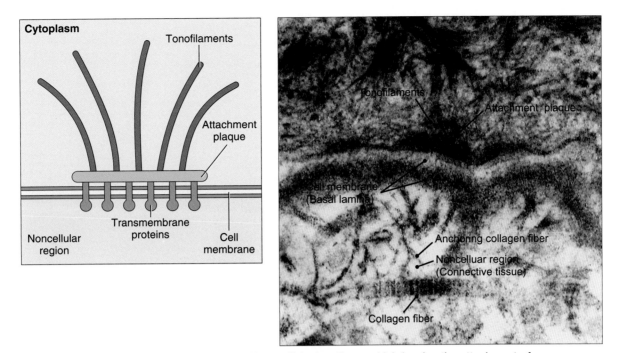

FIGURE 7-6 Hemidesmosomal intercellular junctions, which involve the attachment of cells to an adjacent noncellular surface in a diagram and electron micrograph. This type of intercellular junction occurs at the basement membrane between epithelial and connective tissues (as shown here, see also Figure 8-4), as well as the attachment of the gingiva to the tooth surface. Note the smaller attachment plaques of the hemidesmosomal junction and tonofilaments on the cellular side. Cell adhesion to the noncellular surface is mediated by transmembrane proteins. (From Stevens A, Lowe J: *Human Histology*, ed 3. Mosby, St. Louis, 2005.)

(see Chapter 8). The desmosomal junctions also are released and then reattached in new locations as the cells migrate during tissue turnover.

Another type of intercellular junction is a **hemidesmosome,** which involves an attachment of a cell to an adjacent noncellular surface (Figure 7-6). This type of attachment is present with the gingival epithelium that attaches to the tooth surface (see Chapter 10) as well as in that which occurs between the nails and nail beds. The attachment device of a hemidesmosome

looks like half of a desmosome because it involves a smaller attachment plaque and tonofilaments from only the cellular side. Thus it appears as a thinner disc because the noncellular surface cannot produce the other half of attachment mechanism. Hemidesmosomes are also involved as a mechanism for attaching the epithelium to connective tissue such as in the oral mucosa by way of the basement membrane (see Chapter 8).

Basic Tissues

This chapter discusses the following topics:

- Basic tissues
- Epithelial tissue
  - Histology of epithelial tissue
  - Classification of epithelial tissues
  - Epithelial turnover and repair
- Basement membrane
- Connective tissue
  - Histology of connective tissue
  - Classification of connective tissue
- Specialized connective tissue
  - Cartilage

- Bone
- Blood
- Muscle tissue
  - Classification of muscle tissue
  - Histology of muscle tissue
- Nerve tissue
  - Histology of nerve tissue
  - Nervous system

After studying this chapter, the reader should be able to:

1. Define and pronounce the key terms in this chapter.
2. List and describe each of the basic histological types of tissues.
3. Integrate the knowledge of the basic histology into the specific histology of the orofacial region and the related pathology that may occur.

Key Terms

Adipose connective tissue (ad-i-pose)
Anchoring collage fibers
Appositional growth (ap-oh-zish-in-al)
Basal lamina (bay-sal lam-i-nah)
Basement membrane
Basophil (bay-sah-fil)
Blood
Bone: cancellous (kan-sel-us), compact (kom-pak), immature, marrow (mar-oh), mature, secondary

Calcium hydroxyapatite (hy-drox-see-ap-ah-tite)
Canaliculi (kan-ah-lik-u-lie)
Cartilage (kar-ti-lij)
Cells
Chondroblasts (kon-dro-blasts)
Chondrocytes (kon-dro-sites)
Collagen fibers (kol-ah-jen)
Connective tissue: dense, loose, papillae (pah-pil-ay), proper
Dermis (der-mis)

Elastic fibers (e-las-tik), connective tissues
Endosteum (en-dos-te-um)
Endothelium (en-do-thee-lee-um)
Eosinophil (e-ah-sin-ah-fil)
Epidermis (ep-i-der-mis)
Epithelium (ep-ee-thee-lee-um)
Fibroblast (fi-bro-blast)
Granulation tissue (gran-yoo-lay-shin)
Haversian system (hah-ver-zi-an), canal

Hemidesmosomes (hem-eye-**des**-mo-som)
Howship's lacuna (how-ships)
Immunogen (im-un-ah-jen)
Immunoglobulin (im-u-nah-**glob**-ul-in)
Interstitial growth (in-ter-**stish**-il)
Keratin (**ker**-ah-tin)
Lacuna (plural, **lacunae**) (lah-ku-nah, lah-**ku**-nay)
Lamellae (lah-**mel**-ay)
Lamina propria (lam-i-nah pro-pree-ah)
Lymphocyte (**lim**-fo-site)
Macrophage (**mak**-rah-faje)
Mast cell
Matrix (**may**-triks)
Monocyte (**mon**-ah-site)
Muscle: skeletal
Nerve
Neuron (**noor**-on)
Neutrophil (**noo**-trah-fil)

Odontoclast (o-**don**-to-klast)
Ossification (os-i-fi-**kay**-shun): endochondral (en-do-**kon**-dril), intramembranous (in-trah-**mem**-bran-us)
Osteocytes (os-tee-oh-sites)
Osteoid (**os**-te-oid)
Osteoblasts (**os**-te-oh-blasts)
Osteoclast (**os**-te-oh-klast)
Osteons (**os**-te-onz)
Papillary layer (pap-i-**lar**-ee)
Perichondrium (per-ee-**kon**-dre-im)
Periosteum (per-ee-**os**-te-im)
Plasma (**plaz**-mah)
Plasma cells
Platelets (**plate**-lits)
Polymorphonuclear leukocyte (pol-ee-mor-fah-**noo**-klee-er)
Pseudostratified epithelium (soo-doh-**strat**-i-fide).
Red blood cell

Resorption (re-**sorp**-shun): generalized, localized
Rete ridges (**ree**-tee)
Reticular fibers (re-**tik**-u-ler), lamina, layer
Simple epithelium (ep-ee-**thee**-lee-um)
Squames (skwaymz)
Stratified epithelium (**strat**-i-fide)
Stratified squamous epithelium (skway-mus)
Submucosa (sub-mu-**ko**-sah)
Synapse (**sin**-aps)
Tissues
Turnover time
Trabeculae (trah-**bek**-u-lay)
Tonofilaments (ton-oh-fil-ah-ments)
Volkmann's canals (**volk**-manz)
White blood cell

BASIC TISSUES

Cells with similar characteristics of form and function are grouped together to form tissues. **Tissues** are collections of similarly specialized cells. Tissues are categorized according to four basic histological types. It is during prenatal development that embryonic cell layers differentiate into the various basic histological types. Basic histological tissues include epithelial, connective, muscle, and nerve tissues (Table 8-1). These basic tissues have subcategories that serve specialized functions in the body.

Dental professionals must understand the histology of these basic tissue types before studying the distinct tissues present in the oral cavity and associated regions of the face and neck. An understanding of these basic tissue types helps dental professionals better understand the processes involving wound healing and repair as well as the underlying pathological processes that can occur in these regions.

Most of the tissues of the body can be renewed as their component cells die and are removed from the tissue. The **turnover time** is the time it takes for the newly divided cells to be completely replaced throughout the tissue. This turnover time differs for each of the basic tissues. An understanding of turnover time may be the future basis for how we fight the aging and disease processes in the body, including those that occur in the oral cavity.

EPITHELIAL TISSUE

Epithelium is the tissue type that covers and lines the external and internal body surfaces, including vessels and small cavities. Epithelial tissues not only serve as a protective covering or lining but are also involved in

TABLE 8-1

Classification of Basic Tissues

Tissue	Types
Epithelium	Simple: squamous, cuboidal, columnar, pseudostratified Stratified: squamous (keratinized, nonkeratinized), cuboidal, columnar, transitional
Connective tissue	Solid soft: connective tissue proper, specialized (adipose, fibrous, elastic, reticular) Solid firm: cartilage Solid rigid: bone Fluid: blood, lymph
Muscle	Involuntary: smooth and cardiac Voluntary: skeletal
Nerve	Afferent: sensory Efferent: motor

tissue absorption, secretion, and sensory and specialized functions. Their protection is from physical, chemical, and microbial attack as well as dehydration and heat loss, and includes the formation of an epithelial barrier.

Depending on their classification, epithelial tissues can be derived from any of the three embryonic cell layers: the ectoderm, endoderm, and mesoderm (see Chapter 3). Those of the skin and oral regions are of ectodermal origin. Those lining the respiratory and digestive tract are of endodermal origin, and those of the urinary tract are derived from mesoderm.

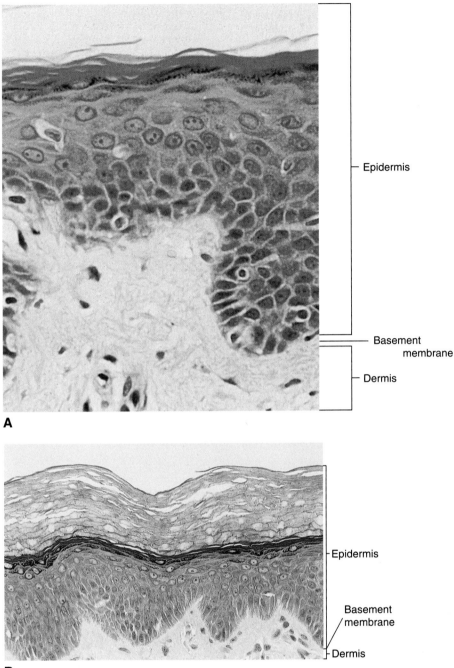

FIGURE 8-1 Microscopic sections of the skin showing the epidermis and dermis, the epithelium and connective tissue portions, respectively. Note the location of the basement membrane between these two tissues. (**A:** From Stevens A, Lowe J. *Human Histology*, ed 3. Mosby, St. Louis, 2005; **B:** Courtesy of Dr. James McIntosh, PhD, Department of Biomedical Sciences, Baylor College of Dentistry, Dallas, TX.)

Histology of Epithelial Tissue

Epithelial tissue consists of closely grouped polyhedral cells surrounded by very little or no intercellular substance or tissue fluid (Figure 8-1). This tissue is capable of rapid turnover. In fact, epithelium is highly regenerative because its deepest and germinal cells are capable of reproduction by mitosis. Epithelial cells usually undergo cellular differentiation as they move to the surface. Epithelial cells are tightly joined by intercellular junctions to one another in the form of desmosomes (except in the more superficial layers) and to nearby noncellular surfaces by hemidesmosomes, such as with the basement membrane (see Chapter 7). These nearby noncellular surfaces also include nails and teeth.

Epithelial tissue is avascular, having no blood supply of its own. Cellular nutrition consisting of oxygen and metabolites is obtained by diffusion from the adjoining connective tissue, which is usually

TABLE 8-2

Types of Epithelial Cells

Cells with Description	Microscopic Appearance in Tissue*
Squamous cells Flattened cells with cell height much less than cell width	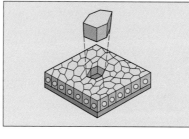
Cuboidal cells Cube-shaped cells with approximately equal cell height and cell width	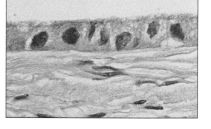
Columnar cells Rectangular or tall cells in which cell height exceeds cell width	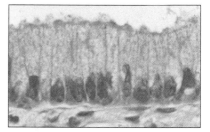

*Note that these epithelial cells are shown in simple epithelium. Diagrams from Stevens A, Lowe J. *Human Histology.* Mosby, St. Louis, 1996.

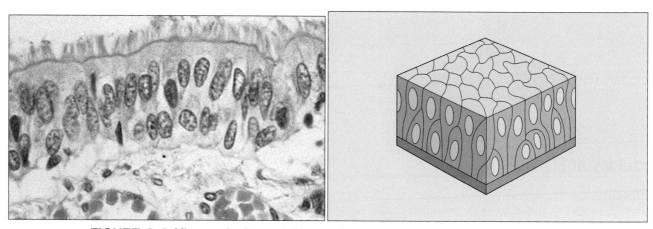

FIGURE 8-2 Microscopic view and diagram of pseduostratified columnar epithelium, such as that present in the respiratory system. This epithelium falsely appears as multiple cell layers when viewed under a low-power microscopic magnification because the cells' nuclei appear at different levels. However, in reality, cells of different heights are seen. Because the cells of different heights all have a direct relationship with the basement membrane, it is still a simple epitheliulm. (From Stevens A, Lowe J. *Human Histology*, ed 3. Mosby, St. Louis, 2005.)

highly vascularized. Between the epithelium and connective tissue in both the skin and oral mucosa is a basement membrane, which is produced by both the epithelium and the adjoining connective tissue (discussed later).

Classification of Epithelial Tissue

Epithelial tissues can be classified into two main categories on the basis of their arrangement into layers of cells: simple and stratified. **Simple epithelium** consists of a single layer of epithelial cells. The further classification of tissue involves different types of epithelial cells according to shape; they can be simple squamous, simple cuboidal, or simple columnar (Table 8-2).

Simple squamous epithelium consists of flattened platelike epithelial cells, or **squames,** lining blood and lymphatic vessels, heart, and serous cavities and important interfaces in the lungs and kidneys (see Table 8-2). The special term **endothelium** is used to refer to the simple squamous epithelium lining these vessels and serous cavities.

Simple cuboidal epithelium consists of cube-shaped cells that line the ducts of various glands, such as certain portions of the salivary gland ducts. Simple columnar epithelium consists of rectangular or tall cells, such as in the lining of other salivary gland ducts, as well as the inner enamel epithelium, whose cells become enamel-forming ameloblasts.

Epithelial tissues can also be classified as **pseudostratified epithelium** (Figure 8-2). This epithelium falsely appears as multiple cell layers when viewed under a low-power microscopic magnification because the cells' nuclei appear at different levels (see Table 8-1 and Chapter 11). However, in reality, with a higher microscopic magnification, cells of different heights are seen. Thus this is a type of simple epithelium because all the cells contact the basement membrane but not all reach the surface. Pseudostratified epithelium lines the upper respiratory tract, including the nasal cavity and paranasal sinuses. This type of epithelial tissue may be ciliated or nonciliated at the tissue surface.

Stratified epithelium consists of two or more layers of cells, with only the lower level contacting the basement membrane (see Table 8-1). Only the shape of the surface layer is used to determine the classification of stratified epithelium. Thus stratified epithelium can consist of cuboidal, columnar, or squamous epithelial cells or a combination of types, as seen in a transitional epithelium.

Most of the epithelial tissues in the body are **stratified squamous epithelium,** which include the superficial portion of the skin and oral mucosa (see Figure 8-1; see also Figure 8-7). Only the more superficial

layers of this portion are flat cells, or squames; the deeper cells vary from cuboidal to polyhedral. The extensions of the epithelium into the connective tissue as they appear on histological section are called **rete ridges**, or rete pegs.

Stratified squamous epithelium can be keratinized or nonkeratinized. **Keratin,** mentioned in Chapter 7, is a tough, fibrous, opaque, waterproof protein that is impervious to bacterial invasion and resistant to friction. Keratin is produced during the maturation of the *keratinocyte* epithelial cells as they migrate to the surface of the keratinized tissue (discussed further in Chapter 9 in relation to oral mucosa). This keratin is less densely packed in the skin and oral cavity, as compared with the densely packed hard keratin of the nails and hair.

An example of keratinized stratified squamous epithelium is the superficial portion of the skin, or **epidermis** (see Figure 8-1; see also Figure 8-7). The epidermis overlies a basement membrane and the adjoining deeper layers of connective tissue (the dermis and hypodermis, discussed later). The epidermis has varying degrees of keratinization depending on the region of the body. Areas such as the palms of the hands and bottom of the feet have large amounts of keratin, which forms calluses.

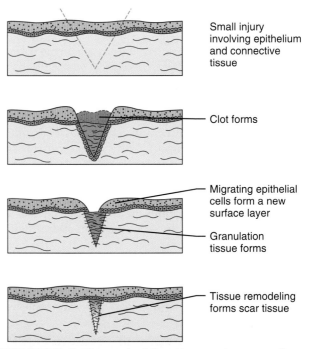

Small injury involving epithelium and connective tissue

Clot forms

Migrating epithelial cells form a new surface layer

Granulation tissue forms

Tissue remodeling forms scar tissue

FIGURE 8-3 The repair of the skin or oral mucosa after an injury. Note the initial formation of the clot. Also note migrating epithelial cells from the surrounding intact tissue and formation of granulation tissue in the later days of repair. Even later, the tissue will remodel and form scar tissue. (From Fehrenbach MJ. Inflammation and repair. In Ibsen OAC, Phelan JA (Editors). *Oral Pathology for Dental Hygienists*, ed 4. WB Saunders, Philadelphia, 2004.)

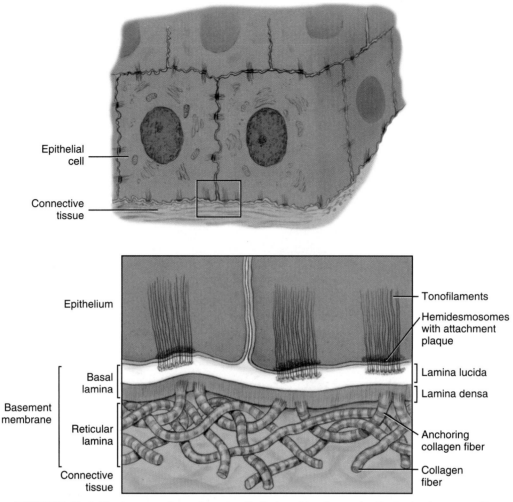

FIGURE 8-4 The basement membrane, with its basal lamina and reticular lamina, as well as the attachment devices from the epithelium (hemidesmosomes and tonofilaments with attachment plaques) and connective tissue (anchoring collagen fibers), respectively.

Epithelial Turnover and Repair

Turnover of epithelium occurs as the newly formed deepest cells migrate superficially. Thus the turnover time is the time taken for a cell to divide and pass through the entire thickness of tissue. In order to migrate, the cells release and then regain their desmosomal intercellular junctions in the more superficial location. The turnover time is high for all epithelial tissues. This high turnover time is a result of the high level of mitotic activity in those deepest dividing cells (see the discussion of oral mucosa in Chapter 9). Thus the older, superficial epithelial cells are being shed or lost at the same rate as the deeper germinal cells are dividing into more cells.

These overall high turnover times vary slightly for the different types of epithelial tissues. However, the epithelium of the oral mucosa has a higher turnover time than the epidermis of the skin. As an example, the epithelium that lines the cheek tissues (buccal mucosa) has a higher turnover time (14 days) than the epithelium that lines the skin (27 days). Clinically, this difference becomes important when dental professionals

sadly note a traumatic superficial injury to the skin of the face lasting for weeks and at the same time happily observe the quicker healing in the cheek area after the patient accidentally superficially bites the tissues (see Chapters 9 and 10 for more discussion).

After an injury to either the skin or oral mucosa, a clot from blood products forms in the area and the inflammatory response is triggered by its white blood cells (Figure 8-3). If the source of injury is removed, tissue repair can begin within the next few days. The epithelial cells at the periphery of the injury will lose their desmosomal intercellular junctions and migrate to form a new epithelial surface layer beneath the clot.

Thus, a clot is very important in repair of the epithelium and must be retained in the first days of repair because it acts as a guide to form a new surface. A clot stays moist in the oral cavity but dries out on the skin (called a *scab* on the skin). Later, after the epithelial surface is repaired, the clot is broken down by enzymes because it is no longer needed. Repair of the epithelium is tied to the repair taking place in the deeper connective tissue (discussed later).

BASEMENT MEMBRANE

The **basement membrane** is a thin, acellular, chemical-based structure always located between any form of epithelium and its underlying connective tissue, as noted in both the skin and oral mucosa (Figure 8-4; see also Figure 7-6 and 8-7). This type of structure is even present embryologically between the two types of tissues of the tooth germ during tooth development (see Chapter 6). The basement membrane is not seen clearly when it is viewed by a scanning or low-power microscopic magnification; only its location can be indicated. A higher power of magnification, such as that afforded by an electron microscope, is needed to see the intricacies of the basement membrane.

The superficial portion of the basement membrane is called the **basal lamina** and is produced by the epithelium. The basal lamina consists of two layers microscopically: The lamina lucida is a clear layer that is closer to the epithelium, and the lamina densa is a dense layer that is closer to the connective tissue. The terms *basement membrane* and *basal lamina,* are sometimes used interchangeably, but the basal lamina is only a portion of the basement membrane. The deeper portion of the basement membrane is called the **reticular lamina**. The reticular lamina consists of collagen and reticular fibers produced and secreted by the underlying connective tissue.

Attachment mechanisms are also part of the basement membrane. These involve **hemidesmosomes** with their attachment plaque, **tonofilaments** from the epithelium (both discussed in Chapter 7), and the **anchoring collagen fibers** from the connective tissue. The tonofilaments loop through the attachment plaque, whereas the collagen fibers of the reticular lamina loop into the lamina densa, forming a flexible attachment between the two tissues.

It is important to note that the interface between the epithelium and connective tissue of the skin and oral mucosa where the basement membrane is located is not two-dimensional, as seen in cross sections of the tissues where there are rete ridges and connective tissue papillae. Instead, the interface consists of three-dimensional *interdigitations* of the two tissues. This complex arrangement increases the amount of surface area for the interface, thus increasing the mechanical strength of the interface as well as the nutrition potential of the avascular epithelium from the vascularized connective tissue.

CONNECTIVE TISSUE

All of the **connective tissue** of the body, when taken together, represents by weight the most abundant type of basic tissue in the body. Connective tissue is derived from the somites during prenatal development. Compared with epithelium, connective tissue is usually

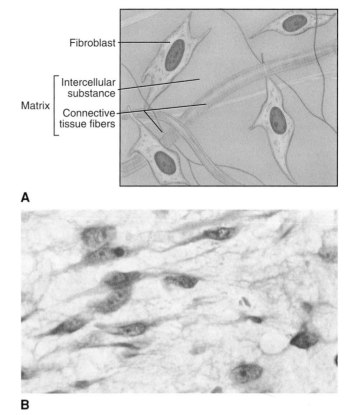

A

B

FIGURE 8-5 Fibroblasts within loose connective tissue showing their spindle or fusiform shape. Note that the fibroblast is the cell that forms the fibers of the connective tissue, as well as the intercellular substance between the tissue components. (Microscopic view from Stevens A, Lowe J. *Human Histology*, ed 3. Mosby, St. Louis, 2005.)

composed of fewer cells spaced farther apart and containing larger amounts of **matrix** between the cells (except in adipose connective tissue). This matrix is composed of intercellular substance and fibers.

Most of the connective tissue is renewable because its cells are capable of mitosis and because most cells can even produce their own matrix of intercellular substance and fibers. In most cases, connective tissues are vascularized (except cartilage), having their own blood supplies. The functions of connective tissue are varied; connective tissues are involved in support, attachment, packing, insulation, storage, transport, repair, and defense.

Histology of Connective Tissue

Many different kinds of cells are found in connective tissue. The most common cell in all kinds of connective tissue is the **fibroblast** (Figure 8-5). Fibroblasts synthesize certain types of protein fibers and intercellular substance. They are flat, elongated cells with cytoplasmic processes at each end. Subpopulations of fibroblasts may be possible in connective tissues. Fibroblasts are considered fixed cells in connective tissue because they do not leave the tissue to enter the blood.

Young fibroblasts that are actively engaged in the production of fibers and intercellular substances appear to have a large amount of cytoplasm, mitochondria, and rough endoplasmic reticulum. Fibroblasts can show aging and inactivity, with a reduction in cytoplasm, mitochondria, and rough endoplasmic reticulum, such as that seen in the later stages of periodontal inflammation. If adequately stimulated during repair, however, fibroblasts can revert to an active state.

Other cells found in connective tissue include migrated white blood cells such as monocytes (macrophages), basophils (mast cells), lymphocytes (including plasma cells), and neutrophils (discussed later). Certain other transient cell types are found in specific classifications of connective tissue and are discussed later.

Many different types of protein fibers are found in various types of connective tissue. **Collagen fibers** are the main connective tissue fiber type found in the body (Figure 8-6). Tissue containing a large amount of collagen fibers is called *collagenous connective tissue*, but all connective tissues (except blood) contain some collagen fibers. Collagen fibers are composed of the protein collagen, many distinct types of which have been shown by immunological study to have great tensile strength. All collagen fibers are composed of smaller subunits, or fibrils, which are then composed of microfibrils, similar to the way that a strong, intact rope is composed of many entwined strands of roping material.

The most common type of collagen protein is Type I collagen, which is found in the dermis of the skin, tendons, bone, teeth, and virtually all connective tissue. Cells responsible for the synthesis of Type I collagen include fibroblasts as well as osteoblasts, which produce bone tissue, and odontoblasts, which produce dentin (see Chapter 6). Twelve other types of collagen are found throughout the mature body or in fetal tissue.

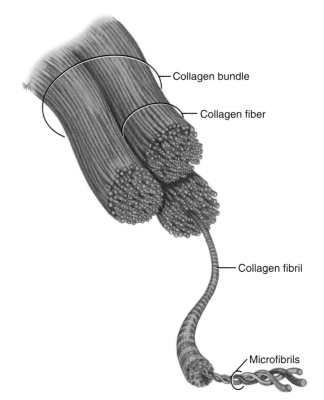

FIGURE 8-6 A collagen bundle, which is composed of smaller portions such as the fibers, fibrils, and microfibrils.

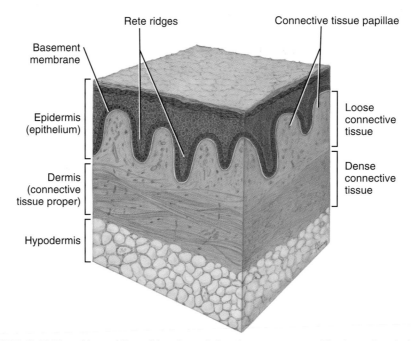

FIGURE 8-7 The skin and its epidermis and dermis components. The hypodermis is present deep to the dermis. Note the interdigitating rete ridges of the epidermis with the connective tissue papillae.

Elastic fibers are another type of fiber. Elastic fibers are composed of microfilaments embedded in the protein elastin, which makes it a very elastic type of tissue. Thus this tissue has the ability to stretch and then to return to its original shape after contraction or extension. Certain regions in the oral cavity, such as the soft palate, contain elastic fibers in their connective tissue portion to allow this type of tissue movement.

Reticular fibers are found in relationship to an embryonic tissue and thus are more rarely found in the body. Reticular fibers are composed of the protein reticulin and are very fine, hairlike fibers. They are branching fibers that form a meshlike network in the tissues that contain them. Reticular connective tissue predominates in the lymph nodes and spleen.

Classification of Connective Tissue

One method of classifying connective tissue is according to texture, which is either soft, firm, rigid, or fluid in nature (see Table 8-1). Soft connective tissue includes those tissues found in the deeper layers of the skin and oral mucosa, such as a connective tissue proper. Firm connective tissue consists of different types of cartilage. Rigid connective tissue consists of bone. Fluid connective tissue consists of blood with all its components and lymph.

CONNECTIVE TISSUE PROPER

Soft connective tissue can be classified as loose connective tissue, dense connective tissue, or specialized connective tissue. Both loose and dense connective tissue are found together in two layers in the form of a **connective tissue proper.** The connective tissue proper is found deep to the epithelium and basement membrane, in the deeper layers of the skin and oral mucosa.

The connective tissue proper in the skin is termed the **dermis** and is found deep to the epidermis (discussed earlier; see Figures 8-1 and Figure 8-7). Deep to the dermis is a hypodermis, which is composed of loose connective tissue and adipose tissue, a specialized connective tissue, as well as glandular tissue, large blood vessels, and nerves. Cartilage, bone, and muscle can be present deep to the hypodermis of the skin, depending on the region of the body. In the oral mucosa, the connective tissue proper is called the **lamina propria**, which is discussed in the next chapter, and the deeper connective tissue is called **submucosa** (both are discussed in Chapter 9).

Loose Connective Tissue

The superficial layer of the dermis of the skin and lamina propria of the oral mucosa is composed of **loose connective tissue** (see Figure 8-7). In the dermis or lamina propria, this layer of loose connective tissue is also called the **papillary layer.** The papillary layer has **connective tissue papillae,** which are extensions of loose connective tissue into the epithelium. This papillary layer has no overly prominent connective tissue element; all the components of the papillary layer are in equal amounts. Thus equal amounts of cells, intercellular substance, fibers, and tissue fluid are in an irregular and looser arrangement. This loose layer of the connective tissue proper serves as padding for the deeper portions of the body.

Dense Connective Tissue

Deep to the loose connective tissue is **dense connective tissue,** such as that found in the deepest layers of the dermis or lamina propria (see Figure 8-7). In contrast to loose connective tissue, dense connective tissue is tightly packed and consists mainly of protein fibers, which give this tissue its strength.

Similar to loose connective tissue, the components of dense connective tissue are still arranged in an irregular manner. The dense connective tissue in the dermis and lamina propria is also called the **reticular layer,** or dense layer. Thus the reticular layer is deep to the papillary layer in these types of a connective tissue proper. In contrast, tendons, aponeuroses, and ligaments are a type of dense connective tissue that has a regular arrangement of strong, parallel collagen fibers with few fibroblast cells.

Connective Tissue Turnover and Repair

Turnover of the connective tissue proper in skin or oral mucosa occurs as a result of the production of fibers and intercellular substance by the fibroblasts. Other types of cells can also undergo mitosis and create additional cells, such as certain white blood cells and endothelial cells. The overall turnover time for a connective tissue proper is slower than its associated epithelial tissues and also varies from region to region.

When injured, the connective tissue proper in the skin or oral mucosa goes through stages of repair that are related to the events in the more superficial epithelium (see Figure 8-3). After a clot forms and an inflammatory response is triggered with white blood cells, fibroblasts migrate to produce an immature connective tissue deep to the clot and newly forming epithelial surface.

This immature connective tissue is called **granulation tissue** and has few fibers and an increased amount of blood vessels. Granulation tissue appears as a redder, soft tissue that bleeds easily. This tissue may become abundant and can interfere with the repair process. Surgical removal of excess granulation tissue may be necessary to allow for optimum repair. This sometimes occurs with the extraction of teeth.

Later, during the repair process, this temporary granulation tissue is replaced by paler and firmer scar tissue in the area. Scar tissue contains an increased

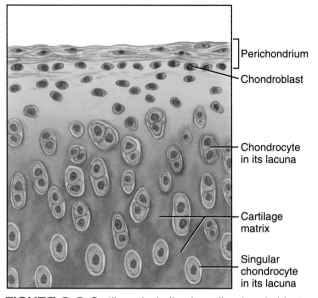

Perichondrium

Chondroblast

Chondrocyte in its lacuna

Cartilage matrix

Singular chondrocyte in its lacuna

FIGURE 8-8 Cartilage, including its cells, chondroblasts, and chondrocytes, and the outer layer of perichondrium, a formative connective tissue sheath.

amount of fibers and fewer blood vessels. The amount of scar tissue varies, depending on the type and size of the wound, amount of granulation tissue, and movement of tissue after injury. Interestingly, the skin shows more scar tissue both clinically and histologically after repair than does the oral mucosa. This difference may be based on differing developmental origins of the tissues producing differing types of fibroblasts and thus different types of fibers.

SPECIALIZED CONNECTIVE TISSUE

Specialized connective tissue includes adipose, elastic, or reticular. **Adipose connective tissue** is a fatty tissue that is found beneath the skin, around organs and various joints, and in portions of the oral cavity. Unlike most connective tissue, this type of connective tissue has cells packed tightly together with little or no matrix. After fibroblasts, the predominant type of cell found in this tissue is the adipocyte, which stores fat intracellularly.

Elastic connective tissue has a large number of elastic fibers in its matrix, which combine strength with elasticity, such as in the tissues of the vocal cords. Reticular connective tissue is a delicate network of interwoven reticular fibers forming a supportive framework for blood vessels and internal organs.

Cartilage

Cartilage is a firm, noncalcified connective tissue that serves as a skeletal tissue in the body (Figure 8-8). Cartilage forms much of the temporary skeleton of the embryo and serves as structural support for certain

soft tissues after birth. Cartilage is also present at articular surfaces of most freely movable joints, such as the temporomandibular joint (see Chapter 19). Unlike rigid bone tissue, cartilage has some flexibility resulting from its fibers in the matrix; however, it has no inorganic or mineralized materials. Additionally, cartilage serves as a model or template in which many of the bones of the body subsequently develop. Further, in regard to the temporomandibular joint, cartilage may form abnormally within an aging articular disc that is normally composed of dense fibrous connective tissue, possibly causing clinical difficulties.

Cartilage, unlike most connective tissue, is avascular. Much like epithelium, this tissue depends on its surrounding connective tissue for its cellular nutrition, such as oxygen and metabolites. The connective tissue surrounding most cartilage is the **perichondrium**, a fibrous connective tissue sheath containing blood vessels. Because it has no vascularity of its own, cartilage takes longer to repair than does vascularized bone tissue. Cartilage also has no nerve supply within its tissue. Thus cartilage subjected to trauma or surgery does not produce overly painful symptoms.

HISTOLOGY OF CARTILAGE

Cartilage is composed of cells and matrix. The matrix is composed of fibers, mainly collagen, and intercellular substance. Thus this matrix is similar to soft connective tissues in composition, except that the matrix of cartilage is firmer.

Two types of cells found in cartilage are the immature **chondroblasts**, which lie internal to the perichondrium and produce cartilage matrix, and the **chondrocytes**, which are mature chondroblasts that maintain the cartilage matrix (see Figure 8-8). After the production of cartilage matrix, the chondrocyte becomes surrounded and enclosed by the matrix. Only a small space surrounds the chondrocyte within the cartilage matrix, the **lacuna** (plural, **lacunae**).

The three types of cartilage—hyaline, elastic, and fibrocartilage—have slightly differing histologies. Most histologists believe that this distinction between types of cartilages is artificial and that most cartilage masses contain a combination of the different types. Hyaline cartilage is the most common type found in the body and contains only collagen fibers as part of its matrix. The associated collagen fibers of hyaline cartilage are much finer than those found in dense connective tissue. Hyaline cartilage can be found in the embryonic skeleton and in growth centers, such as the mandibular condyle. All cartilages start as hyaline cartilage connective tissue and are then modified into the other types of cartilage according to need.

Elastic cartilage is similar to hyaline, except that it has numerous elastic fibers in its matrix in addition to its many collagen fibers. Elastic cartilage is found in the external ear, auditory tube, epiglottis, and portions of the larynx. Fibrocartilage is never found alone and merges gradually with its neighboring hyaline cartilage, such as in portions of the temporomandibular joint (see Chapter 19). Unlike elastic cartilage, fibrocartilage is not merely a modification of hyaline. Rather, it is a transitional type of cartilage between hyaline cartilage and dense connective tissue of tendons and ligaments. The cells of the tissue are enclosed in capsules of matrix, giving it great tensile strength. Unlike elastic or hyaline cartilage, fibrocartilage has no true perichondrium overlying it.

DEVELOPMENT OF CARTILAGE

Cartilage can develop or grow in size in two different ways: interstitial growth and appositional growth (growth during embryological development is discussed in Chapter 3). **Interstitial growth** is growth from deep within the tissue by the mitosis of each chondrocyte, producing a larger number daughter cells within a single lacuna, each of which secretes more matrix, thus expanding the tissue (see Figure 8-8). Interstitial growth is important in the development of bone tissue that uses cartilage as a model for its own formation (endochondral ossification, discussed next).

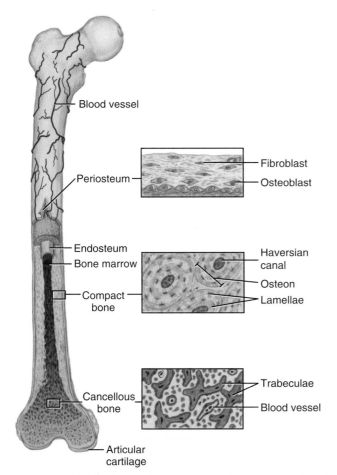

FIGURE 8-9 Anatomy of bone tissue with its compact and cancellous bone, periosteum and endosteum, and bone marrow.

Appositional growth is layered growth on the outside of the tissue from an outer layer of chrondroblasts within perichondrium. This layer of chrondroblasts is always present on the external surface of cartilage to allow appositional growth of cartilage after an injury or remodeling.

AGING AND REPAIR OF CARTILAGE

As cartilage ages, it becomes less cellular and many chondrocytes die. It may start to contain firm fibers in parallel groups, or it may even form calcifications. These calcifications start in scattered areas, which tend to coalesce over time. The cartilage now becomes hard and brittle, losing its flexibility.

Repair of cartilage is slow because the tissue is avascular and is dependent on neighboring connective tissue from the perichondrium to transform into cartilage. With this transformation, the newly formed cartilage slowly proliferates and fills in the defect by appositional growth. In contrast, fractured mature cartilage is often united by dense connective tissue, and if vascularization is initiated, then healing cartilage may eventually be replaced by bone.

Bone

Bone is a rigid connective tissue that constitutes most of the mature skeleton (Figure 8-9). Thus bone serves as protective and structural support for soft tissues and as an attachment mechanism. Bone also aids in movement, manufactures blood cells by way of its red bone marrow, and is a storehouse for calcium and other minerals. Because bone is vascularized with its own blood supply, it repairs quickly compared with cartilage. Thus even though bone is rigid, it is not an inanimate inner rod being moved by the muscles. Bone is a living and functioning tissue in the body. Bone is also the most differentiated of all the connective tissues.

ANATOMY OF BONE

When bone is examined grossly, the outer portion of bone is covered by **periosteum** (see Figure 8-9). Periosteum is a double-layered dense connective tissue sheath. The outer layer of the periosteum contains blood vessels and nerves. The inner layer of the periosteum contains a single layer of cells that give rise to bone-forming cells, the **osteoblasts**.

Deep to the periosteum is a dense layer of **compact bone**. Deep to the compact bone is a spongy bone, or **cancellous bone**. Both compact bone and cancellous bone have the same cellular components, but each has a different arrangement of those components (discussed next). Thus the differences between these two types of bone include the relative amount of solid bone

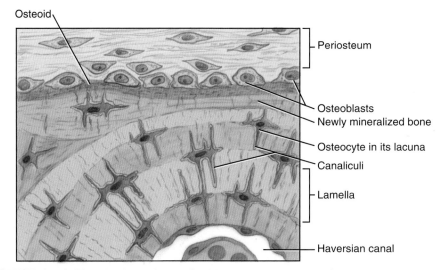

Osteoid

Periosteum

Osteoblasts

Newly mineralized bone

Osteocyte in its lacuna

Canaliculi

Lamella

Haversian canal

FIGURE 8-10 The histology of bone (in this case, compact bone). Note the bone tissue cells, osteoblasts, and osteocytes as well as the periosteum, the outer formative sheath of connective tissue. The initial bone matrix or osteoid mineralizes later into bone tissue.

and also the size and number of soft tissue spaces in each. No sharp boundary exists between these two types of bone. They are located where they best serve the needs for either strength or lightness of weight. Compact bone is strong because it has fewer soft tissue spaces, but it is heavy. In contrast, cancellous bone is light because it is formed by pieces of solid bone that join to form a lattice; it is not as strong because it has more soft tissue spaces.

Lining the medullary cavity of bone on the inside of the layers of compact bone and cancellous bone is the **endosteum**. The endosteum has the same composition as the periosteum but is thinner. On the innermost portion of bone in the medullary cavity is the **bone marrow**. This gelatinous substance is where the blood's stem cells are located and where certain lymphocytes mature (discussed later). These stem cells can produce most of the cells of the blood.

HISTOLOGY OF BONE

Bone consists of cells and a partially calcified matrix that is 50 percent mineralized or inorganic material (Figure 8-10). This inorganic material is packed with matrix between the bone cells. The matrix is composed of organic collagen fibers and intercellular substance. It is this inorganic substance in a crystalline formation of mainly **calcium hydroxyapatite** with the chemical formula of $Ca_{10}(PO_4)_6(OH)_2$ that gives bone its hardness. This same type of inorganic crystal is found in differing percentages in many of the dental tissues, such as enamel, dentin, and cementum (see Table 6-2 for comparison with dental tissues). Smaller amounts of other minerals, such as magnesium, potassium, calcium carbonate, and fluoride, are also present.

Bone matrix is initially formed as **osteoid**, which later undergoes mineralization. The osteoid is pro-

duced by osteoblasts, cuboidal cells that arise from fibroblasts. Osteoblasts are also involved in the later mineralization of osteoid to form bone. Always present in the periosteum is a layer of osteoblasts at the external surface of the compact bone to allow for the remodeling of bone and to allow repair of injured bone.

Within fully calcified bone are **osteocytes**, which are entrapped mature osteoblasts. Similar to the chondrocyte, the cell body of the osteocyte is surrounded by bone except for the space immediately around it, the lacuna (plural, lacunae). The cytoplasmic processes of the osteocyte radiate outward in all directions in the bone and are located in tubular canals of matrix, or **canaliculi**. These canals provide for interaction between the osteocytes. Unlike chondrocytes, osteoblasts never undergo mitosis, and thus only one osteocyte is ever found in a lacuna.

Bone matrix in compact bone is formed into closely apposed sheets, or **lamellae**. Within and between the lamellae are embedded osteocytes with their cytoplasmic processes in the canals. The organized arrangement of concentric lamellae in compact bone is the **Haversian system**.

In the Haversian system, these lamellae form concentric layers of matrix into cylinders or **osteons** around a soft tissue space or **Haversian canal** (Figure 8-11). The osteon is the unit of structure in compact bone and consists of 5 to 20 lamellae. This arrangement in the osteon is similar to the growth rings in a cross section of a tree trunk. However, unlike tree rings that form at a rate of one per year, an entire Haversian system is produced all at the same time, no matter the number of concentric lamellae involved. The Haversian canal is a central vascular canal that contains longitudinally running blood vessels, nerves, and a small amount of connective tissue and is lined by endosteum. The Haversian canals communicate not only with each other but also with the osteocytic processes in the canaliculi. These Haversian canals also provide cellular nutrition for the surrounding bone tissue. The

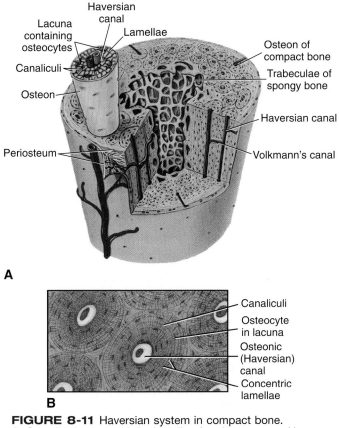

FIGURE 8-11 Haversian system in compact bone. **A:** Overall structure with its lamellae forming osteons. Note Volkmann's canal and its communication with larger blood vessels external to the bone. **B:** Close-up view of the structure, highlighting the individual osteons with their central Haversian canals, osteocytes, and canaliculi. (From Applegate EJ. *The Anatomy and Physiology Learning System,* ed 5. WB Saunders, Philadelphia, 2002.)

Haversian canals are sometimes called *osteonic* or *central canals.*

Located on the outer portion of the Haversian system in compact bone are **Volkmann's canals**, or nutrient canals that contain the same vascular and nerve components as the Haversian canals and are also lined by endosteum. Volkmann's canals pass obliquely or at right angles to the Haversian canals of the osteons and communicate with them as well as with the larger blood supply external to the bone.

Cancellous bone has its bone matrix formed into **trabeculae**, or joined matrix pieces forming a lattice (see Figure 8-9). Lamellae of the matrix of cancellous bone are not arranged into concentric layers around a central blood blood vessel as with the campact bone, but rather their concentric rings are formed into cone-shaped spicules. Osteocytes in lacunae with their cytoplasmic processes are located between the lamellae of the trabeculae. Surrounding the trabeculae are soft tissue spaces that consist of vascular canals with blood vessels, nerves, and varying amounts of connective tissue. These spaces also serve as a nutritional source for the lattice of bone tissue.

DEVELOPMENT OF BONE

Bone development, or **ossification**, has two methods of development: intramembranous and endochondral ossification. The bone produced by both these developmental methods is microscopically the same; only the process of formation is different. **Intramembranous ossification** is formation of osteoid between two dense connective tissue sheets, which then eventually replaces the outer connective tissue (Figure 8-12). During intramembranous ossification, mesenchymal cells differentiate into osteoblasts to form the osteoid.

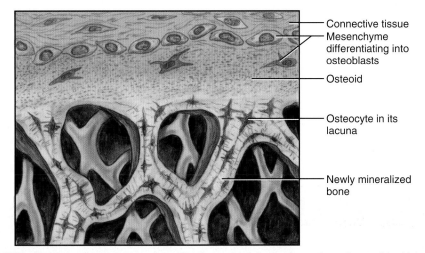

FIGURE 8-12 Intramembranous ossification, which is the formation of osteoid within two dense connective tissue sheets. It eventually replaces the connective tissue. During intramembranous ossification, mesenchyme differentiates into osteoblasts to form osteoid, which later matures into bone.

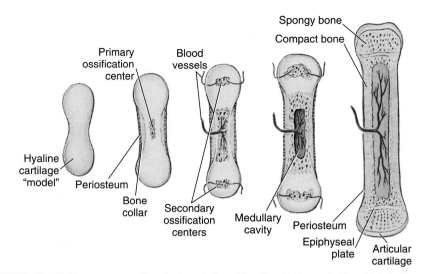

FIGURE 8-13 The process of endochondral ossification (A through E), which is the formation of the osteoid within a cartilage model that subsequently becomes mineralized and dies. Osteoblasts penetrate the disintegrating cartilage and form a primary ossification center that continues forming osteoid toward the ends of the bone during prenatal formation. Later after birth, secondary ossification centers, which allow further growth of bones such as the head of condyle of the mandible, are also formed. (From Applegate EJ. *The Anatomy and Physiology Learning System*, ed 5. WB Saunders, Philadelphia, 2002.)

Intramembranous ossification uses a method of appositional growth similar to that of cartilage, with layers of osteoid being produced. The osteoid later becomes mineralized to form bone. Certain bones in the body, such as the flat bones and clavicle, can form this way, enlarging over time as the appositional growth of bone occurs. The maxilla and the majority of the mandible are formed by intramembranous ossification (see Chapter 14).

Endochondral ossification is the formation of the osteoid within a hyaline cartilage model that subsequently becomes mineralized and dies (Figure 8-13). Osteoblasts penetrate the disintegrating cartilage and form primary ossification centers that continue forming osteoid toward the ends of the bone during prenatal growth. Thus bone matrix eventually replaces the cartilage model. This type of ossification first uses the method of interstitial growth of the initial cartilage tissue to form the model, or pattern, of the future bone's shape. Later, appositional growth of osteoid with layers laid down on the outer perimeter occurs to complete the final bone mass within the model.

Most long bones of the body are formed this way because it allows bone to grow in length from deep within the tissues. Later after birth, secondary ossification centers, which allow further growth of the bones, are also formed. In particular, the head of the mandibular condyle is formed by endochondral ossification (see Chapters 14 and 19).

Regardless of its method of development, bone also goes through specific stages (Figure 8-14). The first bone to be produced by either method of ossification is called woven bone, or **immature bone.** In immature bone, the lamellae are indistinct because of the irregu-

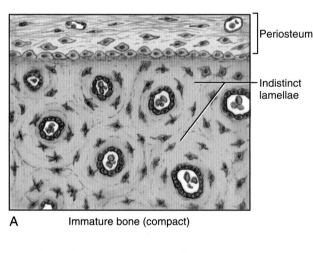

A   Immature bone (compact)

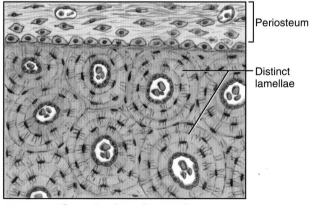

B   Secondary bone (compact)

FIGURE 8-14 The two stages of bone development from immature bone (**A**) to secondary bone (**B**; in this case, compact bone). These stages occur during all methods of ossification as well as during the repair of bone tissue.

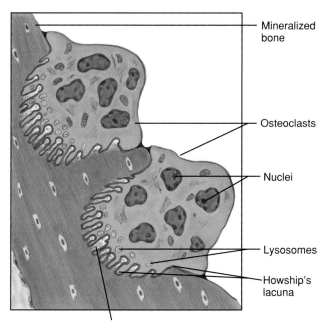

Mineralized bone

Osteoclasts

Nuclei

Lysosomes

Howship's lacuna

Area of bone resorption

FIGURE 8-15 Multinucleated osteoclasts within Howship's lacunae undergoing bone resorption. Note their multiple nuclei within their cytoplasm, which also contains a large number of lysosomes. These are discharged into the tissue, breaking down bone.

lar arrangement of the collagen fibers and lamellae, whether it be the Haversian system or trabeculae.

Immature bone is a temporary tissue that is replaced by a more mature **secondary bone.** Depending on the specific needs of the bone in any given area, secondary bone can be compact or cancellous (see Figure 8-11). In contrast to immature bone, secondary bone has a well organized arrangement of collagen fibers and distinct lamellae.

BONE REPAIR AND REMODELING

After bone fracture and during the repair of bone tissue, bone goes through the stages of bone tissue formation no matter how the bone initially developed. In the area to be repaired, bone tissue forms initially as immature bone, which matures into secondary bone to complete the repair. The repair of bone depends on adequate blood supply, the presence of periosteum with active osteoblasts, and adequate mineral and vitamin levels.

Thus it becomes apparent that bone's overall structure is not static and therefore never remains the same. Throughout life, bone in the body is constantly being remodeled or replaced over time. Bone undergoes removal in some areas and new bone formation in other areas, with the two processes balancing each other. Appositional growth, or layered formation of bone along its periphery, is accomplished by the **osteoblasts,** which later become entrapped as osteocytes (see Figure 8-10).

Resorption can involve the removal of bone tissue (Figure 8-15). The cell that causes resorption of bone tissue is the **osteoclast.** Osteoclasts are large multinucleated cells located on the surface of secondary bone tissue in a large, shallow pit created by resorption called a **Howship's lacuna.** Each osteoclast contains a large number of lysosomes in its cytoplasm, and these are discharged into the tissue when breaking down bone.

Localized resorption occurs in a specific area of a bone as a result of infection, altered mechanical stress, or pressure on the bone so that it adapts by remodeling. This occurs in periodontal disease as well as in a controlled manner in orthodontics (see Chapters 14 and 20). **Generalized resorption** occurs in varying amounts in the entire skeleton as a result of endocrine activity to increase blood levels of calcium and phosphate needed by the body. Excess generalized bone resorption as well as excess bone appositional growth, can occur in certain bone disorders when the two processes are no longer balanced.

Microscopically, cross sections of bone demonstrate layers related to its growth when stained, like growth rings in a tree. When stained, arrest lines, or resting lines, appear as smooth lines between the layers of bone because of osteoblasts having rested, formed bone tissue, and then rested again after appositional growth (see Figures 8-10 and 8-15). Arrest lines show the incremental or layered nature of appositional growth. When stained, reversal lines appear as scalloped lines between the layers of bone. Reversal lines represent areas where resorption has taken place, followed by appositional growth of new bone tissue.

Blood

Blood is a fluid connective tissue that serves as transport medium for cellular nutrients, such respiratory gases, like oxygen and carbon dioxide, and metabolites for the entire body. Blood is carried in endothelium-lined blood vessels and consists of plasma and cells (Table 8-3).

PLASMA

Plasma is the fluid substance in the blood vessels that carries the plasma proteins, blood cells, and metabolites. It is more consistent in composition than tissue fluid and lymph, yet it contains most of the same materials with the addition of red blood cells (tissue fluid is discussed in Chapter 7, lymph in Chapter 11). Serum, another fluid product, is distinguished from the plasma from which it is derived on account of the removal of clotting proteins. If a sample of blood is treated with an agent to prevent clotting and is spun in a centrifuge, the plasma is the superficial layer.

TABLE 8-3

Blood Cells and Related Tissue Cells

Type	Microscopic Appearance	Description	Function
Red blood cell		Biconcave disc without nucleus	Binds and transports oxygen and carbon dioxide
Platelets		Discs without nucleus; cell fragments derived from special line of blood cell	Clotting mechanism
White blood cell	See Table 8-4	Rounded cells with nucleus, many variations (see Table 8-4)	Inflammatory response and immune response

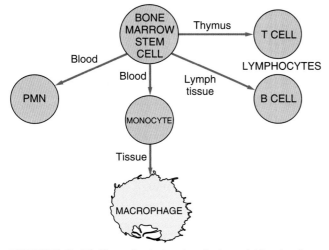

FIGURE 8-16 Flow chart showing that most blood cells possibly come from a common stem cell type in the bone marrow. Some blood cell types mature in the bone marrow (B-cell lymphocyte). Some blood cell types travel and mature in other glands or tissues in the body, such as the thymus (T-cell lymphocyte). PMN = Polymorphonuclear leukocyte or neutrophil. (From Fehrenbach MJ. Immunity. In Ibsen OAC, Phelan JA (editors): *Oral Pathology for Dental Hygienists*, ed 4. WB Saunders, Philadelphia, 2004.)

Blood Cells and Related Tissue Cells

Blood cells and associated derivatives are also called the *formed elements* of the blood. Most blood cells come from a common stem cell in the bone marrow (Figure 8-16). The formed elements of the blood include the red blood cells, platelets, and white blood cells. Not only are these cells present in the blood and its vessels, but also some related components are also present in surrounding connective tissue.

The most common cell in the blood is the **red blood cell (RBC)**, or erythrocyte (see Table 8-3). An RBC is a biconcave disc that contains hemoglobin, which binds and then transports the oxygen and carbon dioxide.

An RBC has no nucleus and does not undergo mitosis because it is formed from the bone marrow's stem cells. There are 5 to 6 million red blood cells per microliter (μl) of blood. In centifuged blood, the RBCs settle to the bottom; this fraction is called the *hematocrit*.

The blood also contains **platelets**, or thrombocytes. Smaller than RBCs, platelets are also disc shaped and have no nucleus. This type of formed element is not a true blood cell but a fragment of another blood cell. Platelets function in the clotting mechanism. There are 250,000 to 400,000 platelets per microliter.

Finally, the blood contains several types of **white blood cell (WBC)**, or leukocyte (see Tables 8-3 and Table 8-4). Like RBCs, WBCs form from the bone marrow's stem cells. WBCs later mature in the bone marrow or in various lymphatic organs. WBCs are involved in the defense mechanisms of the body, including the inflammatory and immune responses. Thus WBCs are also normally found in small numbers in epithelium and connective tissue. WBCs migrate from the blood by moving through openings between the cell junction of the endothelial lining of the vessel to participate in these defense mechanisms.

WBCs differ from RBCs because they possess a nucleus, have more cytoplasm, and have the power of active ameboid movement in order to migrate from the blood to the tissues. Unlike RBCs, WBCs perform their functions not only in the blood but also in other tissues. WBCs are also less numerous than RBCs (only 5000 to 10,000 per cubic milliliter of blood); yet there are five distinct types of WBCs based on their microscopic appearance: neutrophils, lymphocytes, monocytes, eosinophils, and basophils. The fraction of centrifuged blood that settles on the surface of the hemotocrit consists of the WBCs and below the plasma forms the "buffy coat." All WBCs are colorless and are stained so that their differences may be observed.

TABLE 8-4

Blood Cells and Related Tissue Cells

Cells	Microscopic Appearance	Description	Functions
Neutrophil or polymorphonuclear leukocyte (PMN)		Multilobulated nucleus with granules	Inflammatory response: phagocytosis
Lymphocyte		Round nucleus without granules, B,T, and NK types	B and T: Immune response: humoral and cell-mediated NK: Defense against tumor and virally infected cells
Plasma cell		Round nucleus derived from B-cell lymphocytes	Humoral immune response: produces immunoglobulins
Monocyte (blood)/ macrophage (tissue)		Bean-shaped nucleus with poorly staining granules	Inflammatory and immune response: phagocytosis as well as process and present immunogens
Eosinophil		Double-lobed nucleus with granules	Immune response
Basophil		Irregularly shaped double-lobulated nucleus with granules	Immune response
Mast cell (tissue)		Irregularly shaped double-lobulated nucleus with granules	Immune response

The most common WBC in the blood is the **neutrophil**, or **polymorphonuclear leukocyte (PMN)** (Figure 8-17). These are the first cells to appear at an injury site when the inflammatory response is triggered. Large numbers of the PMNs can be present in the suppuration, or pus, sometimes seen locally at the site. PMNs constitute 60 to 70 percent of the total blood WBC count. They have a short life span, contain lysosomal enzymes, are active in phagocytosis (discussed further in Chapter 7), and respond to chemotactic factors. Mature PMNs have a multilobulated nucleus,

and their cytoplasm contains granules. They are therefore classified as one of the granulocytes.

The second most common WBC in the blood is the **lymphocyte**, which makes up 20 to 25 percent of the total WBC count. A lymphocyte has a rounded nucleus. Because its granules do not stain in the cytoplasm, it is classified as an agranulocyte. There are three functional types of lymphocytes: B-cell, T-cell, and NK-cell. B-cells mature in the bone marrow and gut-associated lymphoid tissue such as lymph nodes (see Chapter 11), whereas T-cells mature in the thymus

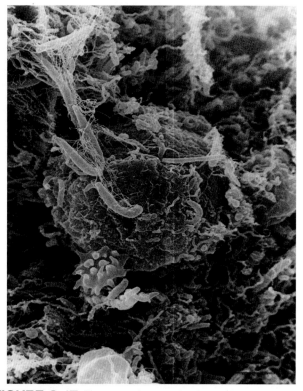

FIGURE 8-17 Electron micrograph of a polymorphonuclear leukocyte (PMN), or neutrophil. The PMN is the most common white blood cell (WBC) and is involved in phagocytosis. It is the first WBC from the blood to the site of injury in the tissues. (Courtesy of Jan Cope, RDH, Instructor, Oregon Institute of Technology, Klamath Falls, OR.)

TABLE 8-5

Known Immunoglobulins (Antibodies)

IgA	Has two subgroups: serous in the blood and secretory in the saliva and other secretions; aids in defense against proliferation of microorganisms in body fluids
IgE	Involved in hypersensitivity reactions because it can bind to mast cells and basophils and bring about the release of bioactive substances such as histamine
IgD	Functions in the activation of B-cell lymphocytes
IgG	Major antibody in blood serum; can pass the placental barrier and forms the first passive immunity for the newborn
IgM	Involved in early immune responses because of its involvement with IgD in the activation of B-cell lymphocytes

(see Figure 8-16). NK-cells also mature in the bone marrow. NK-cells (or natural killer cells) are large cells that are involved in the first line of defense against tumor or virally infected cells by killing them and thus are not considered part of the immune response.

Cytokines are produced by B- and T-cells and are chemical mediators of the immune response. Thus both these types of lymphocytes are involved in the immune response (see Table 8-4). In the past, the immune response was strictly broken into two divisions: humoral and cell-mediated. However, the distinction between the two divisions is less important because they are interrelated.

One important difference between the two divisions remains: The B-cell lymphocytes divide during the immune response to form **plasma cells.** Plasma cells are round cells with a single round nucleus that has a cartwheel appearance. Once mature, plasma cells produce an antibody, or **immunoglobulin (Ig)**, one of the proteins found in the blood. There are five distinct classes of immunoglobulins: IgA, IgE, IgD, IgG, and IgM (Table 8-5). Each plasma cell produces only one specific class of antibody.

Immunoglobulins are formed by plasma cells in response to a specific **immunogen**, or antigen. Immunogens are mainly proteins that are seen by the

body as foreign and are capable of triggering an immune response. An immunoglobulin, along with its specific immunogen, often forms an immune complex in an effort to render the immunogen unable to cause disease. Immunoglobulins can be extracted from the blood of recovering patients and used for passive immunization against certain infectious diseases.

The most common WBC in the connective tissue proper is the **monocyte**, which is termed a **macrophage** after it migrates from the blood into the tissues. A monocyte has a kidney bean–shaped nucleus. Although classified as an agranulocyte, its cytoplasm has small and poorly staining granules. Monocytes contain lysosomal enzymes, are involved in phagocytosis, are actively mobile, and have the ability to respond to chemotactic factors (see Figure 7-4). Monocytes also respond to cytokines. They have a longer life span than PMNs. However, monocytes constitute only 3 to 8 percent of the total WBC count. After migration, macrophages arrive at the site of injury later and in fewer numbers than PMNs when the inflammatory response is triggered. Macrophages also assist in the immune response to facilitate immunoglobulin production. In certain disease states, many macrophages may fuse together, forming giant cells with multiple nuclei. In bone connective tissue, these are called *osteoclasts.*

The fourth type of WBC is the **eosinophil**, a granulocyte with a double-lobed nucleus that looks like a pair of old-fashioned eyeglasses. Normally, eosinophils are 2 to 4 percent of the total WBC count. They increase in numbers during an allergy-induced immune response and in parasitic diseases. Their primary function seems to be the phagocytosis of immune complexes. They have large cytoplasmic granules.

The **basophil** is also normally found in small numbers, 0.5 to 1 percent of the total WBC count. Basophils are also granulocytes, containing granules of histamine and heparin. They have an irregularly shaped double-lobulated nucleus that is often masked by large staining granules. Other WBCs located in the connective tissues include the **mast cell,** which is similar in appearance to the basophil. Like basophils, mast cells are also involved in immune responses with allergies. However, even though both cells are derived from the bone marrow, they probably originate from different stem cells.

Clinical Considerations for Cells in the Blood and Tissue

Dental professionals must understand certain laboratory procedures that have been performed on their patients and that are discussed when recording medical histories. These procedures may also be requested by the supervising dentist if the patient has clinical evidence of unusual periodontal diseases such as agressive periodontitis. These procedures include a complete blood count (CBC), which is an evaluation of both RBC and WBC types to detect infections, anemia, or leukemias. A platelet count can also be performed to determine the number of platelets if bleeding problems are a consideration. A bleeding test can also be performed to test platelet function.

MUSCLE TISSUE

The muscle tissue in the body is part of the muscular system. Like connective tissue, most muscles are derived from somites. Each muscle shortens under neural control, causing soft tissue and bony structures of the body to move. The three types of muscle tissue are classified according to structure, function, and innervation: skeletal, smooth, and cardiac (see Table 8-1).

Classification of Muscle Tissue

Each type of **muscle** has its own type of action, which is the movement accomplished when the muscle cells contract. Smooth muscle and cardiac muscle are considered involuntary muscles because they are under autonomic nervous system control (discussed next). Smooth muscles are located in organs, glands, and the linings of blood vessels. Cardiac muscle is in the wall of the heart (myocardium).

Skeletal muscles are considered voluntary muscles because they are under voluntary control, involving the somatic nervous systems (Figure 8-18). All the major muscles of the body's appendages and trunk are skeletal muscles. Thus skeletal muscles are usually attached to bones of the skeleton. Skeletal muscles also include the muscles of the pharynx, upper esophagus, tongue, facial expression, and mastication.

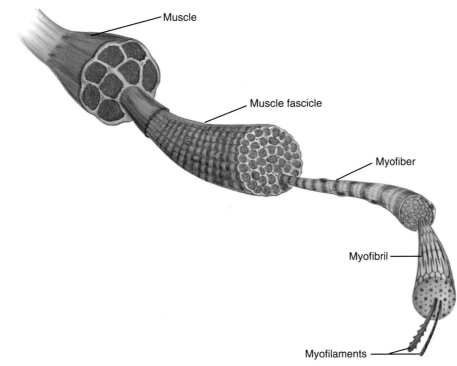

FIGURE 8-18 Skeletal muscle tissue. Its striations and its composition of smaller muscle bundles, fascicles, myofibers, myofibrils, and myofilaments are identified.

Histology of Skeletal Muscle Tissue

Skeletal muscles are also called *striated muscles* because the muscle cells appear striped microscopically. Each muscle is composed of numerous muscle bundles, or fascicles, which then are composed of numerous muscle cells termed *myofibers*. Each myofiber extends the entire length of the muscle and is composed of smaller myofibrils surrounded by the other organelles of the cell. Each myofibril is composed of even smaller myofilaments.

NERVE TISSUE

Nerve tissue forms the nervous system in the body (Table 8-6). Nerves function to carry messages or impulses based on electrical potentials. Nerve tissue in the body causes muscles to contract, resulting in facial expressions and joint movements such as those associated with mastication and speech. Nerve tissue also stimulates glands to secrete and regulates many other systems of the body, such as the cardiovascular system. Nerve tissue also allows for the perception of sensations such as pain, touch, taste, and smell. Nerve tissue is derived from the neuroectoderm in the embryo.

Histology of Nerve Tissue

A **neuron** is the functional cellular component of the nervous system and is composed of three portions: a neural cell body and two types of neural cytoplasmic processes (Figure 8-19). The neural cell body is not involved in the process of impulse transmission but provides the metabolic support for the entire neuron.

One type of process associated with the cell body is an axon, a long, thin, singular cablelike process that conducts impulses away from the cell body. An axon is encased in its own cell membrane. Nerve excitability and conduction are due to changes that develop in

TABLE 8-6

Divisions of the Nervous System

Divisions	Components
Central nervous system	Brain and spinal cord
Peripheral nervous system	Spinal and cranial nerves of the somatic nervous system and autonomic nervous system (sympathetic and parasympathetic)

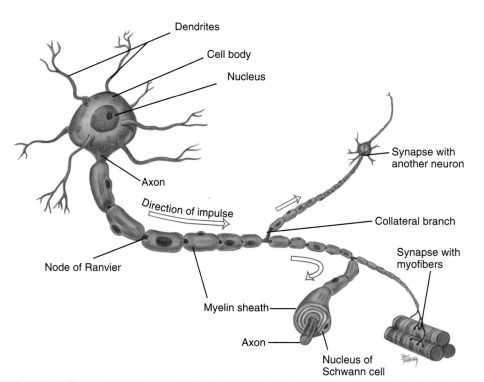

FIGURE 8-19 A neuron, with its cell body, axon, dendrites, and its synaptic relationship with the muscle tissue as well with another neuron.

the nerve membrane. Many axons are additionally covered by layers of a lipid-rich myelin sheath. The myelin sheath consists of tightly wrapped layers of phospholipid-rich membrane of the Schwann cell cytoplasm with very little cytoplasm sandwiched between them. It is only in the outermost layer of the myelin sheath, where the Schwann cell and its nucleus are located. Along a myelinated axon are the nodes of Ranvier, which form a gap between the adjacent Schwann cells. The insulating properties of the myelin sheath and its gaps allow the axon to conduct impulses more quickly. The other type of process associated with the cell body is the dendrite, a threadlike process that usually contains multiple branches, which functions to receive and conduct impulses toward the cell body.

A **nerve** is a bundle of neural processes outside the central nervous system and in the peripheral nervous system. A **synapse** is the junction between two neurons or between a neuron and an effector organ, such as a muscle or gland, where neural impulses are transmitted by chemical means (neurotransmitter substance). To function, most tissues or organs have innervation, a supply of nerves to the part. A nerve allows information to be carried to and from the brain, which is the central information center. An aggregation of neuron cell bodies outside the central nervous system is termed a *ganglion* (plural, *ganglia*).

The two functional types of nerves are afferent and efferent. An afferent nerve, or sensory nerve, carries information or relays impulses from the periphery of the body to the brain (or spinal cord). Thus an afferent nerve carries sensory information, such as taste, pain, or proprioception, to the brain. Proprioception is information concerning the movement and position of the body. This information is sent on to the brain to be analyzed, acted upon, associated with other information, and stored as memory.

An efferent nerve, or motor nerve, carries information away from the brain to the periphery of the body. Thus an efferent nerve carries information to the muscles or glands in order to activate them, often in response to information received by way of the afferent nerve pathway. One motor neuron with its branching fibers may control hundreds of muscle fibers. Autonomic nerves are (by definition) always efferent.

Nervous System

The nervous system has two main divisions: the central nervous system and the peripheral nervous system (see Table 8-6). These two parts of the nervous system are reliant on each other and thus constantly interacting. The central nervous system consists of the brain and spinal cord. The peripheral nervous system consists of the spinal nerves and the cranial nerves and includes both the somatic and the autonomic nervous systems. The spinal nerves extend from the spinal cord to the periphery of the body. The cranial nerves are attached to the brain and pass through openings in the skull. The somatic nervous system operates with conscious control of the individual to move the skeletal muscles.

The autonomic nervous system is a part of the peripheral nervous system. This system operates without conscious control as the caretaker of the body. Autonomic nerves are efferent processes, and they are always in two-neuron circuits. The first neuron carries autonomic impulses to a ganglion, where they are transmitted to the body of the second neuron. The autonomic nervous system itself has two divisions: the sympathetic system and the parasympathetic system. Most tissues or organ systems are supplied by both divisions of the autonomic nervous system.

The sympathetic nervous system is involved in fight-or-flight responses, such as in the shutdown of salivary gland secretion. Such a response by the sympathetic system leads to a dry mouth (xerostomia). Sympathetic neurons arise in the spinal cord and synapse in ganglia arranged in a chain extending nearly the length of the vertebral column on both sides. Therefore all the sympathetic neurons in the head have already synapsed in a ganglion. Sympathetic fibers reach the cranial tissues that they supply by traveling with the arteries.

The parasympathetic nervous system is involved in rest-or-digest responses, such as the stimulation of salivary gland secretion. Such a response by the parasympathetic system leads to salivary flow to aid in digestion. Parasympathetic fibers associated with glands of the head and neck region are carried in various cranial nerves, and their ganglia are located in the head. Therefore parasympathetic neurons in this region may be either preganglionic neurons (before synapsing in the ganglion) or postganglionic neurons (after synapsing in the ganglion).

CHAPTER 9

Oral Mucosa

■ ■ ■

This chapter discusses the following topics:

- Oral mucosa
  - Classification of oral mucosa
  - Epithelium of oral mucosa
  - Lamina propria of oral mucosa
- Regional differences in oral mucosa
  - Labial mucosa and buccal mucosa
  - Alveolar mucosa
  - Floor of the mouth and ventral tongue surface

- Soft palate
- Attached gingiva
- Hard palate
- Tongue
  - Lingual papillae—filiform, fungiform, foliate, circumvallate
- Pigmentation of the oral mucosa
- Turnover time, repair, and aging of the oral mucosa

■ ■ ■

After studying this chapter, the reader should be able to:

1. Define and pronounce the key terms in this chapter.
2. List and describe the types of oral mucosa.
3. Characterize each of the different types of epithelium associated with each type of oral mucosa.
4. Describe the lamina propria of the oral mucosa.
5. List and describe the clinical correlations associated with the regional differences in the oral mucosa.
6. Discuss the turnover times for different tissues in the oral cavity and their clinical correlations.
7. Integrate the knowledge of the histology with the related pathology that may occur within oral mucosa.

■ ■ ■

Key Terms

Basement membrane
Black hairy tongue
Capillary plexus
Connective tissue papillae
  (pah-**pil**-ay)
Fibers: collagen, elastic

Fibroblast (fi-bro-blast)
Fordyce's spots (for-**die**-seez)
Geographic tongue
Granulation tissue (gran-yoo-**lay**-shin)
Hyperkeratinized
  (hi-per-**ker**-ah-tin-izd)

Keratin (**ker**-ah-tin)
Keratohyaline
  granules
  (ker-ah-toe-hi-ah-lin)
Lamina propria
  (lam-i-nah **pro**-pree-ah)

Layer: basal (bay-sal), dense, granular, intermediate, keratin, papillary, prickle, superficial
Lingual papillae (pah-pil-ay)
Melanin pigmentation (mel-a-nin)
Mucogingival junction (mu-ko-jin-ji-val)
Mucoperiosteum (mu-ko-per-ee-os-te-im)

Mucosa (mu-ko-sah): lining, masticatory, oral, specialized
Nonkeratinized stratified squamous epithelium (non-ker-ah-tin-izd)
Orthokeratinized stratified squamous epithelium (or-tho-ker-ah-tin-izd)
Parakeratinized stratified squamous epithelium (pare-ah-ker-ah-tin-izd)

Squames (skwaymz)
Stratified squamous epithelium (strat-i-fide skway-mus)
Stippling
Submucosa
Taste buds, pore
Turnover time
von Ebner's salivary glands (von eeb-ners)

ORAL MUCOSA

Oral mucosa almost continuously lines the oral cavity. Oral mucosa is composed of **stratified squamous epithelium** overlying a connective tissue proper, or **lamina propria** (Figure 9-1; see also Chapter 8). The oral mucosa is perforated in various regions by the ducts of salivary glands (see Chapter 11). Even though each different oral region has an epithelial covering and connective tissue makes up the bulk of lamina propria, regional differences are noted in the oral mucosa throughout the mouth (discussed later). This chapter discusses all the differing oral mucosa of the

oral cavity, except the mucosal tissues associated with the gingival sulcular region (see Chapter 10). A **basement membrane** lies between the epithelial and connective tissues in the oral mucosa. Studies show that this basement membrane serves not as a separation between the two tissues but as a continuous structure linking the two. Today's research focuses on trying to understand the interactions between these two tissues, and the basement membrane may hold many of these answers.

Dental professionals must understand the histology of the oral mucosa, the regional differences, and any clinical considerations that might be related to this information. Only then will they be able to understand

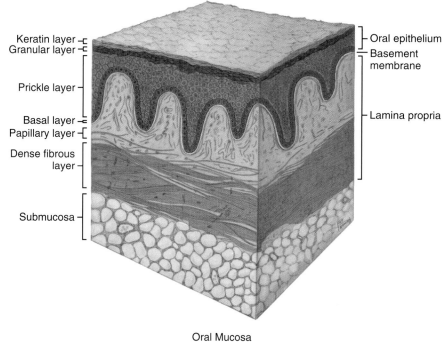

Keratin layer
Granular layer

Prickle layer

Basal layer
Papillary layer

Dense fibrous layer

Submucosa

Oral epithelium
Basement membrane

Lamina propria

Oral Mucosa
(and underlying tissues)

FIGURE 9-1 The general histological features of an oral mucosa composed of stratified squamous epithelium and the lamina propria, the underlying connective tissue proper. A submucosa may be present.

TABLE 9-1

Types of Oral Mucosa

Types	Regions	General Clinical Appearance	General Microscopic Appearance
Lining mucosa	Buccal mucosa, labial mucosa, alveolar mucosa, floor of the mouth, ventral tongue surface, and soft palate	Softer surface texture, moist surface, and ability to stretch and be compressed, acting as a cushion	Nonkeratinized epithelium with smooth interface, few rete ridges, and CT papillae with elastic fibers in the lamina propria and submucosa
Masticatory mucosa	Attached gingiva, hard palate, and dorsal tongue surface	Rubbery surface texture and resiliency, serving as firm base	Keratinized epithelium and interdigitated interface with many rete ridges and CT papillae with thin layer of submucosa or none
Specialized mucosa	Dorsal tongue surface	Associated with lingual papillae	Discrete structures of epithelium and lamina propria (see Table 9-3)

CT = connective tissue.

the clinical considerations involved in injury to the oral mucosa, such as injury that occurs with inflammation, trauma, or periodontal disease as well as with aging.

Classification of Oral Mucosa

Three main types of oral mucosa are found in the oral cavity: lining, masticatory, and specialized mucosa (Table 9-1). This classification of mucosa is based on the general histological features of the tissue. The specific histological features of each oral region are discussed later.

LINING MUCOSA

Lining mucosa is a type of mucosa noted for its softer surface texture, moist surface, and ability to stretch and be compressed, acting as a cushion for the underlying structures. Lining mucosa includes the buccal mucosa; the labial mucosa; the alveolar mucosa; and the mucosa lining the floor of the mouth, the ventral surface of the tongue, and the soft palate.

Histologically, lining mucosa is associated with nonkeratinized stratified squamous epithelium (Figure 9-2). In contrast to masticatory mucosa, the interface between the epithelium and the lamina propria is generally smoother, with fewer and less pronounced rete ridges and connective tissue papillae. In addition to these factors, the presence of elastic fibers in the lamina propria also provides the tissue with a movable base. A submucosa deep to the lamina propria is usually present, overlying muscle, and it allows for compression of the superficial tissue. These general histological features allow this type of mucosa

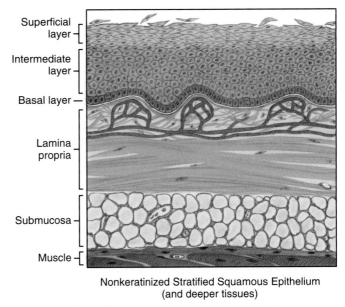

Nonkeratinized Stratified Squamous Epithelium (and deeper tissues)

FIGURE 9-2 Histological features of a nonkeratinized stratified squamous epithelium, which has three layers and is associated with a lining type of oral mucosa. Note the deeper tissues usually present with this tissue.

to serve in regions in the oral cavity where a movable base is needed, as during speech, mastication, and swallowing. Surgical incisions in these tissues frequently require sutures for closure. Local anesthetic injections into these areas are easier to accomplish than others, with less discomfort and easy dispersion of the agent, but infections also spread rapidly.

In many areas of lining mucosa, especially the labial and buccal mucosa, are **Fordyce's spots** or granules (shown in Chapter 2). These spots are a normal variant, visible as small, yellowish elevations on the surface of the mucosa. They correspond to deposits of

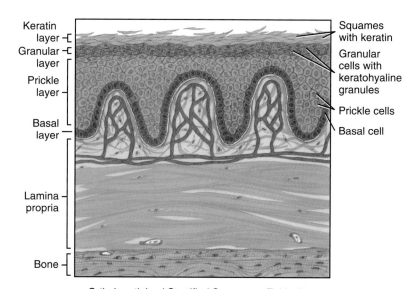

Keratin layer
Granular layer
Prickle layer
Basal layer
Lamina propria
Bone

Squames with keratin
Granular cells with keratohyaline granules
Prickle cells
Basal cell

Orthokeratinized Stratified Squamous Epithelium
(and deeper tissues)

FIGURE 9-3 Histological features of orthokeratinized stratified squamous epithelium, which has four layers and is associated with certain masticatory and specialized types of oral mucosa. Note that the cells in the keratin layer have lost their nuclei and are filled with keratin. The artifact of the spiky look of the prickle layer has not been illustrated. Note the deeper layers that are also usually present with this tissue.

sebum from misplaced sebaceous glands in the submucosa that are usually associated with hair follicles.

MASTICATORY MUCOSA

Masticatory mucosa is noted for its rubbery surface texture and resiliency. Masticatory mucosa includes the attached gingiva, the hard palate, and the dorsal surface of the tongue.

Histologically, masticatory mucosa is associated with keratinized stratified squamous epithelium (Figures 9-3, 9-4, and 9-5). Unlike lining mucosa, the interface between the epithelium and lamina propria in masticatory mucosa is highly interdigitated, with numerous and more pronounced rete ridges and connective tissue papillae, giving it a firm base. In addition, the submucosa is an extremely thin layer or is absent. When masticatory mucosa overlies bone, with or without submucosa, it increases the firmness of the tissue. These general histological features allow this type of mucosa to function in the regions that need a firm base during mastication and speech. Sutures are rarely needed for these tissues after surgery. However, local anesthetic injections are more difficult and cause greater discomfort, as is any swelling from an infectious source in these tissues.

SPECIALIZED MUCOSA

Specialized mucosa is also found on the dorsal and lateral surface of the tongue in the form of the lingual papillae, which are discrete structures composed of

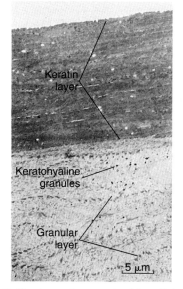

Keratin layer
Keratohyaline granules
Granular layer
5 μm

FIGURE 9-4 Electron micrograph of keratinized epithelium showing the granular and keratin layers. Small keratohyaline granules are visible in the granular layer; the cells of the keratin layer are flattened and contain keratin. It is hard to discern at this lower microscopic power whether this tissue is orthokeratinized or parakeratinized based on the nuclei of the keratin layer. (From Nanci A. *Ten Cate's Oral Histology*, ed 6. Mosby, St. Louis, 2003.)

epithelium and lamina propria (see Chapter 2). This type of oral mucosa is discussed later.

Epithelium of Oral Mucosa

Three types of stratified squamous epithelium are found within the oral cavity: nonkeratinized, ortho-

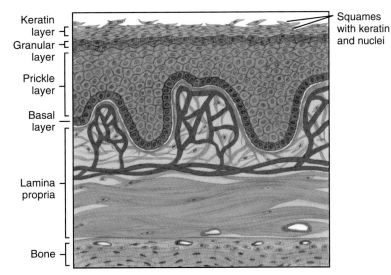

Parakeratinized Stratified Squamous Epithelium
(and deeper tissues)

FIGURE 9-5 Histological features of parakeratinized stratified squamous epithelium, which has three to four layers and is associated with certain masticatory and specialized types of oral mucosa. Note that the cells in the keratin layer have retained their nuclei and are also filled with keratin. Also note the deeper layers that are also usually present with this tissue.

TABLE 9-2

Epithelium of Oral Mucosa

Types of Epitheliulm	Classification	Basic Histological Description
Nonkeratatinized epithelium	Lining mucosa	Basal, intermediate, and superficial layers
Orthokeratinized epithelium	Masticatory mucosa	Basal, prickle, granular, and keratin layers (Note: Keratin layer cells contain only keratin and no nuclei.)
Parakeratinized epithelium	Masticatory mucosa	Basal, prickle, granular, and keratin layers (Note: Keratin layer cells contain keratin and nuclei.)

keratinized, and parakeratinized (Table 9-2). Nonkeratinized epithelium is associated with lining mucosa. Orthokeratinized and parakeratinized epithelium are associated with masticatory mucosa. All forms of epithelium act as a barrier to bacterial invasion and mechanical irritation and offer protection against dryness. These features are accentuated in those epithelial tissues with keratin.

Many researchers use the term *keratinocytes* for the epithelial cells in oral mucosa because they can produce **keratin** either naturally, as in keratinized tissues, or when the tissue is traumatized, as in nonkeratinized tissue. Other non–keratin-producing cells or nonkeratinocytes besides epithelial cells may be present in smaller numbers in the epithelium (Table 9-3). These include melanocytes (discussed later in relation to pigmentation), white blood cells, Langerhans cells, Granstein cells, and Merkel cells. The

polymorphonuclear (PMN) leukocyte is the most commonly occurring white blood cell in all forms of oral mucosa.

NONKERATINIZED STRATIFIED SQUAMOUS EPITHELIUM

Nonkeratinized stratified squamous epithelium is noted in the superficial layers of lining mucosa, such as in the labial mucosa, buccal mucosa, and alveolar mucosa, and the mucosa lining the floor of the mouth, the ventral surface of the tongue, and the soft palate (see Figure 9-2). These lining mucosal tissues have similar epithelial histological traits even though they have some regional differences. Nonkeratinized epithelium is the most common form of epithelium in the oral cavity.

TABLE 9-3

Types of Cells in Epithelium*

Types	Features	Functions
Epithelial cell	Rapidly renewing cell that undergoes a pathway of differentiation with desmosomes	Forms a cohesive sheet that resists physical forces and serves as a barrier to infection
Melanocyte	Dendritic cell of neural crest origin, forms a continuous network near the basement membrane	Synthesis of melanin pigmentation with its transfer to adjacent cells
Langerhans cell	Dendritic bone marrow–derived cell noted near the basement membrane	Immune response with T lymphocytes
Granstein cell	Similar to Langerhans cell	Same as Langerhans cell
Merkel cell	Neural cell noted near the basement membrane	Sensory information

*White blood cells are not included in this table.

Each of these lining mucosal tissues has at least three layers within the epithelium. A **basal layer**, or *stratum basale*, is the deepest of the three layers. The basal layer is a single layer of cuboidal epithelial cells overlying the basement membrane, which in turn is situated superior to the lamina propria. The basal layer produces the basal lamina of the basement membrane.

The basal layer is also considered germinative because mitosis of the epithelial cells occurs within this layer, but this cell division is seen only under higher magnification of the tissue. Future studies may show the existence of an epithelial stem cell in the basal layer that produces other stem and daughter cells, similar to the situation for blood cells in the bone marrow.

The layer of epithelium superficial to the basal layer in nonkeratinized epithelium is the **intermediate layer,** or *stratum intermedium*. The intermediate layer is composed of larger, stacked, polyhedral-shaped cells. These cells appear larger or plumper than the basal layer cells because they have larger amounts of fluid within their cytoplasm. The cells of the intermediate layer have lost the ability to undergo mitosis as they migrated. The intermediate layer makes up the bulk of nonkeratinized epithelium.

The most superficial level in nonkeratinized epithelium is termed the **superficial layer,** or *stratum superficiale*. It is hard to discern the exact division between the superficial layer and the intermediate layers in lining mucosa when viewing histological sections. This layer shows even larger similarly stacked polyhedral epithelial cells with the outer cells flattening into **squames.** The squames show shedding or loss as they age and die during the turnover of the tissue. Thus maturation within this tissue is seen only as

an increase in the size of cells as they migrate superficially.

ORTHOKERATINIZED STRATIFIED SQUAMOUS EPITHELIUM

Orthokeratinized stratified squamous epithelium demonstrates a keratinization of the epithelial cells throughout its most superficial layers (see Figures 9-3 and 9-4). Orthokeratinized epithelium is the least common form of epithelium found in the oral cavity. It is associated with the masticatory mucosa of the hard palate and the attached gingiva. It is also associated with the specialized mucosa of the lingual papillae on the dorsal surface of the tongue. As this tissue matures, it forms keratin within its superficial cells, showing a visible and physiological difference in the cells as they migrate superficially.

Like nonkeratinized epithelium, orthokeratinized epithelium has a single basal layer, or *stratum basale*, undergoing mitosis. This layer also produces the basal lamina of the adjacent basement membrane. Unlike nonkeratinized epithelium, however, orthokeratinized epithelium has more layers superficial to the basal layer: four separate layers with somewhat distinct divisions.

Superficial to the basal layer is the **prickle layer,** or the *stratum spinosum*. This layer is named for an artifact that occurs when the epithelial cells of this layer are dried for microscopic study; the cells shrink as a result of cytoplasmic fluid loss but still maintain their desmosomal cellular junctions. Thus a prickly or spiky look results when the individual dehydrated epithelial cells are still joined at their outer edges. The cells of the prickle layer lose the ability to undergo mitosis as they migrate. The prickle layer makes up the bulk of ortho-keratinized epithelium.

Superficial to the prickle layer is the **granular layer,** or *stratum granulosum.* The epithelial cells in this layer are flat and are stacked in a layer three to five cells thick. In their cytoplasm, these nucleated cells contain prominent **keratohyaline granules**, which stain as dark spots. The keratohyaline granules form a chemical precursor for the keratin found in the more superficial layers.

The most superficial layer in orthokeratinized epithelium is the **keratin layer,** or *stratum corneum,* which shows a variable thickness depending on the region. The cells in the keratin layer are flat and have no nuclei, and their cytoplasm is filled with **keratin.** This soft, opaque, waterproof material is formed from a complex of keratohyaline granules and intermediate filaments from the cells. Keratin and its associated components stain as a translucent dense material. The outer cells of the keratin layer, or squames, show increased flattening and also shedding or loss because they are no longer viable. In addition, portions of the keratin material are also shed as a result of the turnover of the tissue. These squames and their corni-fied cell envelope make up a major part of the epithelial barrier and are continuously being renewed. The epithelial barrier serves as protection from physical, chemical, and microbial attack as well as dehydration and heat loss, that sometimes occurs in the oral cavity environment.

PARAKERATINIZED STRATIFIED SQUAMOUS EPITHELIUM

Parakeratinized stratified squamous epithelium is associated with the masticatory mucosa of the attached gingiva, in higher levels than orthokeratization, and also the tongue's dorsal surface (see Figure 9-5). Most researchers believe that parakeratinized epithelium is an immature form of orthokeratinized epithelium. The presence of this form of keratinization on the skin is considered a disease state; therefore parakeratinization is one of the unique histological features of the healthy oral cavity. Parakeratinized epithelium is also associated with the specialized mucosa of the lingual papillae on the dorsal surface of the tongue.

Parakeratinized epithelium may have all the same layers of epithelium as orthokeratinized epithelium, such as the basal layer, prickle layer, granular layer, and keratin layer, although the granular layer may be indistinct or absent altogether.

The main difference between parakeratinized epithelium and orthokeratinized epithelium is in the cells of the keratin layer. In parakeratinized epithelium, the most superficial layer is still being shed or lost, but these cells of the keratin layer contain not only keratin but also their nuclei, unlike those of orthokeratinized epithelium. This distinction is sometimes difficult to discern at the lower microscopic power used in most histological sections. Studies have shown that even though the epithelial cells have nuclei, they possibly are no longer viable.

Clinical Considerations of Oral Mucosa

Unlike keratinized epithelium, nonkeratinized epithelium normally has no superficial layers showing keratinization. Nonkeratinized epithelium may, however, readily transform into a keratinizing type in response to frictional or chemical trauma, in which case it becomes **hyperkeratinized.**

This change of hyperkeratinization commonly occurs on the usually nonkeratinized buccal mucosa when the linea alba forms, a white ridge of raised calloused tissue that extends horizontally at the level where the maxillary and mandibular teeth come together and occlude (discussed and shown in Chapter 2). Histologically, an excess amount of keratin is noted on the surface of the tissue, and the tissue has all the layers of an orthokeratinized tissue with its granular and keratin layers.

In patients who have habits such as clenching or grinding (bruxism) of their teeth, a larger area of the buccal mucosa becomes hyperkeratinized than just the linea alba (Figure 9-6). This larger white, rough, raised lesion needs to be recorded so that changes may be made in the dental treatment plan in regard to the patient's oral habits (see Chapter 20). Even keratinized tissue can undergo hyperkeratinization; an increase in the amount of keratin is produced as a result of trauma to the region. Changes such as hyperkeratinization are reversible if the source of the injury is removed, but it takes time for the keratin to be shed or lost by the tissue. Thus a baseline biopsy and microscopic study of any whitened tissue for malignant changes may be indicated for patients, especially if they are in high-risk categories, such as smokers or alcoholics. Hyperkeratinized tissue may be associated with the heat from smoking or hot fluids on the hard palate in the form of nicotinic stomatitis (see Chapter 11).

Lamina Propria of Oral Mucosa

All forms of epithelium, whether associated with lining, masticatory, or specialized mucosa, have a lamina propria deep to the basement membrane (see Figure 9-1). The main fiber group in the lamina propria is **collagen fibers,** but **elastic fibers** are present in many regions of the oral cavity. The lamina propria, like all forms of connective tissue proper, has two layers: papillary and dense (Figure 9-7).

The **papillary layer** is the more superficial layer of the lamina propria. The papillary layer consists of loose connective tissue within the **connective tissue papillae,** along with blood vessels and nerve tissue. The tissue has an equal amount of fibers, cells, and intercellular substance. Between the papillary layer and the deeper layers of the lamina propria is a **capillary plexus,** which provides nutrition for all the

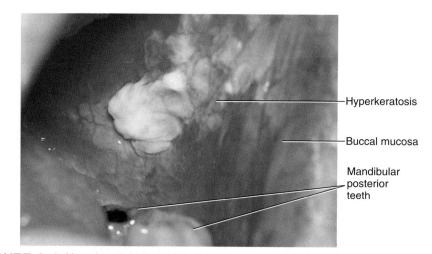

FIGURE 9-6 Hyperkeratinization of the buccal mucosa. The buccal mucosa usually has a nonkeratinized epithelium, but this epithelium has undergone severe physical injury to the area as a result of grinding, or bruxism, of the teeth; the epithelium has thus has become keratinized. Other, more serious lesions of the oral cavity must be ruled out.

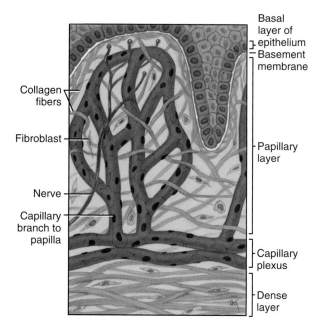

FIGURE 9-7 Histological features of the deeper tissue of the oral mucosa showing the layers and features of the lamina propria.

mucosa and sends capillaries into the connective tissue papillae.

The **dense layer** is the deeper portion of the lamina propria. The dense layer consists of dense connective tissue with a large amount of fibers. A **submucosa** may or may not be present deep to the dense layer of the lamina propria, depending on the region of the oral cavity. The submucosa usually contains loose connective tissue and may contain adipose tissue or salivary glands. The submucosa may overlie bone or muscle within the oral cavity.

Lining mucosa does not have prominent connective tissue papillae and alternating rete ridges. In addition, elastic fibers are present in the papillary layer, thus allowing the tissue to stretch and recoil during speech, mastication, and swallowing. In contrast to lining mucosa, masticatory mucosa has numerous and prominent connective tissue papillae, giving the mucosa a firm base, which is needed for speech and mastication.

The most common cell in the lamina propria, like all types of connective tissue proper, is the **fibroblast.** Fibroblasts synthesize certain types of protein fibers and intercellular substances. Researchers believe that subpopulations of the fibroblast may exist and that controlling the beneficial groups may be the answer to periodontal disease and age-related changes that occur in the lamina propria and other portions of the periodontium. Other cells present in the lamina propria in smaller numbers are white blood cells such as PMNs, mast cells, macrophages, and lymphocytes.

REGIONAL DIFFERENCES IN ORAL MUCOSA

Specific histological features are noted in the different regions of the oral cavity (Table 9-4). These specific histological features are the basis for the differences observed clinically when these regions are examined. One way to integrate these two associated concepts is to review the clinical appearance of the different regions of oral mucosa during an intraoral examination when armed with the new knowledge of the specific underlying histological features. Thus the novice dental professional must look closely at the clinical photographs of the different regions of the oral cavity presented in color in Chapter 2 and compare these with the histological presentation discussed in this chapter as well as in the descriptions of their clinical presentation.

TABLE 9-4

Regional Differences in Oral Mucosa

Region/Appearance	Epithelium	Lamina Propria	Submucosa
Lining Mucosa Labial mucosa and buccal mucosa: opaque pink, shiny, moist; with areas of melanin pigmentation and Fordyce's spots possible	Thick nonkeratinized	Irregular and blunt CT papillae, some elastic fibers, extensive vascular supply	Present with adipose and minor salivary glands, with firm attachment to muscle
Alveolar mucosa: reddish-pink, shiny, moist, extremely mobile	Thin nonkeratinized	CT papillae sometimes absent, many elastic fibers, with extensive vascular supply	Present with minor salivary glands and many elastic fibers, with loose attachment to muscle or bone
Floor of the mouth and ventral tongue surface: reddish pink, moist, shiny, compressible, with vascular blue areas; mobility varies	Extremely thin nonkeratinized	Extensive vascular supply Floor: broad CT papillae Ventral tongue: numerous CT papillae, some elastic fibers, minor salivary glands	Present Floor: adipose with submandibular and sublingual glands, loosely attached to bone/muscles Ventral tongue: extremely thin and firmly attached to muscle
Soft palate: deep pink with a yellow hue and moist surface; compressible and extremely elastic	Thin nonkeratinized	Thick lamina propria with numerous CT papillae and distinct elastic layer	Extremely thin with adipose tissue and minor salivary glands, with a firm attachment to underlying muscle
Masticatory Mucosa Attached gingiva: opaque pink, dull, firm, immobile; with areas of melanin pigmentation possible and varying amounts of stippling	Thick keratinized (mainly parakeratinized, some orthokeratinized)	Tall, narrow CT papillae, extensive vascular supply, and serves as a mucoperiosteum to bone	Not present
Hard palate: pink, immobile, and firm medial portion, with rugae and raphe; cushioned lateral portions	Thick orthokeratinized	Medial portion; rugae and raphe serving as a mucoperiosteum to bone	Present only in lateral portions, with anterior part having adipose and posterior part having minor salivary glands; absent in medial portion, rugae, and raphe

CT = connective tissue.

Labial Mucosa and Buccal Mucosa

CLINICAL APPEARANCE

The labial mucosa and buccal mucosa line the inner lips and cheeks, respectively. Both of these regions appear clinically as an opaque pink, shiny, moist, compressible tissue that stretches easily. Areas of melanin pigmentation may be noted (discussed later). A variable number of Fordyce's spots are scattered throughout the tissue (see Chapter 2). The mucosa of the lips and cheeks is classified as a lining mucosa.

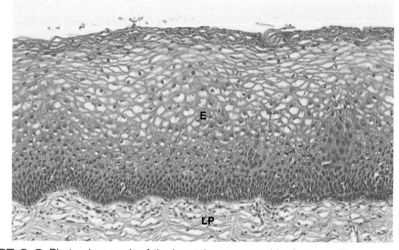

FIGURE 9-8 Photomicrograph of the buccal mucosa and its features. The extremely thick epithelium (*E*) is nonkeratinized and overlies a lamina propria (*LP*) with an extensive vascular supply. The lamina propria has irregular and blunt connective tissue papillae. (From Young B, Heath JW. *Wheater's Functional Histology*, ed 4. Churchill Livingstone, Edinburgh, 2000.)

HISTOLOGICAL FEATURES

The nonkeratinized epithelium of the labial mucosa and buccal mucosa is extremely thick and overlies and obscures a lamina propria with an extensive vascular supply, giving the overall mucosa an opaque and pinkish appearance (Figure 9-8). The lamina propria has irregular and blunt connective tissue papillae but contains some elastic fibers in addition to its collagen fibers, giving the tissue the ability to stretch and return to its original shape. The lamina propria overlies a submucosa that contains adipose tissue and minor salivary glands, giving the tissue its compressibility and moisture, respectively. The submucosa is firmly attached to the underlying muscle in the region of the labial and buccal mucosa, thus preventing any of the tissue from interfering during mastication or speech because the mucosa and muscle function as one unit.

Alveolar Mucosa

CLINICAL APPEARANCE

The alveolar mucosa is a reddish-pink tissue with blue vascular areas. This shiny, moist region is extremely mobile and lines the vestibules of the oral cavity. Alveolar mucosa is classified as a lining mucosa.

HISTOLOGICAL FEATURES

The epithelium of the alveolar mucosa is extremely thin nonkeratinized epithelium that overlies but does not obscure an extensive vascular supply in the lamina propria, making the mucosa redder than the labial mucosa or buccal mucosa. Connective tissue papillae are sometimes absent, and many elastic fibers are present in the lamina propria, thus allowing mobility of the tissue.

The submucosa associated with the alveolar mucosa has minor salivary glands and many elastic fibers in a loose connective tissue, thus giving the tissue its moisture and increased motility, respectively. The submucosa is loosely attached to the underlying muscle or bone, increasing the ability of the tissue to move because the tissue is located between the moving lips and the stationary attached gingiva.

Floor of the Mouth and Ventral Tongue Surface

CLINICAL APPEARANCE

Both the floor of the mouth and the ventral surface (undersurface) of the tongue appear as a reddish-pink tissue with vascular blue areas of veins. The tissue is also moist, shiny, and compressible. Although the tissue of the floor of the mouth has some mobility, the tissue of the ventral surface of the tongue is firmly attached yet allows some stretching along with the tongue muscles. The mucosa of both the floor of the mouth and ventral tongue surface is classified as a lining mucosa.

HISTOLOGICAL FEATURES

Both the floor of the mouth and the ventral tongue surface have an extremely thin nonkeratinized epithelium overlying but not obscuring a lamina propria with an extensive vascular supply, thus making both tissues redder and the veins more apparent.

The connective tissue papillae of the lamina propria are also broad in the tissues of the floor of the mouth. The submucosa deep to the lamina propria consists of loose connective tissue with adipose tissue and includes the submandibular and sublingual salivary glands, giving the tissue its compressibility and moisture, respectively. The submucosa associated with the floor of the mouth is loosely attached to the underlying bone and muscles, thus giving the tissue its movability when the attached tongue moves during mastication and speech.

The connective tissue papillae of the lamina propria of the tongue's ventral surface are numerous. Some elastic fibers and a few minor salivary glands provide the ability to stretch and supply moisture. The submucosa associated with the ventral surface of the tongue is extremely thin and firmly attached to the underlying tongue muscle. This arrangement allows the mucosa and muscles to function as one unit, thus reducing movability during mastication and speech.

Soft Palate

CLINICAL APPEARANCE

The posterior portion of the palate, the soft palate, is deep pink with a yellowish hue and a moist surface. The tissue is compressible and extremely elastic to allow for speech and swallowing. The mucosa of the soft palate is classified as a lining mucosa.

HISTOLOGICAL APPEARANCE

The soft palate has a thin nonkeratinized epithelium overlying a thick lamina propria (Figure 9-9). The lamina propria has numerous connective tissue papillae and a distinct elastic layer for increased mobility. The submucosa associated with the mucosa of the soft palate is extremely thin and has a firm attachment to the underlying muscle to allow for the mechanisms of speech and swallowing. Again, this arrangement allows the mucosa and muscles to function as one unit. The submucosa contains adipose tissue, which gives the tissue its yellow hue and compressibility. The submucosa also has minor salivary glands, giving the tissue its moisture.

Attached Gingiva

CLINICAL APPEARANCE

The attached gingiva that covers the alveolar bone of the dental arches is classified as a masticatory type of mucosa. Healthy attached gingiva is opaque pink, and areas of melanin pigmentation may be seen (discussed later). When dried, the tissue is dull, firm, and immobile.

Stippling is observed clinically as little depressions, which give the surface of the attached gingiva an orange-peel appearance. The amount of stippling varies even within healthy oral cavities. Also noted is the **mucogingival junction,** a sharply defined

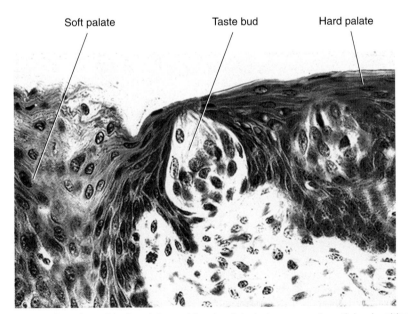

Soft palate   Taste bud   Hard palate

FIGURE 9-9 Junction of soft palate and hard palate between nonkeratinized epithelium and keratinized epithelium and between a lining mucosa and a masticatory mucosa. Note the taste bud located in the epithelium. (From Nanci A. *Ten Cate's Oral Histology*, ed 6. Mosby, St. Louis, 2003.)

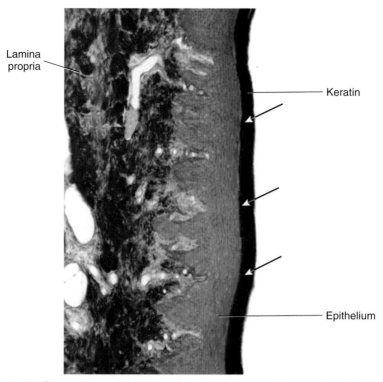

Lamina propria

Keratin

Epithelium

FIGURE 9-10 Photomicrograph of the attached gingiva, which consists of a thick layer of mainly parakeratinized epithelium over a lamina propria with extensive vascularity. Note the keratohyaline granules (*arrows*) in the granular layer deep to the layers of superficial keratin. (From Nanci A. *Ten Cate's Oral Histology*, ed 6. Mosby, St. Louis, 2003.)

scalloped junction between the pinker attached gingiva and the redder alveolar mucosa. Other portions of the gingiva, such as those that face the tooth surface, are discussed in Chapter 10.

HISTOLOGICAL FEATURES

The attached gingiva has a thick layer of mainly parakeratinized epithelium that obscures the extensive vascular supply in the lamina propria, making the tissue appear opaque and pinkish (Figure 9-10). Again, the cells of the keratin layer that have nuclei may be difficult to see in the histological sections. Minor portions of the attached gingiva may be orthokeratinized.

The lamina propria of the attached gingiva also has tall, narrow connective tissue papillae; its stippling is due to a strong attachment or pull of the epithelium toward the lamina propria in these areas, a process that is analogous to the button tufting on upholstery. No submucosa is present. The lamina propria is directly attached to the underlying jawbones, making the attached gingiva firm and immobile. The lamina propria acts as a periosteum to the underlying jawbones and thus is termed a **mucoperiosteum**.

Histologically, the mucogingival junction can be seen as a dividing zone between the keratinized attached gingiva dend the nonkeratinized alveolar mucosa and thus between a masticatory mucosa and a lining mucosa (Figures 9-11 and 9-12). It is also a junction between a tissue with a thick epithelial layer in the pinkish attached gingiva and a tissue with a thin epithelial layer in the redder alveolar mucosa, even though both tissues have a similar extensive vascular supply in the lamina propria.

Hard Palate

CLINICAL APPEARANCE

The anterior portion of the palate, the hard palate, appears pink and is immobile and firm. A cushioned feeling is noted in the lateral portions and a firmer feeling in the medial portion when the hard palate is palpated. The palatal rugae and the median palatine raphe are also firm to the touch. The mucosa of the hard palate is classified as a masticatory type of mucosa.

HISTOLOGICAL FEATURES

The hard palate has a thick layer of orthokeratinized epithelium overlying a thick lamina propria (Figure 9-13). Only the lateral portions of the hard palate have a submucosa, giving the tissue here a cushioned feeling when palpated. The submucosa in the anterior part of

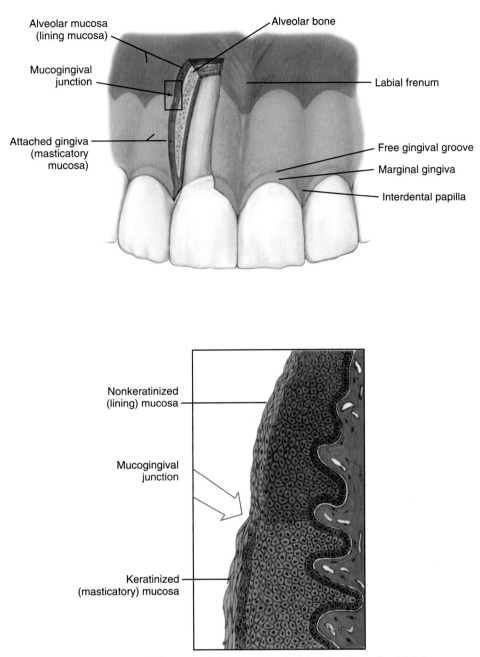

Alveolar mucosa (lining mucosa)

Mucogingival junction

Attached gingiva (masticatory mucosa)

Alveolar bone

Labial frenum

Free gingival groove

Marginal gingiva

Interdental papilla

Nonkeratinized (lining) mucosa

Mucogingival junction

Keratinized (masticatory) mucosa

FIGURE 9-11 Histological features of the mucogingival junction (*arrow*), which is a zone between the keratinized attached gingiva and the nonkeratinized alveolar mucosa and thus between a masticatory mucosa and a lining mucosa.

the lateral portion (from the canines to the premolars) contains adipose tissue. The submucosa in the posterior part of the lateral portion of the hard palate (around the molars) contains minor salivary glands. However, the amount of submucosa in these areas of the hard palate is thinner than that associated with lining mucosa, which becomes apparent when injections of local anesthetic are placed in the area because they can produce slight discomfort.

Submucosa is absent in the medial portion of the hard palate; thus the tissue has a firmer feeling when palpated. This firm feeling is enhanced as a result of the firmness with which the lamina propria is attached to the underlying bone; thus the lamina propria serves as a mucoperiosteum. The landmarks on the hard palate, the palatal rugae and the median palatal raphe, have histological features similar to those of the medial portion of the hard palate.

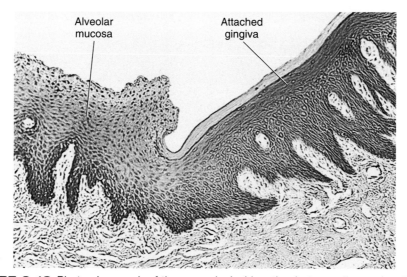

FIGURE 9-12 Photomicrograph of the mucogingival junction between the nonkeratinized alveolar mucosa and the keratinized attached gingiva and thus between a masticatory mucosa and a lining mucosa. (From Nanci A. *Ten Cate's Oral Histology*, ed 6. Mosby, St. Louis, 2003.)

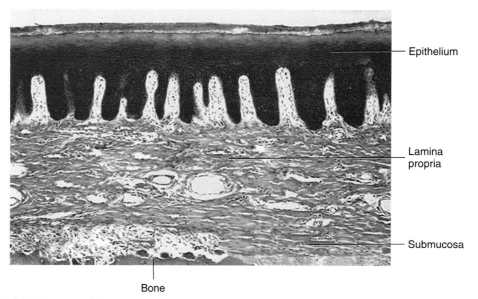

FIGURE 9-13 Photomicrograph of the masticatory mucosa covering the cushioned lateral portion of the hard palate consisting of orthokeratinized epithelium and lamina propria, overlying palatal bone and thin layer of submucosa. (From Nanci A. *Ten Cate's Oral Histology*, ed 6. Mosby, St. Louis, 2003.)

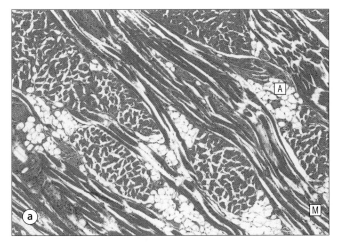

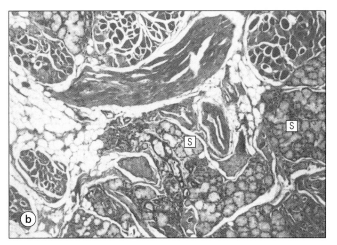

FIGURE 9-14 Photomicrographs of the muscular core of the tongue. **A:** In the anterior, the striated muscle bundles (*M*) are tightly packed with relatively little intervening adipose tissue (*A*). Note that the muscle bundles run in many directions. In the bulkier, less mobile posterio, the adipose tissue is more abundant. **B:** Collections of salivary glands (*S*) are numerous in the submucosa and muscular core of the posterior tongue, particularly close to the junction between the posterior and anterior. (From Stevens A, Lowe J. *Human Histology*, ed 2. Mosby, St. Louis, 1997.)

 Clinical Considerations Concerning Keratinization

When a graft procedure is performed to reduce the amount of gingival recession on the root, keratinization is taken into consideration. Thus the goal of grafting is to increase the amount of attached keratinized tissue. One type of graft, the free gingiva graft, uses a thickness of both keratinized epithelial and lamina propria tissues harvested from the palate and grafted to the root to form a new band of keratinized attached gingiva. This procedure generally is somewhat successful, but the graft tends to be lighter colored, and studies show that the epithelium does not survive the procedure, which means that the donor site requires extra time to heal and produce new epithelium.

In a relatively new procedure for areas of recession, a subepithelial connective tissue graft of only the lamina propria is taken from the surrounding keratinized attached gingiva and is grafted to the root. Epithelial cells from the surrounding tissue migrate to cover the graft and heal the area. This procedure is consistently successful: The new keratinized attached gingival tissue looks more like the surrounding tissues, and healing of the donor site is rapid. Thus the message to form keratin is believed to come from the deeper lamina propria and not directly from the epithelial tissues.

TONGUE

The tongue is a mass of striated muscle tissue in its core, covered by oral mucosa (Figure 19-14). The V-shaped line, the sulcus terminalis, divides the tongue into an anterior two thirds and a posterior one third. In the anterior, the striated muscle bundles are tightly packed, with relatively little intervening adipose tissue in the core. In the bulkier, less mobile posterior, the adipose tissue is more abundant. Collections of salivary glands are numerous in the submucosa and muscular core of the posterior portion of the tongue, particularly close to the junction between the posterior and anterior.

The top surface, or dorsal surface, of the tongue has both a masticatory and specialized type of mucosa present. The masticatory mucosa, an orthokeratinized stratified squamous epithelium, generally covers the surface of the muscle tissue associated with the tongue. The specialized type of oral mucosa found on the dorsal tongue surface, the lingual papillae, has both orthokeratinized and parakeratinized epithelium present. **Lingual papillae** are discrete structures or appendages of keratinized epithelium and lamina propria as described clinically in Chapter 2. Lingual papillae are also found on the lateral surface of the tongue. The four types of lingual papillae are filiform, fungiform, foliate, and circumvallate (Table 9-5). The development of the lingual papillae and the tongue is discussed in Chapter 5.

Three types of lingual papillae are associated with taste buds: fungiform, foliate, and circumvallate. **Taste buds** are barrel-shaped organs of taste derived from the epithelium (Figure 9-15). They are composed of 30 to 80 spindle-shaped cells that extend from the basement membrane to the epithelial surface of the lingual papilla. Turnover of the taste bud cells is fairly rapid, with tissue turnover time approximating 10 days.

The two types of taste bud cells are the supporting and the taste cells. However, the difference between the two is hard to discern on the lower magnification of most histological sections. Many immature forms of the two types are also noted. The supporting cells support the taste bud and are usually located on the

TABLE 9-5

Lingual Papillae

Comparison of	Filiform	Fungiform	Foliate	Circumvallate
Clinical appearance	Most common on body; fine-pointed cones giving the tongue a velvety texture	Lesser numbers on body; mushroom-shaped small red dots	4 to 11 vertical ridges on the lateral surface of the posterior tongue	7 to 15 large, raised mushroom-shaped structures anterior to the sulcus terminalis
Microscopic appearance	Pointed structure with a thick layer of keratinized epithelium, overlying a core of lamina propria; no taste buds	Mushroom-shaped structure with a thin layer of keratinized epithelium overlying a core of lamina propria, with taste buds in the most superficial portion	Leaf-shaped structure of keratinized epithelium overlying a core of lamina propria, with taste buds superficial	Mushroom-shaped structure with similar histology to fungiform—that is, sunken deep to the tongue surface, taste buds in base, and surrounded by a trough, with von Ebner's minor salivary glands in the submucosa
Function	Possibly mechanical	Taste	Taste	Taste

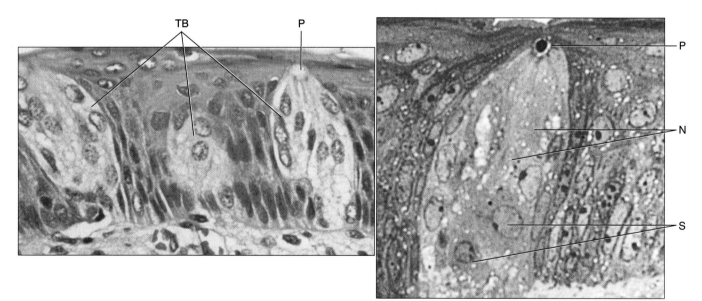

FIGURE 9-15 Histological section of a taste bud (*TB*), with two types of cells: supporting cells (*S*) and taste cells (*N*). Many immature forms are also present. Discerning the associated nerves and differences between the two cell types is difficult at this magnification. Note the taste pore (*P*) at its most superficial portion. (From Stevens A, Lowe J: *Human Histology,* ed 3. Mosby, St. Louis, 2005.)

outer portion of the taste bud. The taste cells are usually located in the central portion of the taste bud and have superficial taste receptors that are responsible for making contact with dissolved molecules of food and producing a taste sensation (see Figures 9-15 and Figure 9-16).

Dissolved molecules of food contact the taste receptors at the **taste pore,** which is an opening in the most superficial portion of the taste bud. Taste cells are also associated with sensory neuron processes in the inferior portion of the taste bud among the cells. These sensory neuron processes receive messages of taste

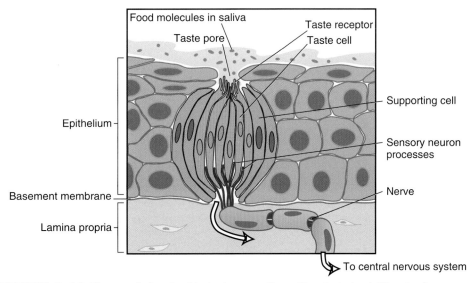

FIGURE 9-16 The events involved in taste sensation with a taste bud. Dissolved molecules of food contact the taste receptors of the taste cells at the taste pore. Taste cells are also associated with sensory neuron processes in the inferior portion of the taste bud, among the cells that receive messages of taste sensation from the taste receptors. This message is then sent by way of the nerve to the central nervous system, where it is identified as a certain type of taste.

sensation by way of the receptors. This message is then sent by way of the nerve to the central nervous system, where it is identified as a certain type of taste.

Evidence suggests that the four fundamental taste sensations—sweet, sour, salty, and bitter—are different on account of four slightly differentiated taste cells. The many tastes that we experience are the result of the blending of the four fundamental taste sensations, the addition of other sensations by the tongue, and the interplay of smell and taste. In the past, the tongue was thought to have a specific mapping of taste sensations, but research studies have proved this assumption to be false.

Filiform Lingual Papillae

CLINICAL APPEARANCE

The filiform lingual papillae are the most common lingual papillae located on the body of the dorsal surface of the tongue. They are shaped like fine-pointed cones of 2 to 3 mm, with the tips naturally turned toward the pharynx. Filiform papillae give the dorsal surface of the tongue its velvety texture. They are sensitive to changes in the body.

HISTOLOGICAL FEATURES

A filiform lingual papilla is a pointed structure with a thick layer of orthokeratinized or parakeratinized epithelium overlying a core of lamina propria (Figure 9-17). An increased amount of keratin is noted also at the surface of each, forming a snow-covered "Christmas tree" arrangement and whiter color of this lingual papilla. No taste buds are present in the epithelium. The filiform possibly have a rudimentary mechanical function as a result of their surface texture, which is related to the increased amount of surface keratinization present. Thus they may aid in guiding food back to the pharynx for swallowing.

Fungiform Lingual Papillae

CLINICAL APPEARANCE

The fungiform lingual papillae are found in lesser numbers than are the filiform on the body of the dorsal surface of the tongue. The fungiform appear as reddish dots that on closer inspection are slightly raised and mushroom shaped and have a 1 mm diameter. Fungiform are not found near the sulcus terminalis, a triangle-shaped landmark that separates the surface of the tongue into its body and base.

HISTOLOGICAL FEATURES

A fungiform lingual papilla is a mushroom-shaped structure with a thin layer of orthokeratinized or parakeratinized epithelium overlying a highly vascularized core of lamina propria, thus producing the redder appearance of this lingual papilla (see Figure 9-17). A variable number of taste buds are located in the most superficial portion of the fungiform's epithelial

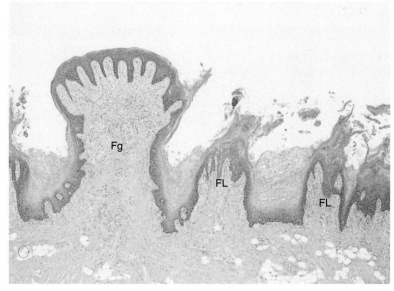

FIGURE 9-17 Histological section of the fungiform lingual papillae (*Fg*) and filiform lingual papillae (*FL*) on the upper or dorsal surface of the tongue. Note the mushroom shape of the fungiform lingual papilla; the taste buds at the superficial surface of this lingual papilla are difficult to discern at this magnification. Notice also the tree shape of the filiform lingual papillae. (From Young B, Heath JW: *Wheater's Functional Histology*, ed 4. Churchill Livingstone, Edinburgh, 2000.)

layer; however, taste buds are not located near the base of the structure. Thus the function of the fungiform is taste sensation.

Foliate Lingual Papillae

CLINICAL APPEARANCE

The foliate lingual papillae appear as 4 to 11 vertical ridges parallel to one another on the lateral surface of the posterior portion of the tongue.

HISTOLOGICAL FEATURES

The foliate lingual papillae are leaf-shaped structures with a layer of orthokeratinized or parakeratinized epithelium overlying a core of lamina propria (Figure 9-18). Taste buds are located in the epithelial layer on the lateral portions of the leaf-shaped structure. Thus the function of the foliate is taste sensation. Some researchers believe that the foliate are not true lingual papillae because of their rudimentary appearance, developmental background, and location.

Circumvallate Lingual Papillae

CLINICAL FEATURES

When the tongue is arched and extended, the circumvallate lingual papillae appear as 7 to 15 large, raised,

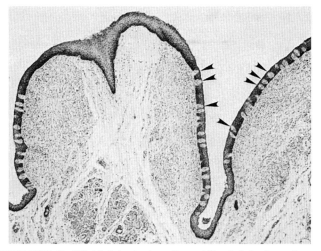

FIGURE 9-18 Histological section of the foliate lingual papillae on the lateral surface of the tongue. Taste buds (*arrows*) are located in the epithelial layer on the lateral portions of the leaf-shaped structure. (From Nanci A. *Ten Cate's Oral Histology*, ed 6. Mosby, St. Louis, 2003.)

mushroom-shaped structures just anterior to the sulcus terminalis. With the tongue in a more relaxed and natural position, the circumvallate are sunken as deep as the tongue surface because they are surrounded by a circular trough or trench. The circumvallate are lined up in an inverted V-shaped row facing the pharynx, mimicking the shape of the sulcus terminalis. The circumvallate have a larger diameter than the fungiform, measuring from 3 to 5 mm.

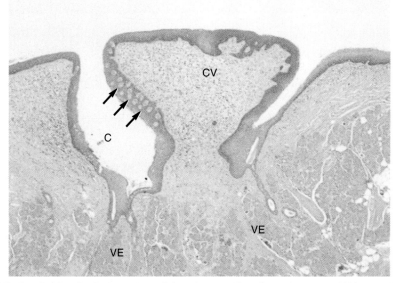

FIGURE 9-19 Histological section of the circumvallate lingual papillae (*CV*) with their taste buds (*arrows*) within the epithelial layer and surrounded by a circular trough (*C*). Notice von Ebner's salivary glands (*VE*), which flush the trough. (From Young B, Heath JW. *Wheater's Functional Histology*, ed 4. Churchill Livingstone, Edinburgh, 2000.)

HISTOLOGICAL FEATURES

The circumvallate lingual papillae are mushroom-shaped structures with orthokeratinized or parakeratinized epithelium overlying a core of lamina propria (Figure 9-19). Hundreds of taste buds are located in the epithelium surrounding the entire base of each circumvallate, opposite the circular trough lined by the surrounding tongue surface tissue.

It is important to note that **von Ebner's salivary glands** are also present in the submucosa deep to the lamina propria of the circumvallate lingual papillae. These serous types of minor salivary glands have ducts that open into the trough, flushing the area near the taste pores so as to introduce new taste sensations from several sequential food molecules (see Chapter 11 for more discussion). Thus the function of the circumvallate is taste sensation.

Clinical Considerations with the Tongue

Two commonly found lesions are associated with the dorsal surface of the tongue and involve the lingual papillae. Neither lesion is serious, but both should be recorded on the patient's chart if such lesions are present. One of these tongue lesions is a **geographic tongue,** which appears as red and then paler pink to white patches on the body of the tongue. These patches change shape with time, resembling a geographic map (Figure 9-20). This lesion is found in all age groups and shows the sensitivity of the filiform lingual papillae to changes in their environment. These red and white surface patches of geographic tongue correspond to groups of filiform papillae undergoing changes from parakeratinized epithelium, which appears redder, to orthokeratinized epithelium, which appears whiter. This lesion is sometimes associated with soreness or slight burning on the surface of the tongue. No treatment is needed for geographic tongue, although dental personnel should reassure the patient and rule out any other more serious tongue lesion.

A less common change noted on the dorsal tongue surface is **black hairy tongue** (Figure 9-21). With this disturbance, normal shedding of epithelium of the filiform lingual papillae does not occur. As a result, a thick layer of dead cells and keratin builds up on the tongue surface, which becomes extrinsically stained by tobacco, medicines, or chromogenic (colored) oral bacteria. Some studies show that this condition might be an effect of fungal overgrowth, possibly as a result of high doses of antibiotics or radiation. Brushing the tongue is recommended in this case to promote tissue shedding and remove debris. Generally, brushing the dorsal surface of the tongue is important for overall good hygiene of the oral cavity and to reduce malodor, or halitosis. Studies show that microbial colonization on the tongue's surface is an important factor in the development of bad breath.

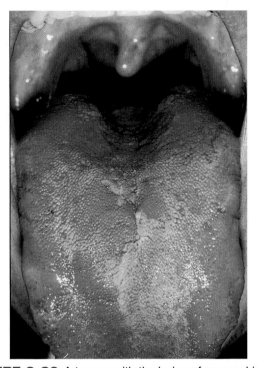

FIGURE 9-20 A tongue with the lesion of geographic tongue, showing the sensitivity of the filiform lingual papillae. Red and then paler pink to white patches appear on the body of the tongue.

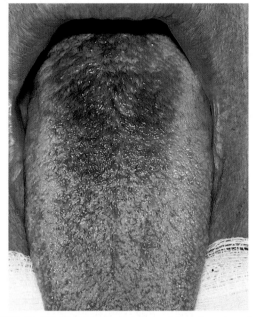

FIGURE 9-21 Black hairy tongue on the dorsal surface of the tongue, where normal shedding of epithelium of the filiform lingual papillae is lacking. This results in a thick layer of dead cells and keratin, which becomes stained.

PIGMENTATION OF THE ORAL MUCOSA

The oral mucosa can range in color from pink to reddish pink (see Chapter 1). The presence of **melanin pigmentation** in the epithelium may give rise to localized flat areas of the oral mucosa that range in color from brown to brownish black (Figure 9-22). This condition is distinct from the nevus or mole that is a benign tumor of melanin, which appears in the oral cavity usually as one small macule or papule.

Melanin is a pigment formed by melanocytes, which are derived from the neural crest cells. Melanocytes are clear cells that occupy a position in the basal layer of the stratified squamous epithelium between the dividing epithelial cells (Figure 9-23). The melanocytes have small cytoplasmic granules, or inclusions, called *melanosomes,* which store the melanin pigment. The melanocytes inject these melanosomes into the neighboring newly formed epithelial cells of the basal layer.

As the tissue ages, the injected cells migrate to the surface of the oral mucosa and appear clinically as a group of localized flat pigmented areas or macules. Because melanocytes are evenly distributed throughout the oral mucosa, clinical signs of pigmentation are based on the degree of melanin-producing activity of the melanocytes, which is controlled by genetic programming.

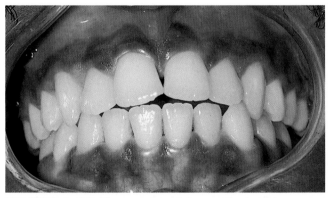

FIGURE 9-22 Pigmentation of the attached gingiva associated with the permanent dentition. It is most abundant at the base of the interdental gingiva. Because the melanocytes that form the melanin throughout the oral mucosa are evenly distributed, differences in pigmentation are based on the degree of melanin-producing activity of the melanocytes, which is controlled by genetic programming.

If pigmentation is present in the oral cavity, it appears most abundant at the base of the interdental gingiva associated with both dentitions. The pigmentation of both the oral mucosa and skin may increase with some endocrine diseases. Biopsy and histological study are recommended to rule out any malignancies if dramatic localized pigment changes are noted in the oral tissues.

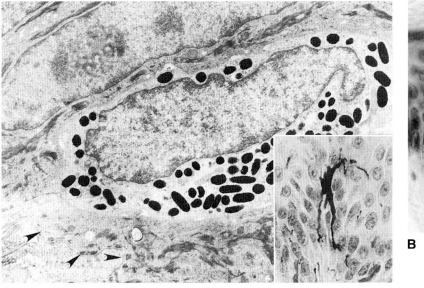

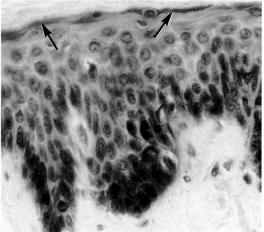

A

B

FIGURE 9-23 A: Electron micrograph of melanocyte in the basal layer of pigmented oral epithelium. The dense melanosomes are abundant. Arrowheads indicate the basal lamina. **Inset:** Photomicrograph of histological section showing a melanocyte. The cell appears dark because it has been stained histochemically to reveal the presence of melanin. **B:** Photomicrograph of the attached gingiva showing the pigmentation process within the oral mucosa. Note the granular layer (*arrows*) and the deposits of melanin, particularly in the basal layer. Melanin is a pigment formed by melanocytes, which are clear cells in the basal layer. Pigment is stored within these cells as melanosomes. The melanocytes inject these melanosomes into the neighboring cells. As the tissue ages, the injected cells migrate to the surface and appear clinically as a group as localized flat pigmented areas or macules. (A: From Nanci A. *Ten Cate's Oral Histology*, ed 6. Mosby, St. Louis, 2003. B: Courtesy of TS Leeson, Professor Emeritus, Cell Biology and Anatomy, Medicine and Oral Health, University of Alberta, Alberta, Canada.)

TABLE 9-6

Median Turnover Times for Oral Tissues*

Hard palate	24 days
Floor of mouth	20 days
Buccal and labial mucosa	14 days
Attached gingiva	10 days
Taste buds	10 days
Junctional epithelium (attached to tooth)	4–6 days

*Note that for comparison the turnover time for the skin is 27 days.

TURNOVER TIME, REPAIR, AND AGING OF THE ORAL MUCOSA

Overall, the **turnover time** for the oral mucosa is higher than for the skin (concept discussed in Chapter 8). Regional differences in the turnover times do, however, exist within the oral cavity (Table 9-6). The gingival epithelium that attaches to the tooth surface (junctional epithelium) has the highest turnover time, 4 to 6 days, of all the oral tissues (see Chapter 10). One of the lowest turnover times is for the hard palate, at 24 days. All other oral mucosal tissue turnover times fall between these two low and high rates,

thus between 4 and 24 days. Regional differences in the pattern of epithelial maturation or keratinization appear to be associated with different turnover times; nonkeratinized buccal mucosa turns over faster than keratinized attached gingiva, about 1.5 times faster.

Generally, the epithelial portion of any region of oral mucosa has a higher turnover time than cells of the lamina propria, although the turnover time of matrix, both fibers and intercellular substance, is fairly rapid. All tissues of the oral cavity have a higher turnover time than the skin, which has a turnover time of 27 days. Such differences noted in turnover times for oral mucosal tissues can have important implications for healing and rate of recovery time from damage.

The repair process of the oral mucosa is similar to that of the skin (see Chapter 8). After an injury to the oral mucosa, a moist clot from blood products forms in the area and the inflammatory response is triggered with its white blood cells. In the next days as tissue repair begins, the epithelial cells at the periphery of the injury will lose their desmosomal junctions and migrate to form a new epithelial surface layer beneath the clot. Thus the clot is highly important in repair of the epithelium and must be retained in the first days of repair because it acts as guide to form a new surface. Later, after the epithelial surface is repaired, the clot

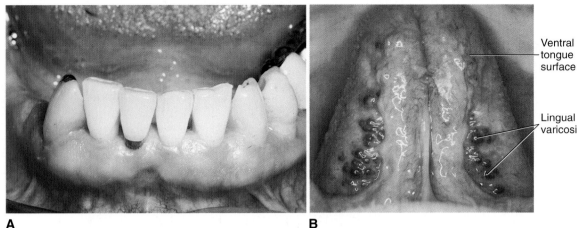

A   **B**

FIGURE 9-24 Various changes resulting from aging in the oral cavity. **A:** Loss of stippling of the attached gingiva. **B:** Lingual varicosities on the ventral surface of the tongue.

breaks down from enzymes because it is no longer needed.

At the same time, fibroblasts migrate to produce an immature connective tissue in the injured lamina propria deep to the clot and newly forming epithelial surface. This immature connective tissue is called **granulation tissue** and has fewer fibers and an increased amount of blood vessels. Granulation tissue appears as a soft, bright red tissue that bleeds easily. This tissue may become abundant and may actually interfere with the repair process. Surgical removal of excess granulation tissue may be necessary to allow for optimal repair, such as in a tooth extraction or certain periodontal surgical techniques.

This temporary granulation tissue is later replaced by firmer and paler scar tissue in the area. The replacement tissue is characterized by an increased amount of fibers and fewer blood vessels. The amount of scar tissue varies depending on the type and size of the wound, amount of granulation tissue, and movement of tissue after injury. The oral mucosa shows less scar tissue either clinically or histologically after repair than does the skin because fewer fibers are located in this area than in the skin when it undergoes a similar injury. The minimal scar tissue formation in oral mucosa after repair is similar to fetal tissue repair.

This difference in the amount of scar tissue formation in the skin and oral mucosa is useful both aesthetically and functionally when oral or periodontal surgery is performed. Researchers believe it may be linked to the different embryological origins of the fibroblasts from the two tissues. The skin fibroblasts are derived from the mesoderm, and the oral mucosal fibroblasts are derived from neural crest cells.

After the source of injury is removed, the repair of the oral mucosa generally follows times similar to its turnover time. Studies show that epithelial cells possess receptors for growth factors and also respond to chemical mediators of the inflammatory process. Further studies may show a way to speed repair and also prevent aging in the oral mucosa.

Aging of the oral mucosa mirrors some of the changes observed in the skin, lips, and mucosa of other areas of the body (Figure 9-24). As with those of the skin, it is also difficult to separate changes caused by aging in the oral mucosa from changes caused by chronic disease.

Aging of the oral mucosa is seen clinically as a reduction of stippling on the attached gingiva, an increase in Fordyce's spots in the labial and buccal mucosa, and enlargement of the lingual veins to form lingual varicosities on the ventral surface of the tongue. The number of lingual papillae, especially the foliate lingual papillae, and associated taste buds is also reduced. Many of the changes in the oral cavity may be due to changes in the salivary glands (see Chapter 11 for more discussion) that make the oral mucosa drier (xerostomia) and less protective, but these changes are not directly due to aging.

Histologically, the thickness and number of rete ridges in the epithelium diminish as the oral mucosa ages. Epithelial mitotic activity is reduced, as is the surface area of the epithelium. In addition, the degree of keratinization of the masticatory mucosa declines, especially in the attached gingiva. Cell division at the basal layer of the epithelium does not slow down, but recent studies show that the turnover times slow down for all tissues.

Exposure of the dental tissues from recession of attached gingiva in the aged population is argued to be more a sign of disease than of age (see Chapter 10). Also thought to be a sign of disease in the aged is creasing and then cracking at the labial commissures, which possibly results from a loss of vertical dimension of the dentition and jaws (see Chapters 14 and 20).

Histologically, changes also occur in the composition of the matrix of the lamina propria and in a less-defined division between the papillary and dense layers in older oral mucosa. Collagen fibers appear thickened and are arranged into dense bundles resembling those found in tendons or ligaments. Elastic fibers, if present in the lamina propria, appear changed even though more of them are present. This change in elastic fibers may explain the loss of resiliency found in aged oral mucosa.

The fibroblasts decrease in quantity, appear smaller, and are less active in older oral mucosa. The entire lamina propria has a slower collagen turnover time. Overall, with aging, the ability of the oral mucosa to repair itself is reduced and the length of the repair time is increased, just as turnover time is increased.

Clinical Considerations Concerning Oral Mucosa Turnover Time

Dental personnel must consider the shorter turnover time for oral tissues when diagnosing lesions of the oral mucosa. Should the lesion be traumatic, complete healing takes up to approximately 2 weeks, depending on the region involved, if the source of the injury is removed. Although possible sources of injury to the oral mucosa may be physical, chemical, or infectious, assumptions should never be made about the source of any lesion of the oral mucosa. Biopsy with histological study is the only way actually to diagnose any lesion.

Thus a delay of approximately 2 weeks to allow a lesion to undergo healing before obtaining a referral does not adversely affect a patient's health. However, a longer delay (e.g., until the next recall visit) before the lesion is checked is not in the best interests of a patient because malignant changes do not heal but grow in size and may metastasize. A larger lesion with metastasis gives the patient a poorer prognosis if the lesion is later determined to be malignant after histological study.

Turnover times have implications during the treatment of cancer by surgical, chemical, and radiological means because these methods can damage the oral mucosal tissues as they halt the cancerous growth. Healing varies according to the turnover times of the tissue. Thus the buccal mucosa heals faster than the hard palate when subjected to cancer therapy methods.

With the increasing age of the patient base, dental professionals must consider the associated effects of aging on the oral mucosa during dental treatment. Age-associated changes such as lingual varicosities and loss of stippling should be distinguished from conditions resulting from oral or systemic disease.

In the future, many changes associated with aging may be prevented. With present knowledge, gingival recession might be prevented by correct tooth-brushing techniques, placement of a protective guard against occlusal forces, or institution of crown-lengthening procedures. Other changes, such as a drier mouth and loss of resiliency, should be considered and complications prevented when treatment is performed on older patients. (See Chapter 11 for a discussion of xerostomia, or dry mouth.)

CHAPTER 10

Gingival and Dentogingival Junctional Tissues

■ ■ ■

This chapter discusses the following topics:

- Gingival tissues
  - Clinical appearance of gingival tissues
  - Histological features of gingival tissues
- Dentogingival junctional tissues
  - Histological features of dentogingival junctional tissues
- Development of dentogingival junctional tissues
- Turnover time in dentogingival junctional tissues

■ ■ ■

After studying this chapter, the reader should be able to:

1. Define and pronounce the key terms in this chapter.
2. List and describe each of the types of gingival tissues.
3. Describe the histological features of the different types of gingival tissues.
4. Describe the composition and development of the dentogingival junctional tissues.
5. Discuss turnover of the dentogingival junction tissues.
6. Integrate the knowledge of the histology of the gingival and dentogingival junctional tissues with the related pathology that may occur.

■ ■ ■

Key Terms

Basal lamina, external, internal
Col (kohl)
Dentogingival junction, junctional tissues (den-to-jin-ji-val)
Epithelial attachment
Free gingival crest, groove
Gingiva: attached, interdental, marginal

Gingival fluid, hyperplasia (hi-per-**play**-ze-ah), recession (re-**sesh**-un), sulcus
Gingivitis (jin-ji-vie-tis)
Junctional epithelium (jungk-shun-al)
Lamina propria (lam-i-nah pro-pree-ah)

Masticatory mucosa (mass-ti-**ka**-tor-ee)
Melanin pigmentation (mel-a-nin)
Periodontal pocket
Periodontitis (pare-e-oh-*don*-tie-tis)
Sulcular epithelium (sul-ku-lar)

GINGIVAL TISSUES

Surrounding the maxillary and mandibular teeth in the alveoli and covering the alveolar processes is the **gingiva** (Figure 10-1). Different types of gingiva are present in the oral cavity. The gingiva that tightly adheres to the bone around the roots of the teeth is the **attached gingiva.** The gingiva between adjacent teeth is an extension of attached gingiva and is called the **interdental gingiva,** or interdental papilla.

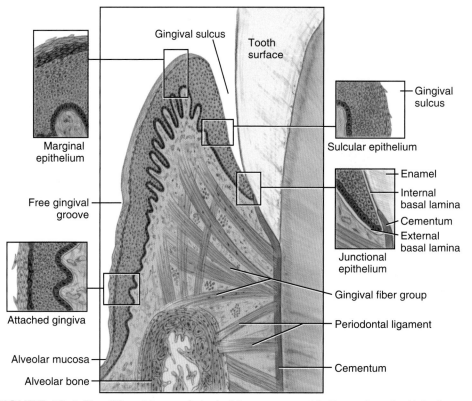

FIGURE 10-1 The different types of gingival tissues present in the oral cavity. Note the marginal gingival and attached gingiva as well as the sulcular epithelium and junctional epithelium.

At the gingival margin of each tooth is the free gingiva, or **marginal gingiva,** which is continuous with the attached gingiva. The gingiva that faces the tooth, the dentogingival junctional tissues, is discussed later.

Apical to the contact area, the interdental gingiva assumes a nonvisible concave form between the facial and lingual gingival surfaces, called the **col.** The col varies in depth and width, depending on the expanse of the contacting tooth surfaces. The epithelium covering the col consists of the marginal gingiva of the adjacent teeth, except that it is nonkeratinized. The col is mainly present in the broad interdental gingiva of the posterior teeth and generally is not in those interproximal tissues associated with anterior teeth. In the absence of contact between adjacent teeth, the attached gingiva extends uninterrupted from the facial to the lingual aspect. The col may be important in the formation of periodontal disease but is seen clinically only when posterior teeth are extracted.

The gingival tissues are the most important tissues of the orofacial region for dental professionals to know and understand. All the periodontal therapy performed, and oral hygiene instruction given, are for the purpose of creating a healthy environment for these gingival tissues. Even with restorative care, the impact on the gingival tissues must be considered. When healthy, these tissues present an effective barrier to the

barrage of periodontal insults. Dental professionals also must understand the histology of the healthy, normal gingival tissues. This helps in understanding the pathological changes that occur during the disease states involving the gingival tissues.

When these gingival tissues are not healthy, they provide a gateway for periodontal disease to advance into the deeper tissues of the periodontium, leading to a poor prognosis for long-term retention of the teeth. Thus both the type of periodontal therapy and instructions given to patients by dental professionals and restorative care are based on the clinical conditions of these tissues. Overall, the clinical appearance of the tissues reflects their underlying histology, both in health and disease.

Clinical Appearance of Gingival Tissues

Both the attached gingiva and the marginal gingiva are easily seen in the oral cavity, whether the gingival tissues are healthy or not. The gingival margin, or **free gingival crest,** at the most superficial portion of the marginal gingiva, is also easily seen clinically, and its location should be recorded on a patient's chart.

The attached gingiva is a **masticatory mucosa** (see Chapter 9). Healthy attached gingiva is pink in color, with some areas of **melanin pigmentation** possible.

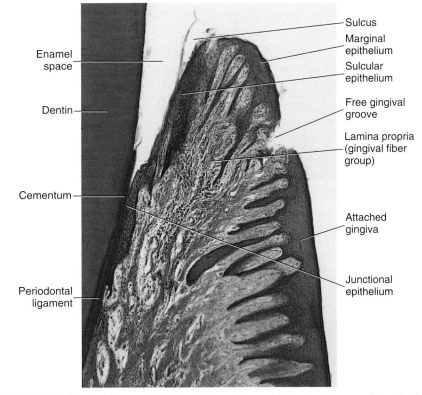

Enamel space

Dentin

Cementum

Periodontal ligament

Sulcus

Marginal epithelium

Sulcular epithelium

Free gingival groove

Lamina propria (gingival fiber group)

Attached gingiva

Junctional epithelium

FIGURE 10-2 Photomicrograph of the different types of gingival tissues. Deep to the epithelium is the underlying lamina propria, which is continuous with the periodontal ligament, which is adjacent to the cementum on the tooth surface. (Courtesy of Dr. James McIntosh, PhD, Department of Biomedical Sciences, Baylor College of Dentistry, Dallas, TX.)

The tissue when dried is dull, firm, and immobile, with varying amounts of stippling. The width of the attached gingiva varies according to its location. However, certain levels of attached gingiva may be necessary for the stability of the underlying root of the tooth.

The interdental papillae fill in the area between the teeth up to their contact areas to prevent food impaction. The interdental papillae assume a conical shape for the anterior teeth and a blunted shape buccolingually for the posterior teeth.

A **free gingival groove** separates the attached gingiva from the marginal gingiva. This is a slight depression on the gingiva corresponding to the depth of the gingivalsulcus. This groove varies in depth according to the area of the oral cavity; the groove is very prominent on the mandibular anterior and premolar regions.

The marginal gingiva varies in width from 0.5 to 2.0 mm from the free gingival crest to the attached gingiva. The marginal gingiva follows the scalloped pattern established by the contour of the cementoenamel junction of the teeth. The marginal gingiva has a more translucent appearance than the attached gingiva yet has a similar clinical appearance, including pinkness, dullness, and firmness. In contrast, the marginal gingiva lacks the presence of stippling, and the tissue is mobile or free from the underlying tooth

surface, as can be demonstrated with a periodontal probe.

Histological Features of Gingival Tissues

The attached gingival and the marginal gingival tissues have some similar histological features, yet each has features specific to the tissue (Figure 10-2). The attached gingival tissue has a thick layer of mainly parakeratinized epithelium, which obscures its extensive vascular supply in the **lamina propria,** making the tissue pinkish (see Chapter 9). The lamina propria also has tall, narrow papillae, giving the tissue its varying amounts of stippling. The interface between the epithelium and lamina propria is highly interdigitated. The lamina propria is directly attached to the underlying jawbones, making the attached gingival firm and immobile, and thus serves as a mucoperiosteum.

Similar to the attached gingiva, the marginal gingiva has a surface layer of keratinized stratified squamous epithelium. The associated lamina propria also has tall, narrow papillae, but this lamina propria is continuous with the lamina propria of the gingival tissues that face the tooth. Unlike the attached gingiva, the marginal gingiva is not attached to the underlying jawbones, making this tissue firm but mobile.

Clinical Considerations for Gingival Tissues

With active periodontal disease, the marginal and attached gingival tissues can become enlarged, especially the interdental papillae (Figure 10-3). This growth results from edema occurring in the lamina propria of these tissues cauased by the inflammatory response. Tissue fluid from the lamina propria's capillaries flows out to flush the area of its injurious agents. The gingival tissues can also become redder with active periodontal disease because hyperemia, or increased blood flow, occurs in the capillaries of the lamina propria. The gingival tissues may also lose their stippling because the inflammatory edema reduces the strong attachment between the epithelium and lamina propria.

The location of the free gingival crest can also change with periodontal disease (Figure 10-4). As the tissues become inflamed, the gingival margin can become higher or more occlusal. **Gingival recession**, with its lower, or more apical, gingival margin, can also result from periodontal disease, tooth position, abrasion by incorrect toothbrushing methods, and possibly strong frenal attachments, abfraction from occlusal stresses such as parafunctional habits, and changes caused by the aging process. All changes in these gingival tissues should be recorded in a patient's chart. The width of the attached gingival may also decrease with periodontal disease and should be recorded as well.

Within the gingival tissues, **gingival hyperplasia** can affect both the epithelium and lamina propria. Gingival hyperplasia is overgrowth of the interproximal gingival resulting from the intake of certain drugs for seizure control (phenytoin sodium), certain antibiotics, and specific heart medications (Figure 10-5). According to some theories, these drugs increase the populations or output of certain types of fibroblasts. The amount of gingival overgrowth is related to the drug dose and amount of inflammation induced by bacterial plaque biofilm. Gingival overgrowth can interfere with proper oral hygiene and thus may need to be periodically removed by surgery.

The gingival contours form a silhouette around the cervical section of a tooth, a fact that should be acknowledged when considering smile design. The cervical peak of the gingival contour is referred to as the *gingival apex of the contour*. The apex of maxillary central incisors and canines is distal to a line drawn through the midline or long axis of the tooth. The maxillary lateral incisor apex is equal to the midline or long axis of the tooth. The gingival apex of a lateral incisor is also 1 mm short of the central incisor and canine's apex heights. The canine and central incisor gingival apex are equal in height.

The gingival contour is also related to its position in regard to the lip line. Some cases of "gummy smile," or an excessive display of gingiva, are not ideal, such as when the maxillary central incisors and canines barely touch the lip line or border of the upper lip. The lateral incisor may touch the lip line or be 1- to 2-mm coronal to the lip line, revealing some gingiva. In most cases, orthodontics, in conjunction with periodontal surgery, can alter the gingival contours for a more pleasing smile.

Note that the gingival fiber group is found in the lamina propria of the marginal gingiva (see Chapter 14 for more discussion). Some histologists consider the gingival fiber group part of the periodontal ligament, but this fiber group supports only the gingival tissues and not the tooth in relation to the jaws. The lamina propria of the marginal gingiva is also continuous with the adjacent connective tissue, which includes the lamina propria of the attached gingival, as well as the periodontal ligament.

DENTOGINGIVAL JUNCTIONAL TISSUES

The **dentogingival junction** is the junction between the tooth surface and the gingival tissues. Together the sulcular epithelium and junctional epithelium form the **dentogingival junctional tissues.** Both the sulcular epithelium and junctional epithelium are difficult to see in clinical examination of healthy gingival tissues.

The crevicular epithelium, or **sulcular epithelium,** stands away from the tooth, creating a **gingival sulcus,** or space that is filled with **gingival fluid** or crevicular fluid (see Figure 10-1). The depth of the healthy gingival sulcus varies from 0.5 to 3 mm, with an average of 1.8 mm. A normal gingival fluid flow rate is fairly slow and has been calculated at 1 to 2 microliters per tooth

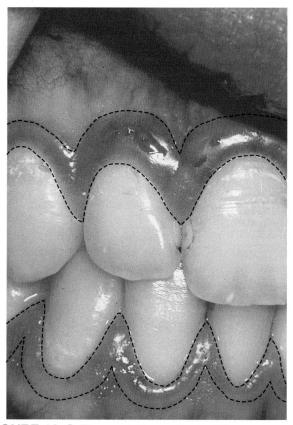

FIGURE 10-3 The marginal and attached tissues undergoing active periodontal disease (*dashed lines*) with its tissue enlargement.

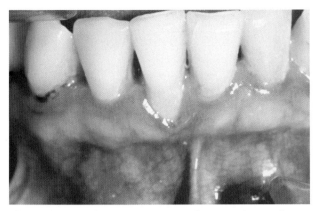

FIGURE 10-4 Gingival recession of an anterior tooth as a result of unknown sources.

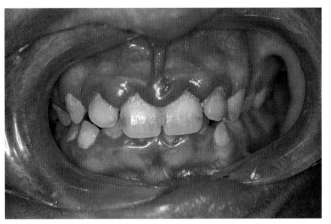

FIGURE 10-5 Gingival hyperplasia caused by the intake of a certain drug and poor oral hygiene.

per hour. Thus the amount of gingival fluid in the healthy state is considered minimal.

The gingival fluid seeps between the epithelial cells and into the gingival sulcus. It allows the components of the blood to reach the tooth surface through the junctional epithelium from the blood vessels of the adjacent lamina propria. The gingival fluid contains both the immunological components and cells of the blood, although in lower amounts and in different proportions.

The gingival fluid includes WBCs, especially PMNs, as well as IgG and IgM and serum IgA, which have a role in the specific defense mechanism against disease. Thus any immunological reactions in the blood are directly relevant to those found in the gingival fluid and may affect the health of the tooth and associated gingival tissues. Gingival fluid passes from the gingival sulcus into the oral cavity, where it mixes with saliva.

A deeper extension of the sulcular epithelium is the **junctional epithelium (JE).** The JE lines the floor of the gingival sulcus and is attached to the tooth surface. The junctional epithelium is attached to the tooth surface by way of an **epithelial attachment (EA).** The attachment of the JE to the tooth surface can occur on enamel, cementum, or dentin. The position of the EA on the tooth surface is initially on the cervical half of the anatomical crown when the tooth first becomes functional after eruption (discussed later).

The probing depth of the gingival sulcus is measured by a calibrated periodontal probe. In a healthy-case scenario, the probe is gently inserted, slides by the sulcular epithelium, and is stopped by the EA. However, the probing depth of the gingival sulcus may be considerably different from the true histological sulcus depth. Probing measurements are subject to variations depending on the operator's insertion pressure, the accuracy of the readings, and the ability of the probe tip to penetrate tissues that are ulcerated or inflamed.

Histological Features of Dentogingival Junctional Tissues

Histologically, the sulcular epithelium consists of stratified squamous epithelium similar to the epithelium of the outer marginal gingival and attached gingiva (Figure 10-6). In contrast, the sulcular epithelium is of a nonkeratinized type, with its cells tightly packed, unlike the keratinized marginal gingival and attached gingiva. In addition, the interface between the sulcular epithelium and the lamina propria that it shares with these outer gingival tissues is relatively smooth compared with the other's strongly interdigitated interface.

The deeper interface between the JE and the underlying lamina propria is also relatively smooth, without rete ridges or connective tissue papillae (Figures 10-7 and 10-8). The JE cells are loosely packed, with fewer desmosomal junctions between cells, as compared with other gingival tissues. The number of intercellular spaces between the epithelial cells of the JE is also more than other gingival tissues. Overall, the JE is more permeable than other gingival tissues.

This increased permeability allows for emigration of large numbers of mobile WBCs from the blood vessels in the deeper lamina propria into the JE, even in healthy tissues. This mainly involves the PMNs, with those cells actively undergoing phagocytosis. The PMNs also enter the gingival fluid in the gingival sulcus in healthy mouths. The presence of these WBCs may keep the tissue healthy by protecting it from microorganisms within the bacterial plaque biofilm and associated toxins.

The JE is also thinner than the sulcular epithelium, ranging coronally from 15 to 30 cells thick at the floor of the gingival sulcus and tapering to a final thickness of 3 to 4 cells at its apical portion. The superficial, or suprabasal, cells of the JE serve as part of the EA of the gingival to the tooth surface.

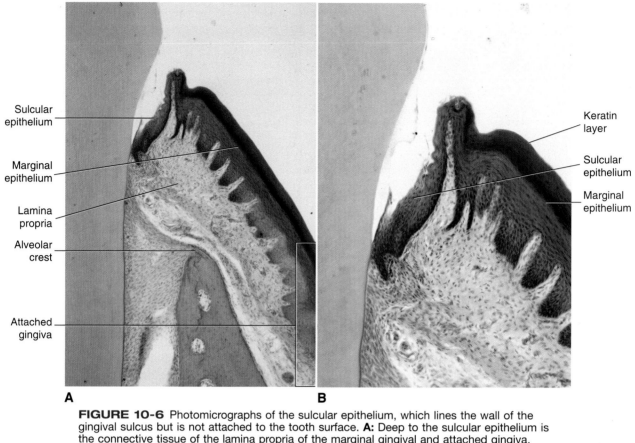

Sulcular epithelium

Marginal epithelium

Lamina propria

Alveolar crest

Attached gingiva

Keratin layer

Sulcular epithelium

Marginal epithelium

A   **B**

FIGURE 10-6 Photomicrographs of the sulcular epithelium, which lines the wall of the gingival sulcus but is not attached to the tooth surface. **A:** Deep to the sulcular epithelium is the connective tissue of the lamina propria of the marginal gingival and attached gingiva. Note that deeper still is the alveolar crest of the alveolar bone. **B:** Close-up view of the sulcular epithelium. The sulcular epithelium is nonkeratinizeds, and the interface between it and the lamina propria that it shares with the keratinized marginal gingival and attached gingiva is relatively smooth compared with the other's strongly interdigitated interface. (Courtesy of Dr. James McIntosh, PhD, Department of Biomedical Sciences, Baylor College of Dentistry, Dallas, TX.)

These superficial, or suprabasal, epithelial cells of the JE provide the hemidesmosomes and an **internal basal lamina** that create the EA because this is a cell-to-noncellular type of intercellular junction (see Chapter 7 for a discussion of hemidesmosomes and Chapter 8 for a discussion of basal lamina). The structure of the EA is similar to that of the junction between the epithelium and subadjacent connective tissue. The internal basal lamina consists of a lamina lucida and lamina densa (Figures 10-8 and 10-9).

This internal basal lamina of the EA is continuous with the **external basal lamina** between the junctional epithelium and the lamina propria at the apical extent of the JE. The EA is very strong in a healthy state, acting as a type of seal between the soft gingival tissues and the hard tooth surface.

The deepest layer of the JE, or basal layer, undergoes constant and rapid cell division, including mitosis. This process allows a constant coronal migration as the cells die and are shed into the gingival

sulcus. The few layers present in the JE—from its basal layer to the surprabasal, or superficial, layer—does not show change in cellular appearance related to maturation, unlike other gingival tissues. They do not mature into a granular layer or intermediate layer. Thus the JE does not mature like keratinized tissue, which fills its matured superficial cells with keratin. Nor does JE mature like nonkeratinized tissue, which enlarges its cells as they mature and migrate superficially.

The JE cells have many organelles in their cytoplasm, rough endoplasmic reticulum, Golgi complex, and mitochondria, indicating a high metabolic activity. However, the JE cells remain immature or undifferentiated until they die and are shed or lost in the gingival sulcus. The key to this state of cellular immaturity of the JE may be found in future studies of the adjoining lamina propria; this lamina propria appears to be functionally different from the connective tissues underlying the other types of oral epithelium that do mature.

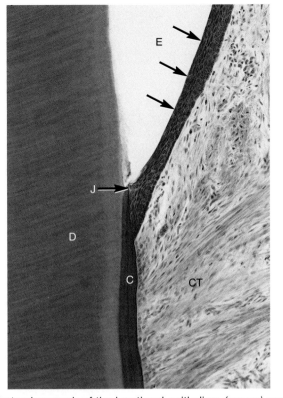

FIGURE 10-7 Photomicrograph of the junctional epithelium *(arrows)* overlying the enamel *(E)*, which is a space created by fixation. Note the cementoenamel junction *(J)* and the cementum *(C)* and dentin *(D)* of the tooth. Deep to the junctional epithelium is the connective tissue *(CT)* of the periodontal ligament. Note also that this is an initial junctional epithelium before the eruption of the tooth into the oral cavity. (Courtesy of Dr. James McIntosh, PhD, Department of Biomedical Sciences, Baylor College of Dentistry, Dallas, TX.)

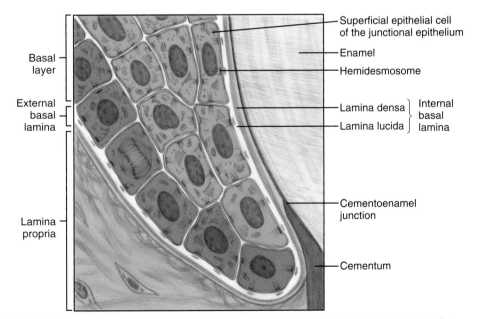

FIGURE 10-8 The epithelial attachment that attaches the junctional epithelium to the tooth surface.

Development of Dentogingival Junctional Tissues

Before the eruption of the tooth and after enamel maturation, the ameloblasts secrete a basal lamina on the surface that serves as a portion of the primary EA. As the tooth actively erupts, the coronal portion of the fused reduced enamel epithelium and surrounding epithelial tissues peels back off the crown (see Chapter 6). The ameloblasts also develop hemidesmosomes for the primary EA and become firmly attached to the enamel surface (see Figure 10-7).

However, the cervical portion of the fused tissue remains attached to the neck of the tooth by the primary EA. This fused tissue that remains near the cementoenamel junction after the tooth erupts serves as the initial JE of the tooth, creating the first tissue attached to the tooth surface.

This tissue is later replaced by a definitive JE as the root is formed (see Figures 10-8 and 10-9). The definitive JE is formed from all the cell types present in the reduced enamel epithelium as a result of mitosis of the cells, except for the ameloblasts, which are forever lost. This proliferating tissue now can provide both the basal lamina and hemidesmosomes for the secondary EA to the tooth surface. After eruption of the tooth, 3 or 4 years may pass before the initial tissue becomes the definitive JE.

Although controversial, many studies show that the ameloblasts undergo cellular changes that make them indistinguishable from the other newly formed JE cells. These transformed ameloblasts are eventually replaced by these new cells.

Clinical Considerations for Junctional Epithelium

The increased permeability of the JE that allows emigration of the PMN type of white blood cell also allows microorganism from the bacterial plaque biofilm and associated toxins to enter this tissue from the deeper lamina propria (Figure 10-10). When these damaging agents can enter the JE, the tissue undergoes the initial signs of active periodontal disease with **gingivitis**. These signs include acute inflammation and epithelial ulceration or tissue thinning and also an increased number of WBCs. This ulceration of the JE allows even more damaging agents to enter the even deeper periodontium, advancing the disease. The interface between the dentogingival junctional tissues and the lamina propria with inflammation shows the formation of rete pegs and connective tissue papillae. The lamina propria also shows breakdown of the collagen fibers as the disease advances.

Bleeding after gentle probing also occurs at this time and is due to the periodontal probe damaging the lamina propria's increased blood vessels, which are close to the surface because of the ulceration of the JE (Figure 10-11). Bleeding can also occur with flossing. The presence of bleeding is one of the first signs of active periodontal disease in uncomplicated cases and should be recorded in a patient's chart. However, in patients who smoke, the tissues rarely bleed because of unknown factors not related to bacterial plaque biofilm and calculus formation.

Periodontal inflammation is also accompanied by an increase in the amount of gingival fluid, either of a serous (clear) or suppurative nature, distending the tissue further. Thus relatively large amounts of fluid pass through the more permeable epithelial wall. This gingival fluid is clinically noted only when it involves whiter suppuration, or pus, resulting from the presence of cellular debris and extensive populations of PMNs. Current clinical practice does not allow measurement of these increased fluid levels. In the future, however, this measurement may be possible chairside; it is now used in research to show the level of activity of the disease. Gingival fluid also supplies the minerals for subgingival calculus formation.

When the deeper tissues of the periodontium are affected by periodontal disease, further damage can occur and the disease can become chronic in nature; this condition is considered to be **periodontitis**. With the advancement of periodontal disease, the prognosis for retention of the tooth becomes risky, then guarded, as alveolar bone is lost and the periodontal ligament become increasingly disorganized. As the disease progresses, exposed furcations (areas between the roots) are noted around the posterior teeth (see Chapter 17) and the teeth become mobile.

True apical migration of the EA also occurs with advanced periodontal disease, causing a deeper gingival sulcus. A gingival sulcus that is deeper than 3 mm is considered a **periodontal pocket**. The depth of the periodontal pockets must be recorded in a patient's chart for proper monitoring of the progress of the periodontal disease. Unlike in clinically healthy situations, portions of the sulcular epithelium can sometimes be seen in periodontally involved gingival tissues if air is blown into the periodontal pocket, exposing the newly denuded roots of the tooth.

A periodontal pocket can become an infected space and result in an abscess formation with a papule on the gingival surface. Incision and drainage of the abscess may be necessary as well as systemic antibiotics. Placement of local antimicrobial delivery systems within the periodontal pocket to reduce localized infections is now becoming a reality in private practice. Endoscopic photographic evaluation is also becoming available in practice. The dental endoscope facilitates subgingival visual examination without reliance on tactile sense and without surgical flap access. The clinician views a video monitor that displays the magnified image transmitted by a fiberoptic bundle attached to a subgingival instrument. This direct, real-time visualization of the hard and soft tissues within the gingival pocket region may aid the clinician in diagnosis and therapy of periodontal disease. Techniques for identification and interpretation of the hard and soft tissue images as well as the location of root deposits and caries are being developed.

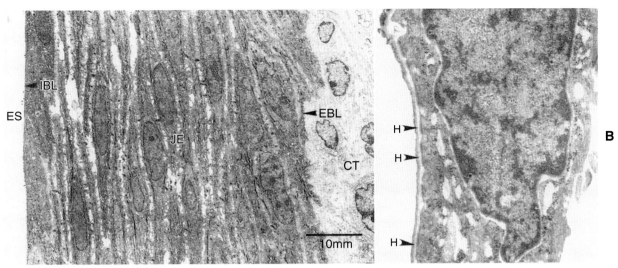

FIGURE 10-9 Electron micrographs of junctional epithelium *(JE)* and epithelial attachment. **A:** Shows the attachment of the JE to the enamel surface at the internal basal lamina *(IBL)* and to the connective tissue *(CT)* of the lamina propria by the external basal lamina *(EBL)*. The lack of differentiation of the epithelium and the wide intercellular spaces are notable. *ES,* Enamel space. **B:** Structure of the attachment of a single JE cell to the enamel surface by way of the internal basal lamina. Hemidesmosomes *(H)* are evident at the surface of the cell. (**A** and **B:** From Nanci A. *Ten Cate's Oral Histology*, ed 6. Mosby, St. Louis, 2003.).

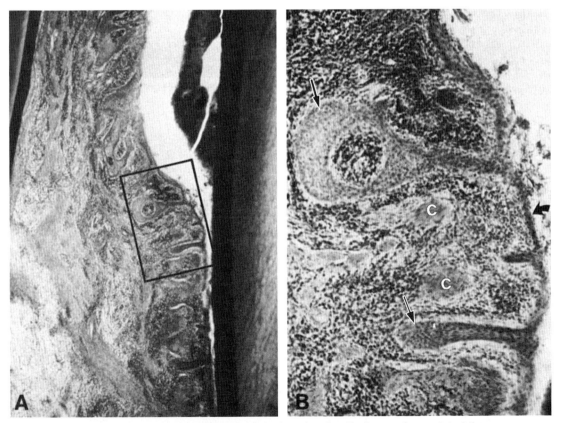

FIGURE 10-10 A: Photomicrograph of the junctional epithelium and associated tissues with the advancement of periodontal disease. This area acts as a gateway to periodontal toxins because of the increased intercellular spaces and reduced numbers of desmosomes. **B:** Higher magnification of the area within the rectangle in **A.** Note the ulceration of junctional epithelium *(curved arrow),* increased numbers of blood vessels in the lamina propria, and formation of rete pegs and connective tissue papillae *(straight arrows)* at the interface between the dentogingival junctional tissues and the lamina propria. Note also the breakdown of the collagen fibers *(C)* of the lamina propria, a result of periodontal disease. (From Newman MG, Takei HH, Carranza FA. *Clinical Periodontology*, ed 9. WB Saunders, Philadelphia, 2002.)

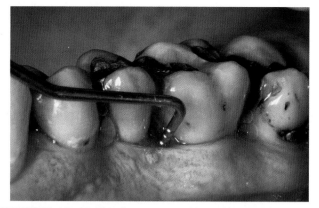

FIGURE 10-11 Bleeding upon probing of a periodontal pocket. This bleeding is due to increased blood vessels in the lamina propria. The blood vessels are close to the surface because of ulceration of the junctional epithelium caused by periodontal inflammation.

Turnover Time of the Dentogingival Junctional Tissues

Both the sulcular epithelium, outer marginal epithelium, and attached epithelium turnover process occurs in a manner similar to that of the epithelium of the attached gingiva; the basal cells migrate superficially after cell division, undergo maturation, and take the place of the superficial cells, which are shed or lost in the oral cavity as they die.

In JE, even though it does not undergo cellular maturation, its basal cells migrate superficially upon dividing and continuously replace the dying suprabasal or superficial cells that are desquamated into the gingival sulcus. The migratory route of the cells, as turnover takes place in the JE, is in a coronal direction, parallel to the tooth surface. Such cells continuously dissolve and reestablish their hemidesmosomal attachments on the tooth surface. The JE has the highest turnover time in the entire oral cavity, which is 4 to 6 days (see comparison chart of turnover times in Chapter 9).

Clinical Considerations with Gingival Tissue Turnover Time

Given that the turnover time of the JE is approximately 1 week, evaluation of periodontal therapy must occur after this time to allow full healing of the area. Thus scheduling of patients should follow this biological temporal factor of turnover time. In addition, patients must have the information and skills necessary to enact a change in their oral hygiene methods to allow for optimal healing during this period.

Finally, if methods could be devised for allowing a more coronal reattachment of the JE and total periodontal regeneration in a patient with periodontal tissue damage, changes would also occur in the way periodontal treatment is performed and oral hygiene instructions are given. Thus practicing dental professionals must keep up with changes in this area of information to remain current in periodontal treatment and oral hygiene instructions.

CHAPTER 11

Head and Neck Structures

This chapter discusses the following topics:

- Head and neck structures
- Glands
  - Salivary glands
  - Thyroid gland
- Lymphatics
  - Lymph nodes
  - Intraoral tonsillar tissue
- Nasal cavity
  - Histology of the mucosa of the nasal cavity
- Paranasal sinuses
  - Histology of the mucosa of the paranasal sinuses
  - Development of the paranasal sinuses

After studying this chapter, the reader should be able to:

1. Define and pronounce the key terms in this chapter.
2. Describe the location of each head and neck structure.
3. Discuss the histological features and embryological development of each head and neck structure.
4. Integrate the knowledge of the histology of head and neck structures with the related pathology that may occur.

Key Terms

Acinus (plural, acini) (as-i-nus, as-i-ny): serous, mucoserous, mucous
Afferent vessels (af-er-int)
Capsule (kap-sule)
Colloid (kol-oid)
Duct: excretory (ex-kreh-tor-ee), intercalated (in-turk-ah-lay-ted), parotid, striated (stri-ate-ed), sublingual, submandibular
Efferent vessel (ef-er-ent)
Erectile tissue (e-rek-tile)
Follicles (fol-i-kls)
Foramen cecum (for-ay-men se-kum)
Germinal center (jurm-i-nil)

Gland: exocrine (ek-sah-krin), endocrine (en-dah-krin)
Goblet cells
Goiter (goy-ter)
Hilus (hi-lus)
Lobes
Lobules (lob-ules)
Lumen (loo-men)
Lymph (limf), nodes
Lymphadenopathy (lim-fad-uh-nop-ah-thee)
Lymphatic ducts, nodules (nah-jools), vessels
Lymphatics (lim-fat-iks)
Mucous cells (mu-kis)
Mucocele (mu-kah-sele)

Myoepithelial cells (my-oh-epee-thee-lee-al)
Nasal cavity (nay-zil kav-it-ee), conchae (kong-kay), septum
Naris (plural, nares) (nay-ris, nay-rees)
Nicotinic stomatitis (nik-ah-tin-ik sto-mah-ti-tis)
Paranasal sinuses (pare-ah-na-zil sy-nuses)
Parathyroid glands (par-ah-thy-roid)
Parotid papilla
Ranula (ran-u-lah)
Respiratory mucosa
Saliva (sah-li-vah)

HEAD AND NECK STRUCTURES

Dental professionals must have a sound understanding of the histology and development not only of the oral mucosa, gingiva, and dentogingival junctional tissues but also of the associated head and neck structures. The clinical functioning of the head and neck structures is related to the underlying histology. In addition, many of the pathological lesions that are encountered in the oral cavity can be associated with changes in these associated structures of the head and neck and thus are reflected in changes in their underlying histology. The head and neck structures to be discussed include the salivary glands, thyroid gland, lymphatics, nasal cavity, and paranasal sinuses.

GLANDS

The glands to be discussed include the salivary glands and thyroid gland. Dental professionals must be able to locate and identify these glands. This information helps dental professionals determine if the glands are involved in a disease process and the extent of that involvement.

A **gland** is a structure that produces a chemical secretion necessary for normal body functioning. An **exocrine gland** is a gland having a duct associated with it. A **duct** is a passageway that allows the glandular secretion to be emptied directly into the location where the secretion is to be used. An **endocrine gland** is a ductless gland with its secretions conveyed directly into the blood and then carried to some distant location to be used. Motor nerves associated with both types of glands help regulate the flow of the secretion. Sensory nerves are also present in the gland.

Salivary Glands

The **salivary glands** produce **saliva**. Saliva contains minerals, electrolytes, buffers, enzymes, immunoglobulins (secretory IgA), and metabolic wastes. The secretion by these glands is controlled by the autonomic nervous system. Saliva lubricates and cleanses the oral mucosa, protecting it from dryness and potential car-

cinogens. This secretory product also helps in digestion of food by enzymatic activity. Additionally, saliva serves as a buffer protecting the oral mucosa against acids from food and bacterial plaque biofilm. Saliva is also involved in antibacterial activity. Finally, saliva helps maintain tooth integrity because it is involved in remineralization of the tooth surface. However, because it contributes to the formation of the pellicle on the tooth and mucosal surfaces, saliva is also involved in the first step in bacterial plaque biofilm formation. Saliva also supplies the minerals for supragingival calculus formation.

Salivary glands are classified as either major or minor, depending on their size, but both types have similar histological features. Both the major and minor salivary glands are exocrine glands and thus have associated ducts that help convey the saliva directly into the oral cavity, where it is used.

HISTOLOGY OF SALIVARY GLANDS

Both major and minor salivary glands are composed of both epithelium and connective tissue (Figure 11-1). Epithelial cells both line the duct system and produce the saliva. Connective tissue surrounds the epithelium, protecting and supporting the gland. The connective tissue of the gland is divided into the **capsule**, which surrounds the outer portion of the entire gland, and the septa. Each **septum** (plural, **septa**) helps divide the inner portion of the gland into the larger **lobes** and smaller **lobules**. Both the capsule and septa carry nerves and blood vessels that serve the gland.

SECRETORY CELLS AND ACINI

Epithelial cells that produce the saliva are called **secretory cells** (Figure 11-2). The two types of secretory cells are classified as either mucous or serous cells, depending on the type of secretion produced. **Mucous cells** have a cloudier-looking cytoplasm and produce mucous secretory product. In contrast, **serous cells** have a clear cytoplasm and produce serous secretory product. A combination of secretory cells present in the gland can produce a mixed secretory product. In some glands, one type of cell predominates so that the product is either more mucous or more serous.

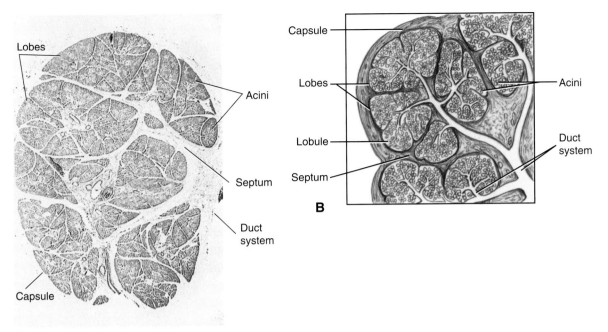

FIGURE 11-1 The composition of a salivary gland. **A:** Micrograph of salivary glands. **B:** Diagramic representation. (**A** from Nanci A. *Ten Cate's Oral Histology*, ed 6. Mosby, St. Louis, 2003.)

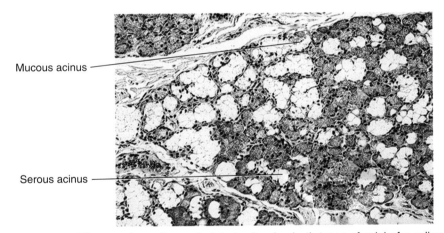

FIGURE 11-2 Microscopic sections of a lobule showing both types of acini of a salivary gland: mucous acinus and serous acinus. (From Nanci A. *Ten Cate's Oral Histology*, ed 6. Mosby, St. Louis, 2003.)

Secretory cells are found in a group, or **acinus** (plural, **acini**), which resembles a cluster of grapes. Each acinus is located at the terminal portion of the gland connected to the ductal system, with many acini within each lobule of the gland. Each acinus consists of a single layer of cuboidal epithelial cells surrounding a **lumen,** a central opening where the saliva is deposited after being produced by the secretory cells.

The three forms of acini are classified in terms of the type of epithelial cell present and the secretory product being produced. The major and minor salivary glands have different types of acini (Table 11-1). The different types of acini are often difficult to classify on histological sections of the glands.

Serous acini are composed of serous cells producing serous secretory product and have a narrow lumen (Figure 11-3). In contrast, **mucous acini** are composed of mucous cells producing mucous secretory product, and their lumen is wider. **Mucoserous acini** have both a group of mucous cells surrounding the lumen and a

TABLE 11-1

Comparison of Major Salivary Glands

	Parotid	Submandibular	Sublingual
Size	Largest, encapsulated	Intermediate, encapsulated	Smallest, no capsule
Location	Behind mandibular ramus, anterior and inferior to ear	Beneath the mandible	Floor of the mouth
Excretory ducts	Parotid duct (Stenson's): opens opposite maxillary second molar on buccal mucosa	Submandibular duct (Wharton's): opens near lingual frenum on floor of mouth	Sublingual duct (Bartholin's): opens at same area as the submandibular duct; may have additional ducts at the submandibular folds
Striated ducts	Short	Long	Rare or absent
Intercalated ducts	Long	Short	Absent
Acini	Mainly serous	Serous and mucoserous	Mainly mucous, with some mucoserous

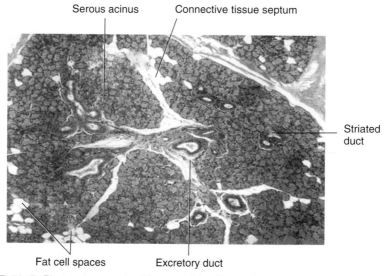

Serous acinus Connective tissue septum

Striated duct

Fat cell spaces Excretory duct

FIGURE 11-3 Photomicrograph of the parotid salivary gland. Note that the connective tissue septae divide the serous acini into lobules. A serous secretory product is produced. (From Nanci A. *Ten Cate's Oral Histology*, ed 6. Mosby, St. Louis, 2003.)

serous demilune, or "bonnet" of serous cells superficial to the group of mucous secretory cells (Figures 11-4 and 11-5). Because the mucoserous acini contain both types of secretory cells, they produce a mixed secretory product. However, the major distinctions between serous and mucous cells have become less important with additional studies of their cellular functioning.

To facilitate the flow of saliva out of each lumen into the connecting ducts, **myoepithelial cells** are located on the surface of some of the acini as well as on portions of the ductal system, the intercalated ducts (Figure 11-6). Each myoepithelial cell consists of a cell body with four to eight cytoplasmic processes radiating outward. The myoepithelial cells are specialized epithelial cells that resemble an octopus on a rock; they are situated on the surface of the acini and have a contractile nature. When these cells contract, they squeeze the acinus, forcing the saliva out of the lumen and into the connecting duct. More than one myoepithelial cell can sometimes be found on a single acinus. When associated with the ducts, the cells orient themselves lengthwise and contract to shorten or widen the ducts to keep them open. New studies are showing additional functions for the myoepithelial cells, such as sig-

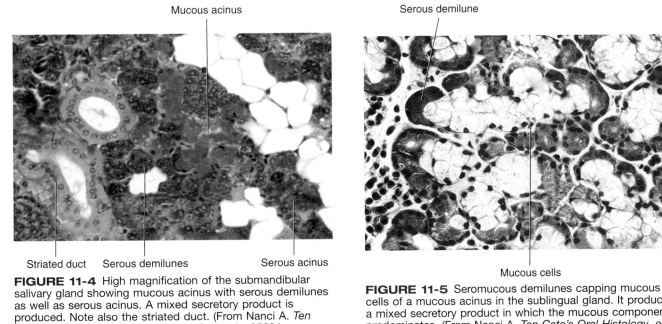

FIGURE 11-4 High magnification of the submandibular salivary gland showing mucous acinus with serous demilunes as well as serous acinus. A mixed secretory product is produced. Note also the striated duct. (From Nanci A. *Ten Cate's Oral Histology*, ed 6. Mosby, St. Louis, 2003.)

FIGURE 11-5 Seromucous demilunes capping mucous cells of a mucous acinus in the sublingual gland. It produces a mixed secretory product in which the mucous component predominates. (From Nanci A. *Ten Cate's Oral Histology*, ed 6. Mosby, St. Louis, 2003.)

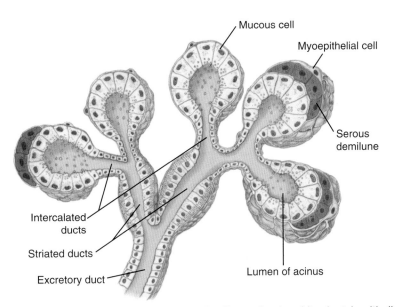

FIGURE 11-6 Diagram of microscopic view of salivary gland and its ductal epithelium. Note the myoepithelial cell on top of an acinus.

nalling the secretory cells or protecting the salivary gland tissue.

DUCTAL SYSTEM

The ductal system of salivary glands consists of hollow tubes connected initially with the acinus and then with other ducts as the ducts progressively grow larger from the inner to the outer portions of the gland (see Figure 11-6). Each type of duct is lined by different epithelium, depending on its location in the gland. In comparison, each major salivary gland displays differences in the length or types of ducts present (see Table 11-1). The ductal system is not just a pipeline for the passageway of saliva; it also actively participates in the production and modification of saliva.

The duct associated with an acinus or terminal portion of the gland is the **intercalated duct**. Thus this duct is attached to the acinus much as a stalk is attached to a cluster of grapes. The intercalated duct consists of a hollow tube lined with a single layer of cuboidal epithelial cells. Many intercalated ducts are found in each lobule of the gland. These ducts not only serve as a passageway for saliva; they also contribute many macromolecular components, which are stored in their secretory granules, to the saliva. These include lysozyme, lactoferrin, and other currently unknown components.

The **striated duct** is a portion of the ductal system that is connected to the intercalated ducts in the lobules of the gland. The overall diameter of this duct is greater than that of each acinus, and its lumen is larger than those of the acini and intercalated ducts. The striated duct consists of a hollow tube lined with a single layer of columnar epithelial cells characterized by what appear to be basal striations. These basal striations are due to the presence of numerous elongated mitochondria in narrow cytoplasmic partitions separated by highly folded and interdigitated cell membranes. Not only does the striated duct serve as a passageway for saliva; it is also involved in the modification of saliva. Its cells actively resorb and secrete electrolytes into the saliva from the adjacent blood vessels near the striated regions.

In the final portion of the salivary gland ductal system is the **excretory duct,** or secretory duct, which is located in the septum of the gland. These ducts are larger in diameter than the striated ducts. Saliva exits by way of this duct into the oral cavity. The excretory duct is a hollow tube lined with a variety of epithelial cells. The cells lining the excretory duct initially consist of pseudostratified columnar epithelium, which then undergoes a transition to stratified cuboidal as the duct moves to the outer portion of the gland.

On the outer portion of the ductal system that empties into the oral cavity, the excretory duct lining becomes stratified squamous epithelium, blending with surrounding oral mucosal tissues at the ductal opening. Thus the excretory duct serves as a passageway for saliva; however, it may be found to have more functions as it is studied further.

MAJOR SALIVARY GLANDS

The **major salivary glands** are three large paired glands that have ducts named for them (Figure 11-7 and see Table 11-1). These major salivary glands are the parotid, the submandibular, and the sublingual glands. The submandibular and sublingual glands can be palpated as nontender, firm masses in a healthy patient, but only a portion of the parotid gland can be palpated because part of the gland is deep to the overlying musculature and skin.

Although the **parotid salivary gland** is the largest encapsulated major salivary gland, it provides only 25 percent of the total salivary volume. It is located in an area behind the mandibular ramus, anterior and inferior to the ear. The serous cell predominates in the

parotid, making its saliva mainly a serous secretory product (see Figure 11-3). The duct associated with the parotid gland is the **parotid duct,** or Stenson's duct. This long duct emerges from the gland and then opens up into the oral cavity on the inner surface of the buccal mucosa, usually opposite the maxillary second molar, at the **parotid papilla.**

The **submandibular salivary gland** is the second-largest encapsulated major salivary gland, but it provides 60 to 65 percent of the total salivary volume. It lies beneath the mandible in the submandibular fossa, posterior to the sublingual salivary gland.

Because the secretory cells in the submandibular gland are both serous and mucous, its saliva is a mixed secretory product (see Figure 11-4). The gland also contains serous demilunes. The duct associated with the submandibular gland is the **submandibular duct,** or Wharton's duct. This long duct travels anteriorly on the floor of the mouth and opens into the oral cavity at the **sublingual caruncle.**

The **sublingual salivary gland** is the smallest, most diffuse, and only unencapsulated major salivary gland. It provides only 10 percent of the total salivary volume. It is located in the sublingual fossa, anterior to the submandibular salivary glands, in the floor of the mouth.

The secretory cells in the sublingual gland are both serous and mucous, but the mucous cells predominate. Thus its saliva is a mixed secretory product, in which the mucous component predominates (see Figure 11-5). The short ducts associated with the sublingual gland sometimes combine to form the **sublingual duct,** or Bartholin's duct. The sublingual duct then opens directly into the oral cavity through the same opening as the submandibular duct, the **sublingual caruncle.** Some other smaller ducts of the sublingual gland may open along the **sublingual fold.**

MINOR SALIVARY GLANDS

The **minor salivary glands** are much smaller than the major salivary glands but are more numerous. The minor salivary glands are also exocrine glands, but their unnamed ducts are shorter than those of the major salivary glands. These short ducts open directly onto the mucosal surface. These glands are scattered in the tissues of the buccal, labial, and lingual mucosa; the soft palate; the lateral portions of the hard palate; and the floor of the mouth.

There are also minor salivary glands, **von Ebner's salivary glands,** associated with the large circumvallate lingual papillae, on the posterior portion of the tongue's dorsal surface (see Chapter 9). Most minor salivary glands have mostly mucous cells, with a few serous cells. As a result, most minor salivary glands secrete a mainly mucous secretory product, with some serous components. The exception is von Ebner's

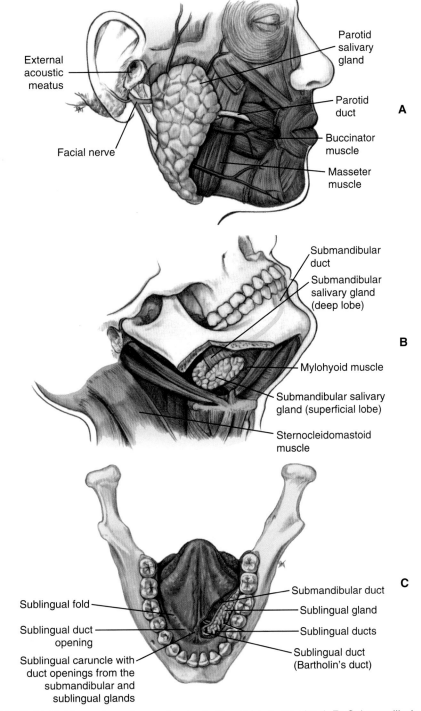

FIGURE 11-7 The major salivary glands. **A:** Parotid salivary gland. **B:** Submandibular salivary gland. **C:** Sublingual salivary gland (note that the tongue is elevated and the tissues sectioned in the highlighted area). (**A** and **B** from Fehrenbach MJ, Herring SW. *Illustrated Anatomy of the Head and Neck*, ed 2. WB Saunders, Philadelphia, 2002.)

glands, which contain only serous cells and thus secrete only a serous secretory product.

DEVELOPMENT OF SALIVARY GLANDS

Between the sixth and eighth weeks of prenatal development, the three major salivary glands begin as epithelial proliferations, or buds, from the ectodermal lining of the primitive mouth. The rounded terminal ends of these epithelial buds grow into the underlying mesenchyme, producing the secretory cells, or glandular acini, and the ductal system.

The portions of the glands that contain supporting connective tissue, such as the outer capsule and inner septa, are produced from the mesenchyme, which is influenced by neural crest cells. It is important to note that interaction between the developing components of the epithelium, mesenchyme, nerves, and blood vessels is necessary for complete development of the salivary glands.

The parotid salivary glands appear early in the sixth week of prenatal development and are the first major salivary glands formed. The epithelial buds of these glands are located on the inner portion of the cheek, near the angles of the primitive mouth. These buds will grow posteriorly toward the otic placodes of the ears and branch to form solid cords with rounded terminal ends near the developing facial nerve.

Later, at approximately 10 weeks of prenatal development, these cords are canalized and form ducts, with the largest becoming the parotid duct for the parotid gland. The rounded terminal ends of the cords form the acini of the glands. Secretion by the parotid glands via the parotid duct begins at approximately 18 weeks of gestation. Again, the supporting connective tissue of the gland develops from the surrounding mesenchyme.

The submandibular salivary glands develop later than the parotid glands and appear late in the sixth week of prenatal development. They develop bilaterally from epithelial buds in the sulcus surrounding the sublingual folds on the floor of the primitive mouth. Solid cords branch from the buds and grow posteriorly, lateral to the developing tongue.

The cords of the submandibular gland later branch further and are canalized to form the ductal portion. The submandibular gland acini develop from the cords' rounded terminal ends at 12 weeks, and secretory activity via the submandibular duct begins at 16 weeks. Growth of the submandibular gland continues after birth with the formation of more acini. Lateral to both sides of the tongue, a linear groove develops and closes over to form the submandibular duct.

The sublingual salivary glands appear in the eighth week of prenatal development, later than the other two major salivary glands. They develop from epithelial buds in the sulcus surrounding the sublingual folds on the floor of the mouth, lateral to the developing submandibular gland. These buds branch and form into cords that canalize to form the sublingual ducts associated with the gland. The rounded terminal ends of the cords form acini.

Much like the major salivary glands, the minor salivary glands arise from both the ectoderm and endoderm associated with the primitive mouth, similar to the major glands. They remain as small, isolated acini and ducts within the oral mucosa or submucosa lining the mouth.

The contractile myoepithelial cells, which are important in the secretion of saliva from each acinus, arise from neural crest cells and thus are ectodermal in origin. They surround the developing acini, as well as portions of the ductal system, and become active between the twenty-fourth to thirty-fifth weeks of prenatal development.

Clinical Considerations for Salivary Glands

Certain medications, disease processes, or destruction of salivary tissue by radiation may result in decreased production of saliva by these glands. Decreased production of saliva is called **xerostomia**, or dry mouth. Xerostomia can result in increased trauma to a nonprotected oral mucosa, increased cervical caries, and problems in speech and mastication (Figure 11-8). Thus many changes must be made in the dental treatment plan of patients with dry mouth. Such alterations in care include the recommendation of sipping water, use of artificial saliva, fluoride rinses, avoidance of alcohol-containing products, and increased recall visits. Medications that stimulate salivary production are available for nondrug-related xerostomia. Transplanting lost salivary tissue is now being performed. Aging does not seem to influence the production of resting saliva, or unstimulated saliva production, but some current studies show that stimulated saliva production may be less than normal in older individuals.

The salivary glands may also become blocked, stopping the drainage of saliva from the duct. This blockage can cause glandular enlargement and tenderness resulting from retention of saliva in the gland. This blockage of the duct can result from stone (or sialolith) formation or trauma to the duct opening.

This retention of saliva in the gland can result in a **mucocele** if it involves a minor salivary gland or in a **ranula** if it involves the submandibular salivary gland (Figures 11-9 and 11-10). These two salivary gland lesions are treated by removal of the stone or surgical removal of the gland. The submandibular duct's tortuous travel to its ductal opening for a considerable upward distance may be the reason this gland is the salivary gland most commonly involved in stone formation.

Another oral lesion associated with salivary glands is **nicotinic stomatitis** (Figure 11-11). With this lesion, the hard palate is whitened by hyperkeratinization caused by the heat from tobacco use or hot liquid consumption (see Chapter 9). This heat also causes inflammation of the duct openings of the minor salivary gland of the palatal area, and thus they become dilated. This inflammation of the ductal epithelium is seen clinically in the red macules scattered on the whiter background of the palatal mucosa.

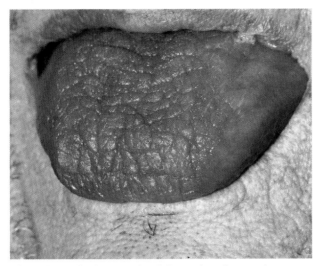

FIGURE 11-8 Xerostomia of the oral cavity causing inflammation of the oral mucosa, including the tongue tissues.

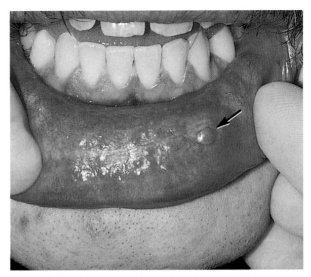

FIGURE 11-9 Mucocele *(arrow)* on the lower lip involving the severance of the associated minor salivary gland duct and enlargement of the gland.

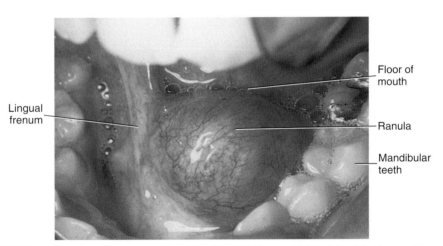

Floor of mouth

Lingual frenum

Ranula

Mandibular teeth

FIGURE 11-10 Ranula on one side of the floor of the mouth involving blockage of the submandibular salivary gland duct from stone formation resulting in enlargement of the gland.

Thyroid Gland

The **thyroid gland** is the largest endocrine gland and is located in the anterior and lateral regions of the neck, inferior to the thyroid cartilage (Figure 11-12). Because it is ductless, the thyroid gland produces and secretes its products, **thyroxine** and other hormones, directly into the blood. Thyroxine is a hormone that stimulates the metabolic rate. The gland consists of two lateral lobes connected anteriorly by an isthmus. In a healthy patient, the gland is not visible but can be palpated and is mobile, moving superiorly when a person swallows.

The **parathyroid glands** typically consist of four to eight small endocrine glands, two on each side, usually close to the thyroid gland or even inside it on its posterior surface. The parathyroid glands are not visible or palpable during an extraoral examination of a patient. However, the parathyroid glands may alter the thyroid gland as a result of their involvement in a disease process.

HISTOLOGY OF THE THYROID GLAND

The thyroid gland is covered by a connective tissue capsule that extends into the gland by way of septa (Figure 11-13). The septa divide the gland into larger lobes and smaller lobules. Each lobule is composed of **follicles**, irregularly shaped spheroidal masses that are embedded in a meshwork of reticular fibers. Each follicle consists of a layer of simple cuboidal epithelium enclosing a cavity that is usually filled with a stiff

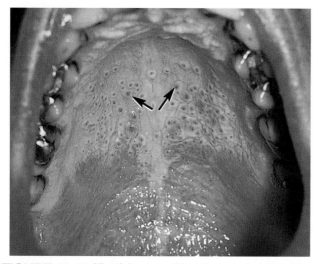

FIGURE 11-11 Nicotinic stomatitis with hyperkeratinization of the palatal mucosa and ductal inflammation of the minor salivary glands *(arrows)*. This palatal lesion is due to smoking or contact with hot liquids.

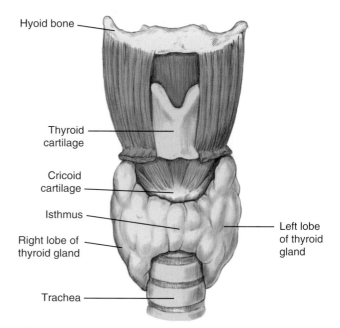

FIGURE 11-12 The location of the thyroid gland. (From Fehrenbach MJ, Herring SW. *Illustrated Anatomy of the Head and Neck,* ed 2. WB Saunders, Philadelphia, 2002.)

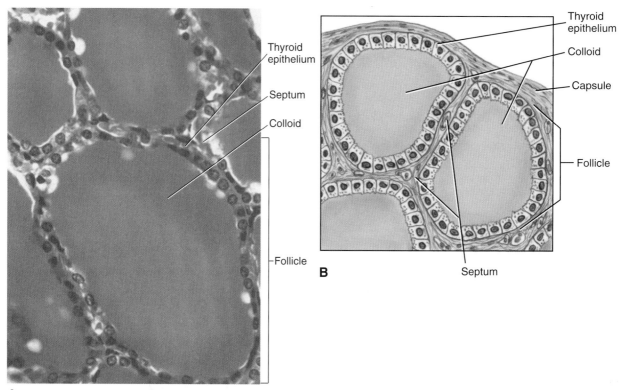

FIGURE 11-13 The histology of the thyroid gland. **A:** Photomicrograph showing the portions of the gland **B:** Diagramic representation. (**A** from Young B, Heath JW. *Wheater's Functional Histology*, ed 4. Churchill Livingstone, Edinburgh, 2000.)

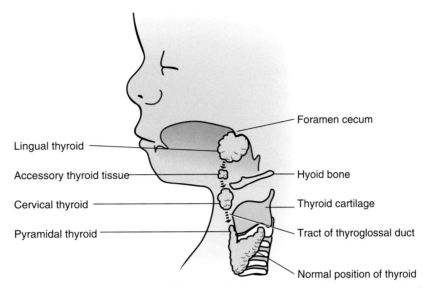

FIGURE 11-14 The development of the thyroid gland from a median downgrowth of the tongue, connected by a thyroglossal duct (path is shown by the broken line). Note that remnants of thyroid tissue can remain at all these original sites and become cystic.

material called **colloid**, which is the reserve for the production of thyroxine.

DEVELOPMENT OF THE THYROID GLAND

The thyroid gland is the first endocrine gland to appear in embryonic development and develops from endoderm invaded by mesenchymal cells. At approximately the twenty-fourth day of prenatal development, the thyroid gland develops. It forms from a median downgrowth at the base of the tongue, connected by a **thyroglossal duct**, a narrow tube that later becomes obliterated (Figure 11-14).

The **foramen cecum,** which is the opening of the thyroglossal duct, is a small, pitlike depression located where the sulcus terminalis points backward toward the oropharynx. This duct shows the origin of the thyroid and the pathway of the thyroid gland's migration into the neck region.

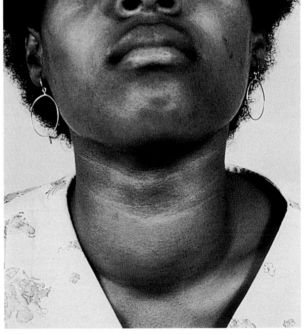

FIGURE 11-15 Goiter or enlarged thyroid gland caused by an endocrine disorder.

Clinical Considerations for the Thyroid Gland

During a disease process involving the thyroid gland, the gland may become enlarged and possibly may be viewed during an extraoral examination. This enlarged thyroid gland is called a **goiter** (Figure 11-15). A goiter may be firm and tender when palpated and may contain hard masses. Any patient who has any undiagnosed changes in the thyroid gland should be referred to a physician.

LYMPHATICS

The **lymphatics** are a part of the immune system and help fight disease processes. They also serve other functions in the body. The lymphatic system consists of a network of lymphatic vessels linking lymph nodes throughout most of the body. Tonsillar tissue located in the oral cavity and pharynx is also part of the lymphatic system. This chapter describes the intraoral tonsillar tissue in detail; the pharyngeal and tubal tonsillar tissue is not discussed.

The **lymphatic vessels** are a system of endothelial-lined channels that are mostly parallel to the venous blood vessels in location but are more numerous. Tissue fluid drains from the surrounding region into the lymphatic vessels as **lymph**. Lymph is similar in composition to tissue fluid and plasma.

Each lymphatic vessel drains its particular region, and all of these vessels communicate with one another. Lymphatic vessels are lined with endothelium-like blood vessels, but the lymphatic vessels are larger and thicker in diameter than the blood system's capillaries. Lymphatic vessels are found within most of the oral tissues, even within the tooth's pulp tissue.

Smaller lymphatic vessels containing lymph converge into the larger endothelial-lined **lymphatic ducts,** which empty into the venous system of the blood in the chest area. The drainage pattern of the lymphatic vessels into the lymphatic ducts depends on the side of the body involved, right or left, because the lymphatic ducts are different on each side.

Lymph Nodes

The **lymph nodes** are bean-shaped bodies grouped in clusters along the connecting lymphatic vessels, positioned to filter toxic products from the lymph to prevent their entry into the blood system (Figure 11-16). Lymph nodes are located in various regions of the head and neck area (see Chapter 1 for these regions).

In healthy patients, lymph nodes are usually small, soft, and free or mobile in the surrounding tissue. The lymph nodes can be superficial in position with the superficial veins or deep in the tissue with the deep blood vessels. Normally, lymph nodes cannot be seen or palpated during an extraoral examination of a healthy patient.

The lymph flows into the lymph node by way of many **afferent vessels.** On one side of the node is a depression, or **hilus,** where the lymph flows out of the node by way of fewer or even a single **efferent vessel.** Lymph nodes can be classified as either primary or secondary nodes. Lymph from a particular tissue region drains into primary nodes or regional nodes. Primary nodes, in turn, drain into secondary nodes or central nodes.

HISTOLOGY OF LYMPH NODES

Each lymph node is composed of organized lymphoid tissue and contains lymphocytes that actively filter toxic products from the lymph (Figure 11-16). The entire node is surrounded by a connective tissue capsule. Bands of connective tissue called **trabeculae** extend from the capsule into the node. The trabeculae separate the node into masses of lymphocytes, called

lymphatic nodules, or follicles. The lymph flows between the lymphatic nodules and other tissue spaces or sinuses.

Each lymphatic nodule has a **germinal center** containing many immature lymphocytes. As they mature, these lymphocytes enter either the area of the nodule surrounding the germinal center or the lymph. These mature lymphocytes are of the B-cell type and are involved in the humoral immune response with immunoglobulin production (discussed further in Chapter 8).

DEVELOPMENT OF LYMPH NODES

Lymphatic vessels develop from the blood vessels by a process of budding and fusion of isolated groups of mesenchymal cells. Peripherally located mesenchymal cells form the lymphatic nodules in the connective tissue associated with the developing lymphatic vessels. These nodules become surrounded by sinuses and complete the lymph node. A capsule and trabeculae later form around the developing lymphatic nodules from the surrounding mesenchyme.

Intraoral Tonsillar Tissue

Intraoral **tonsillar tissue** consists of nonencapsulated masses of lymphoid tissue located in the lamina propria of the oral mucosa. It is covered by stratified squamous epithelium that is continuous with the surrounding oral mucosa. Tonsils, like lymph nodes, contain lymphocytes that remove toxic products and then move to the epithelial surface as they mature. Unlike lymph nodes, tonsillar tissue is not located along lymphatic vessels but is situated near airway and food passages to protect the body against disease processes from the related toxic products (see Chapter 2).

The **palatine tonsils** are two rounded masses of variable size located between the anterior and posterior faucial pillars (see Chapter 2). Histologically, each mass contains fused-together lymphatic nodules that generally have germinal centers (Figure 11-17). Each tonsil also has 10 to 20 epithelial invaginations, or grooves, which penetrate deeply into the tonsil to form tonsillar crypts. These crypts contain shed epithelial cells, mature lymphocytes, and oral bacteria.

The **lingual tonsil** is an indistinct layer of diffuse lymphoid tissue located on the base of the dorsal surface of the tongue, posterior to the circumvallate lingual papillae (see Chapter 2). The lymphoid tissue consists of many lymphatic nodules, usually each with a germinal center and only one associated tonsillar crypt.

Behind the uvula, on the superior and posterior walls of the nasopharynx, are the **pharyngeal tonsils.** They form an incomplete tonsillar ring, Waldeyer's ring. When they become enlarged, as is common in children, they are called the *adenoids*.

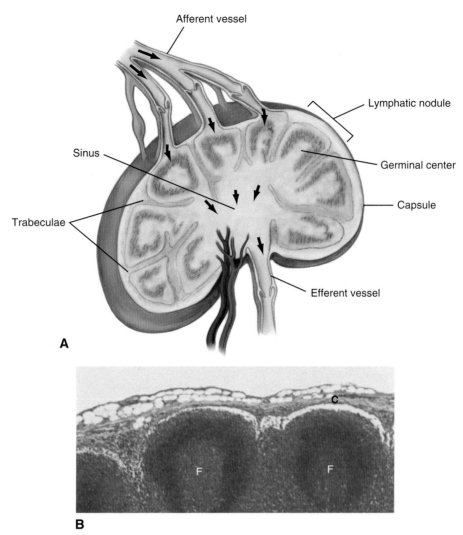

FIGURE 11-16 A lymph node and its features. **A:** Diagramic representation. **B:** Photomicrograph of the node showing the nodule or follicle with its germinal center *(F)* and capsule *(C)*. (**A** from Fehrenbach MJ, Herring SW. *Illustrated Anatomy of the Head and Neck,* ed 2. WB Saunders, Philadelphia, 2002. **B** from Young B, Heath JW. *Wheater's Functional Histology,* ed 4. Churchill Livingstone, Edinburgh, 2000.)

Clinical Considerations for Lymph Nodes

When a patient has an active disease process, such as cancer or infection, in a specific region, the region's lymph nodes respond. The resultant increase in size and change in consistency of the lymphoid tissue are termed **lymphadenopathy**. Lymphadenopathy results from an increase in both the size of each individual lymphocyte and the overall cell count in the lymphoid tissue. With more and larger lymphocytes, the lymphoid tissue is better able to fight the disease process.

This lymphadenopathy may allow the node to be viewed during an extraoral examination. More important, changes in consistency from firm to bony hard allow the lymph node to be palpated during the extraoral examination. Palpation of an involved node may be painful, and the node can become fixed and attached to the surrounding tissues.

Lymphadenopathy can also occur in the intraoral tonsils, causing tissue enlargement that can be viewed on an intraoral examination (Figure 11-18). The intraoral tonsils may also be tender when palpated. Lymphadenopathy of tonsils in the oral cavity may cause airway obstruction with its complications and lead to infection of the tonsillar tissue. If any lymph nodes are palpable or if there is an enlargement or infection of intraoral tonsillar tissue, these findings should be recorded in the patient's chart and appropriate physician referrals should be made.

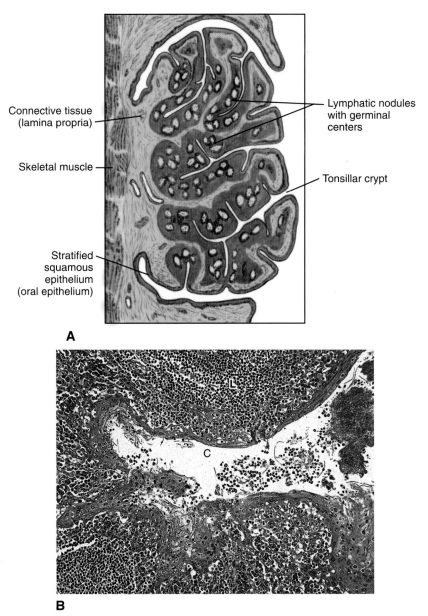

Connective tissue (lamina propria)

Skeletal muscle

Lymphatic nodules with germinal centers

Tonsillar crypt

Stratified squamous epithelium (oral epithelium)

A

B

FIGURE 11-17 Histological features of the palatine tonsillar tissue. **A:** Diagramic representation. **B:** Photomicroph of the tissue showing the crypt *(C)* lined by squamous epithelium and lymphoid nodule *(L)*. Note that the crypt contains oral bacteria, which is a normal finding. (From Stevens A, Lowe J. *Human Histology*, ed 3. Mosby, St. Louis, 2005.)

NASAL CAVITY

The **nasal cavity** is the inner space of the nose (Figure 11-19). The nasal cavity communicates with the exterior by two nostrils, or **nares.** The nares are separated by the midline **nasal septum,** which consists of both bone and cartilage. The nasal septum also divides the internal nasal cavity into two portions.

Each lateral wall of the nasal cavity has three projecting structures, or **nasal conchae**, which extend inward. Beneath each concha are openings through which the paranasal sinuses or nasolacrimal ducts communicate with the nasal cavity. The posterior portion of the nasal cavity communicates with the nasopharynx and then with the rest of the respiratory system. The development of the nasal septum and cavity is described in Chapter 5.

Histology of the Mucosa of the Nasal Cavity

The nasal cavity is lined by a **respiratory mucosa** like the rest of the respiratory system (see Chapter 8). Respiratory mucosa is different from oral mucosa lining the oral cavity but similar to that lining the trachea and bronchi. Respiratory mucosa consists of pseudostratified columnar epithelium with cilia (Figure 11-20).

Within the epithelium and surrounded by mucous and serous glands are **goblet cells,** which rest on the basement membrane. Fluids or mucus from the goblet cells and glands keep this mucosa moist, provide humidity, and trap any foreign materials from the inspired air.

The moist mucus forms a superficial coating on the respiratory mucosa. This coating is moved by ciliary action posteriorly to the nasopharynx, where it is either expectorated or swallowed. In this manner, foreign materials are trapped and removed. Because the lamina propria of the mucosa is very vascular, it also warms the air. In the roof of each portion of the nasal cavity is a specialized area containing the olfactory mucosa, which carries the receptors for the sense of smell.

Overlying the conchae is an extensive, superficial plexus of large, thin-walled vessels termed **erectile tissue**. This tissue is capable of considerable engorgement. This engorgement happens at periodic intervals of 30 to 60 minutes, thus closing off the involved side of the nasal cavity to enable the respiratory mucosa to recover from the effects of dryness during respiration. The deepest portions of the lamina propria are continuous with the periosteum of the nasal bone or perichondrium of the nasal cartilage.

The respiratory mucosa of the nasal cavity and septum is continuous and similar to that of the nasopharynx. The respiratory mucosa of the nasopharynx gives way to the stratified squamous epithelium of the oropharynx. The stronger stratified squamous epithelium of the oropharynx, with its soft palate and posterior wall of the pharynx, allows for the mechanical stress of swallowing.

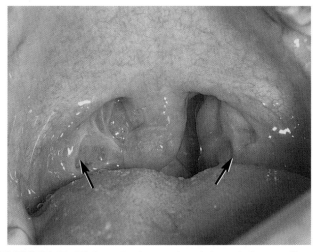

FIGURE 11-18 Lymphadenopathy of the palatine tonsils showing enlargement. (From Fehrenbach MJ, Herring SW. *Illustrated Anatomy of the Head and Neck*, ed 2. WB Saunders, Philadelphia, 2002.)

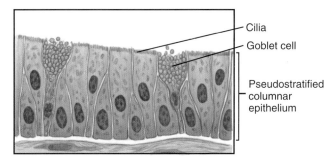

FIGURE 11-20 The histological features of the respiratory mucosa of the nasal cavity.

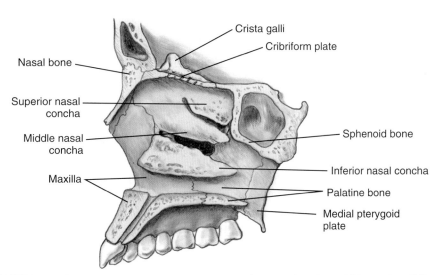

FIGURE 11-19 The nasal cavity and its features. (From Fehrenbach MJ, Herring SW. *Illustrated Anatomy of the Head and Neck*, ed 2. WB Saunders, Philadelphia, 2002.)

PARANASAL SINUSES

The **paranasal sinuses** are paired air-filled cavities in bone (Figure 11-21). The paranasal sinuses include the frontal, sphenoid, ethmoid, and maxillary sinuses. The sinuses communicate with the nasal cavity through small openings in the lateral nasal wall. The openings mark the outpouchings from which the paranasal sinuses develop. The sinuses serve to lighten the skull bones, act as sound resonators, and provide mucus for the nasal cavity.

Histology of the Mucosa of the Paranasal Sinuses

The paranasal sinuses are lined with respiratory mucosa consisting of pseudostratified ciliated columnar epithelium continuous with the epithelial lining of the nasal cavity (see Figure 11-20, see also Figure 8-2). The epithelium of the sinuses, although it is similar to that of the nasal cavity, is thinner and contains fewer goblet cells. The respiratory mucosa of the sinuses also shows a thinner underlying lamina propria that is continuous with the deeper periosteum of the bone and has fewer associated glands. No erectile tissue is present in the paranasal sinuses.

Development of the Paranasal Sinuses

Some paranasal sinuses develop during late fetal life; the rest develop after birth. They form as outgrowths of the wall of the nasal cavity and become air-filled extensions in the adjacent bones. The original openings of the outgrowths persist as orifices of the adult sinuses.

The maxillary sinuses are small at birth, and only a few of the ethmoid sinuses are present. The maxillary sinuses grow until puberty and are not fully developed until all the permanent teeth have erupted in early adulthood. The ethmoid sinuses do not start to grow until 6 to 8 years of age.

The frontal sinuses and sphenoid sinuses are not present at birth. At approximately 2 years of age, the

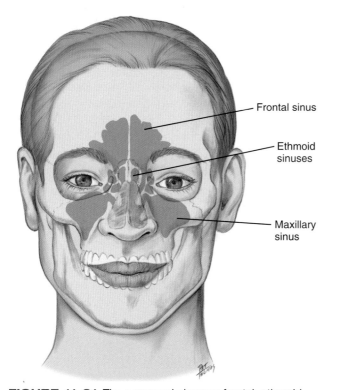

— Frontal sinus

— Ethmoid sinuses

— Maxillary sinus

FIGURE 11-21 The paranasal sinuses: frontal, ethmoid, maxillary. (The sphenoid sinus is not shown in this view because it is deep to the ethmoid sinus.) (From Fehrenbach MJ, Herring SW. *Illustrated Anatomy of the Head and Neck*, ed 2. WB Saunders, Philadelphia, 2002.)

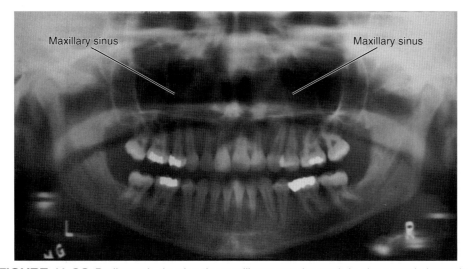

Maxillary sinus   Maxillary sinus

FIGURE 11-22 Radiograph showing the maxillary posterior teeth in close proximity to the maxillary sinuses.

two most anterior ethmoid sinuses grow into the frontal bone, forming the frontal sinus on each side, and are visible on radiographs by the seventh year. At the same time, the two most posterior ethmoid sinuses grow into the sphenoid bone and form the sphenoid sinuses. Growth of sinuses in the size and shape of the face is important during infancy and childhood and adds resonance to the voice during puberty.

Clinical Considerations for the Nasal Cavity and Paranasal Sinuses

The respiratory mucosa of the nasal cavity and paranasal sinuses can become inflamed and the space congested with mucus as a result of allergies or respiratory tract infection. This inflammation can lead to a stuffed-up feeling in the nasal cavity and **sinusitis** in the sinus. The symptoms for both are discomfort caused by the pressure of the increased mucus production with nasal or pharyngeal discharge.

With blocked nasal passages and with sinusitis, medications are used to effect vasoconstriction in the blood vessels while reducing the amount of mucus produced. In cases of chronic sinusitis, surgical treatment may be needed. Patients undergoing these respiratory difficulties may not be able to use nitrous oxide adequately; may feel uncomfortable with the use of a rubber dam; and may breathe through the mouth, causing gingivitis of the maxillary anterior teeth.

Because the maxillary posterior teeth are in close proximity to the maxillary sinus, maxillary sinusitis can sometimes result as infection spreads from a periapical abscess associated with a maxillary posterior tooth (Figure 11-22). As the infection spreads, the sinus floor is perforated and the sinus mucosa becomes involved in the infection. During an extraction, a contaminated tooth or root fragments can also be surgically displaced into the maxillary sinus. In addition, the pain from a maxillary sinusitis can sometimes be misinterpreted by the patient as involving the maxillary teeth because of their close proximity. Differential diagnosis of the symptoms and radiographs can aid in determining the cause of this facial pain.

CHAPTER 12

Enamel

■ ■ ■

This chapter discusses the following topics:

- Enamel
- Apposition of enamel matrix
- Maturation of enamel matrix
- Components of mature enamel
- Further microscopic features of mature enamel

■ ■ ■

After studying this chapter, the reader should be able to:

1. Define and pronounce the key terms in this chapter.
2. Describe the properties of enamel.
3. Discuss the apposition and maturation of enamel.
4. Demonstrate and discuss the microscopic features of enamel.
5. Integrate the knowledge of the histology with the clinical considerations involved with enamel.

■ ■ ■

Key Terms

Abfraction (ab-**frak**-shen)
Abrasion (uh-**brey**-zhun)
Ameloblast (ah-**mel**-oh-blast)
Amelogenesis
  (ah-mel-oh-**jen**-i-sis)
Apposition stage (ap-oh-**zish**-in)
Attrition (ah-**trish**-un)
Calcium hydroxyapatite
  (hy-drox-see-**ap**-ah-tite)

Caries
Dentinoenamel junction
Enamel (ih-**nam**-l): dysplasia
  (dis-**play**-ze-ah), erosion
  (e-ro-zhun), lamellae, matrix, pearl,
  rods, spindles, tufts
Imbrication lines (im-bri-**kay**-shun)
Interprismatic region (in-ter-
  priz-mat-ik)

Lines of Retzius (ret-**zee**-us)
Maturation stage (ma-cher-**ray**-shin)
Neonatal line (ne-oh-**nate**-l)
Perikymata (per-ee-ki-**maht**-ah)
Reduced enamel epithelium
Tomes' process

ENAMEL

Mature **enamel** is a crystalline material that is the hardest calcified tissue in the human body (see Table 6-2). In its mature state, it is noted for its almost total absence of organic matrix. Enamel in a healthy state, precluding trauma or disease, can be removed only by rotary cutting instruments or rough files such as those used in dentistry. Enamel is avascular and has no nerves within it. Although enamel is the hardest calcified tissue in the body, it can be lost forever because it is nonvital and therefore not a renewable resource. However, it is not a static tissue because it can undergo mineralization changes (discussed later).

Clinical Considerations for Enamel Tissue

One way that enamel and other hard tissues of the tooth are lost is through **attrition**, which is the wearing away of hard tissue as a result of tooth-to-tooth contact (Table 12-1). This tooth wear increases with age. Permanent first molars wear more than seconds; seconds more than thirds. Attrition is discussed in Chapters 16 and 17 with regard to specific teeth and in Chapter 20 with regard to parafunctional habits. The relationship between the loss of the vertical dimension of the face and alveolar bone loss is discussed in Chapter 14. Enamel loss may also result from friction caused by excessive toothbrushing and abrasive toothpaste. This wear is considered **abrasion.**

Enamel can also be lost by **erosion** through chemical means. Erosion is particularly apparent in patients with the eating disorder of bulimia, in which patients force themselves to vomit to remove their stomach contents in pursuit of weight loss (Figure 12-1). The lingual surface of the anterior teeth and the occlusal surface of all the teeth are eroded by the acid content of the vomit. The yellow underlying dentin is thereby exposed and can undergo attrition because it is less mineralized than enamel. Treatment of bulimia is multifactorial and includes behavior

changes. Similar erosion can be caused by gastric reflux. If facial enamel lesions of the anterior teeth are evident, the patient may be overusing acid-containing carbonated soft drinks or sport drinks (especially idiet formulations and those containing enamel-eroding citric acid).

Another way that enamel and other hard tissues of the tooth can be lost is by **caries.** Caries is a process by which a cavity is created by demineralization, or loss of minerals. This demineralization is due to acid production by cariogenic bacteria (discussed later) and occurs when the pH is less than 5.5. Caries is discussed further in this chapter in relation to enamel structure.

Finally, enamel can be lost as a result of **abfraction** (see Figure 12-1, B). Abfraction may be caused by tensile and compressive forces during tooth flexure, which possibly occurs during parafunctional habits with their occlusal loading (see Chapter 20). It consists of cervical lesions that cannot be attributed to any particular cause, such as erosion or toothbrush abrasion; abfraction causes the enamel to pop off starting at the cervical region, thus exposing the area to possible further wear, dentin hypersensitivity, or caries.

Mature enamel is by weight 96 percent mineralized or inorganic material, 1 percent organic material, and 3 percent water. This crystalline formation of mature enamel consists of mainly **calcium hydroxyapatite** with the chemical formula of $Ca_{10}(PO_4)_6(OH)_2$. This calcium hydroxyapatite is similar to that found in lesser percentages in bone, dentin, and cementum.

Other minerals, such as carbonate, magnesium, potassium, sodium, and fluoride, are also present in smaller amounts. Studies have challenged this composition of enamel and instead maintain that it is mainly carbonated hydroxyapatite because of its relationship with fluoride uptake. Whatever the formation, the crystals of enamel are set at different angles throughout the crown area. Discussion of the elegant crystalline nature of enamel is awkward at best, but this chapter is an attempt to do justice to this beautiful jewel-like material.

Enamel is usually the only portion of a tooth that is seen clinically in a healthy mouth because it covers the anatomical crown. Enamel provides a hard surface for mastication and speech. Enamel also provides the pleasing whiteness of a healthy smile. Enamel alone is various shades of bluish white, which is seen on the incisal tips of newly erupted incisors, but it turns various shades of yellow-white elsewhere because of the underlying dentin. The enamel on primary teeth has a more opaque crystalline form and thus appears whiter than on permanent teeth.

Because the overall shade of enamel varies in each person and possibly within a dentition, a shade value is taken when integrating tooth-colored restorative materials or artificial teeth or crowns within an individual dentition. The goal is to match as closely as pos-

sible the color of the patient's other teeth. This shade value is selected by comparing the patient's natural teeth to a shade guide of plastic model crowns that have been moistened and are viewed in natural light. These shade guides are provided by various manufacturers. New technology allows a digital read-out of the color of the enamel. (The whitening process is discussed later.)

On radiographs, the differences in the mineralization of different portions of the tooth can be noted. Enamel appears more radiopaque (lighter) than dentin and pulp, both of which appear more radiolucent (darker).

Preservation of the enamel of every tooth during a patient's lifetime is one of the goals of every dental professional. Dental professionals must take into consideration the properties of enamel when deciding the caries risk for patients, counseling patients and communities on fluoride use, applying enamel sealants, and using and recommending polishing agents. All these considerations are discussed throughout this chapter.

APPOSITION OF ENAMEL MATRIX

Amelogenesis is the process of enamel matrix formation that occurs during the **apposition stage** of tooth development. The exact time of the apposition stage varies according to the tooth that is undergoing development. Many factors can affect amelogenesis (see Chapter 6).

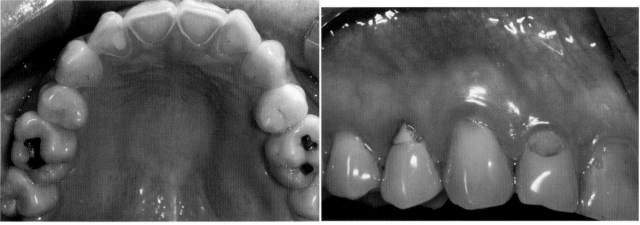

FIGURE 12-1 Clinical loss of enamel. **A:** Lingual erosion in a patient with a past history of bulimia. Note that the permanent maxillary central incisors have been covered using a veneer restoration because of the amount of hard tissue loss. **B:** Abfraction of the upper right quadrant is noted, especially on the lateral incisor. The first premolar has been repaired with restorative materials but has secondary caries around the margins.

TABLE 12-1

Hard Tissue Loss

Term	Definition	Clinical Appearance
Attrition	Loss through tooth-to-tooth contact (mastication or parafunctional habits)	Matching wear on occluding surfaces Shiny facets on amalgam contacts Enamel and dentin wear at the same rate Possible fracture of cusps or restorations
Erosion	Loss through chemical means (acid) not involving bacteria	Broad concavities within smooth surface enamel Cupping of occlusal surfaces, (incisal grooving) with dentin exposure (dentin hypersensitivity possible) Increased incisal translucency Wear on nonoccluding surfaces (location depends on acid intake type) Raised and shiny amalgam restorations Preservation of enamel cuff in gingival crevice common Pulp exposure and loss of surface characteristics of enamel in primary teeth
Abrasion	Loss through friction from toothbrushing and/or toothpaste	Usually located at facial cervical areas Lesions more wide than deep Canines commonly affected because of tooth position
Caries	Loss through chemical means (acid) from cariogenic bacteria	All surfaces can be affected Occlusal surfaces more commonly affected, especially in the pits and grooves Possibly rapid progression of interproximal lesions if progress goes unchecked Cervical lesions sometimes secondary to other forms of hard tissue loss or gingival recession
Abfraction	Possible loss through tensile and compressive forces during tooth flexure (parafunctional habits)	Can affect both facial and lingual cervical areas Deep, narrow V-shaped notch Commonly affects single teeth that have occlusal loads

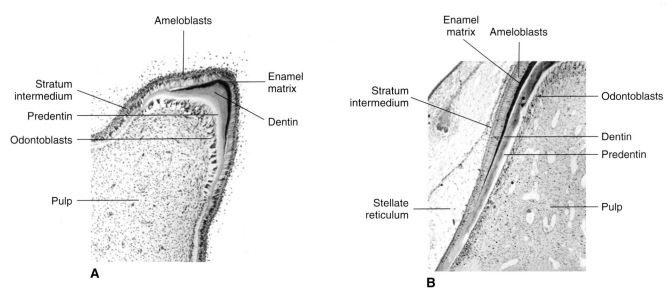

FIGURE 12-2 Photomicrographs of a tooth undergoing matrix formation of both enamel and dentin. The inset shows ameloblasts producing enamel matrix from their Tomes' processes. (From Nanci A. *Ten Cate's Oral Histology*, ed 6. Mosby, St. Louis, 2003.)

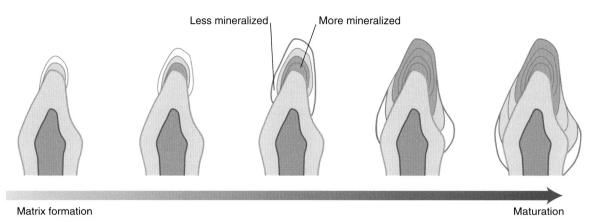

FIGURE 12-3 Wave patterns of enamel matrix formation in the crown during apposition. This pattern is repeated during the maturation of enamel.

Enamel matrix is produced by ameloblast cells (Figure 12-2). Each **ameloblast** is approximately 4 micrometers in diameter, 40 micrometers in length, and hexagonal in cross section. The ameloblasts are columnar cells that differentiate during the apposition stage in the crown area. Ameloblasts are not differentiated in the root area; thus the enamel is confined to the crown of the tooth.

The enamel matrix is secreted from each ameloblast from its **Tomes' process** (see Figure 12-2, B). Tomes' process is the secretory surface of the ameloblast that faces the dentinoenamel junction (DEJ), unlike the process associated with the odontoblast, which is a true cytoplasmic process from a cell body. With a one-to-one relationship to each ameloblast, Tomes' process has a six-sided pyramidal shape. Tomes' process is responsible for the way the enamel matrix is laid down; thus it is the guiding factor.

Enamel matrix is an ectodermal product because ameloblasts are derived from the inner enamel epithe-lium of the enamel organ, which was originally derived from the ectodermal layer of the embryo. Enamel matrix initially is composed of proteins and carbohydrates and only a small amount of calcium hydroxyapatite crystals.

Early enamel matrix is therefore only partially mineralized, as compared with fully matured enamel (discussed later). Ameloblasts are also responsible for this partially mineralized state of the enamel matrix because they actively pump calcium hydroxyapatite into the forming enamel matrix as it is secreted by Tomes' processes.

Enamel matrix is first formed in the incisal/occlusal portion of the future crown near the forming DEJ (Figure 12-3). This is the first wave of enamel apposition, which moves to the future outer enamel surface. The second wave of enamel apposition overlaps the first wave, and this entire process then moves cervically to the cementoenamel junction (CEJ).

Clinical Considerations with Enamel Structure

Certain developmental disturbances, such as an **enamel pearl** and types of **enamel dysplasia** (see Chapter 6), can occur in enamel during the apposition stage. Another common developmental disturbance is deepened pits and grooves on the occlusal surface of posterior teeth and lingual surface of anterior teeth (as discussed and shown in Chapters 16 and 17). These are created when ameloblasts back into one another during the apposition stage, cutting off their source of nutrition. This loss of nutritional support causes incomplete maturation of enamel matrix, making it weak or even absent in that area.

These weak areas of pits and grooves are target areas for caries (Figure 12-4). Bacterial plaque biofilm can become sheltered in these irregular areas and cannot be reached by careful oral hygiene. The bacterial plaque biofilm produces acids that slowly demineralize the weak enamel areas, producing caries. There is a "tug-of-war" between demineralization and remineralization at the surface; when demineralization outweighs remineralization, caries results. Remineralization is the deposition of minerals into enamel from salivary minerals and fluoride (discussed later). However, with the cariogenic process, the surface enamel of the pit or groove remains intact as the subsurface zones become further demineralized. Thus caries remains in the subsurface, working its way to the dentin/pulp area.

Protection against this type of caries is provided by the use of enamel sealants that cover the pits and grooves on the teeth (discussed in Chapters 16 and 17 in relation to specific teeth and later in this chapter in relation to tooth preparation). Educating patients about the importance of enamel sealants in caries prevention is an important responsibility for dental professionals. Many clinicians are even recommending these sealants for adults past the usual age of caries risk because of the possibility of future caries at these sites.

Similar to the caries that occurs in pits and grooves, smooth surface caries, which occurs interproximally, does not involve the breakdown or demineralization of the surface layers of enamel (see Figure 12-4). Zones are also present with smooth surface caries as they are with caries of pits and grooves.

Both caries in the pits and grooves and smooth surface caries are first noted clinically as a white-spot lesion wherein the enamel appears whiter and rougher as a result of slight surface demineralization. However, this lesion may be difficult to see clinically and may only be detected through the use of a "sticky" explorer for both types of caries. Thus the enamel surface is finally undermined, and the explorer falls into already destroyed subsurface. Early subsurface lesions cannot be detected on radiographs until they spread at least 200 micrometers into the dentin, a process that can take 3 to 5 years. Certain light-induced devices now allow dental professionals to better diagnose early lesions involving the enamel.

If caries is only in the enamel, it does not cause pain to the patient because the enamel has no nerves within it. For the same reason, initial cavity preparation during removal of enamel only is usually painless. Pain occurs only when the deeper layers of dentin and then pulp are involved (see Chapter 13 for a discussion of tooth pain). Thus it is important to emphasize to patients the need for recall examinations for early detection of decay before pain is involved. Pain is a late finding in caries, and the risk of tooth loss increases while waiting for this symptom to appear.

The type of polishing agent used by dental professionals and by patients at home is also a very important consideration. Older toothpastes and professional polishing agents abraded the enamel surface, removing valuable tooth layers to obtain temporary aesthetic results. Selective polishing methods are now used only to remove stain on natural enamel surfaces. The use of less abrasive professional and patient polishing agents helps preserve the limited enamel on the crowns. It is also not necessary to polish the teeth to remove bacterial plaque biofilm before topical fluoride application or, in many cases, enamel sealant placement.

MATURATION OF ENAMEL MATRIX

During the **maturation stage** of tooth development, enamel matrix completes its mineralization process after the apposition of enamel matrix when it is only approximately 30 percent mineralized. Thus mineralization of enamel matrix to a fully matured tissue covers two stages of tooth development, both the apposition and maturation stages. Enamel mineralization also continues after eruption of the tooth (discussed next).

During the maturation of enamel matrix, ameloblasts actively pump even more calcium hydroxyapatite into the already partially mineralized enamel matrix and withdraw an equal amount of the organic materials at the same time. Thus the ameloblast is specifically responsible for maturation of enamel matrix into mature enamel.

Two waves of maturation in the tooth follow the same pattern as enamel matrix formation (see Figure 12-3). The first wave of enamel mineralization occurs in the occlusal portion of the future crown near the forming DEJ and moves to the future outer enamel surface. The second wave of enamel mineralization overlaps the first wave as the process moves cervically to the forming CEJ.

After the ameloblasts are finished with both enamel apposition and maturation, they become part of the **reduced enamel epithelium** (REE), along with the other portions of the compressed enamel organ. The REE fuses with the oral mucosa, creating a canal to allow the enamel cusp tip to erupt through the oral mucosa into the oral cavity. Unfortunately, the ameloblasts are lost forever as the fused tissues

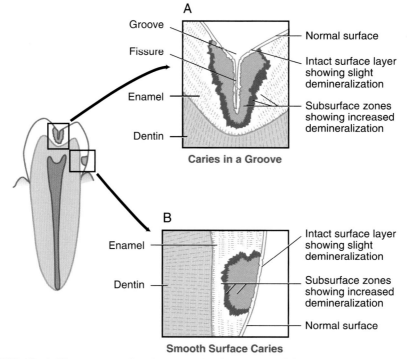

FIGURE 12-4 The process of caries occurring in a groove **(A),** and smooth surface caries **(B),** with both showing the different zones. Note that both types of caries have an intact surface layer and demineralization is in the subsurface zones.

disintegrate during tooth eruption, preventing any further enamel apposition. (Tissues can become part of Nasmyth's membrane, as described in Chapter 6.) Enamel is not a renewable resource because there is no way to retrieve the lost ameloblasts. New research involves the study of amelogenins, the principal extra-cellular matrix protein component involved in this process of the mineralizing of enamel; amelogins may play a substantial role in controlling the growth and organization of enamel crystals.

After the tooth erupts into the oral cavity, how-ever, the mineralization of enamel continues. This

Clinical Considerations with Enamel

Fluoride can enter the enamel systemically through the blood supply of developing teeth by ingestion of fluoride in drops, tablets, or treated water, all of which are considered preeruptive methods. It can also enter topically by direct contact on exposed teeth surfaces by ingestion of fluoridated water or professional application or directed use of prescription or over-the-counter rinses, gels, foams, chewable tablets, and fluoridated toothpastes, all of which are considered posteruptive methods. Fluoride in prophylaxis pastes provides only brief action and must not take the place of topical applications of fluoride in dental offices.

The most recent theory of systemic fluoride action proposes that fluoride enters the crystalline formation of enamel during tooth development. This action may produce differences in the morphology of the teeth, resulting in more caries-resistant teeth, which are slightly smaller in their occlusal surfaces and have shallow grooves. Further studies in this area are necessary for a complete understanding of the role of fluoride during tooth development.

In contrast, new studies have shown that topical (as opposed to systemic) uses of fluoride have a more important role in caries control than previously thought. Use of topical fluoride results in an increased level of remineralization of any demineralized regions at the surface, which can actually reverse the carious process. Remineralization is the deposition of minerals into enamel in a way that resembles that of posteruptive maturation, although the minerals are deposited into previously demineralized enamel. This remineralization may produce an enamel crystal that is larger and thus more resistant to acid attack. In addition to its direct mineralizing effect on enamel, fluoride may affect oral bacteria by interfering with the actual microbial acid production, reducing potential enamel destruction. Thus the need for daily topical fluoride exposure through the use of a combination of fluoride therapies has been demonstrated for all age groups.

Just as important, excess fluoride taken systemically during tooth development can cause a type of enamel dysplasia (see Chapter 6 for more information). This type of enamel dysplasia is called *dental fluorosis,* and its intrinsic staining can occur in areas where the water naturally has too much fluoride (Figure 12-5). Affected teeth appear mottled in coloration. It can also occur with younger children who ingest too much sweetly flavored fluoridated toothpaste.

posteruptive maturation is due to a depositing of minerals such as fluoride and calcium from saliva into hypomineralized areas of enamel (see discussion of fluoride, next).

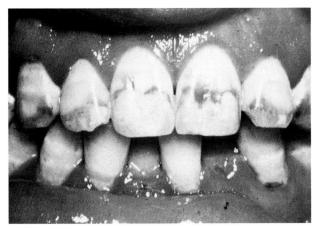

FIGURE 12-5 Dental fluorosis with its intrinsic staining caused by ingestion of excess amounts of fluoride that occurred naturally in a certain water system.

COMPONENTS OF MATURE ENAMEL

Enamel rods, or enamel prisms, are the crystalline structural unit of enamel (Figure 12-6). The enamel rods and associated structures are best viewed under a microscope to obtain the best understanding of them. Most enamel rods extend the width of the enamel from the DEJ to the outer enamel surface. Consequently, each enamel rod is oriented somewhat perpendicular to the DEJ and the outer enamel surface (from less than 90 degrees to 60 degrees). Thus each enamel rod varies in length because the width of enamel varies in different locations of the crown area. Those near the cusps or incisal edges, where the enamel is the thickest, are quite long compared with those near the CEJ. However, the course of the rods from these two end points is not an overall straight course. Rather, the rods show varying degrees of curvature from the DEJ to the outer enamel surface. This curved course of the enamel rods reflects the movements of the ameloblasts during enamel production.

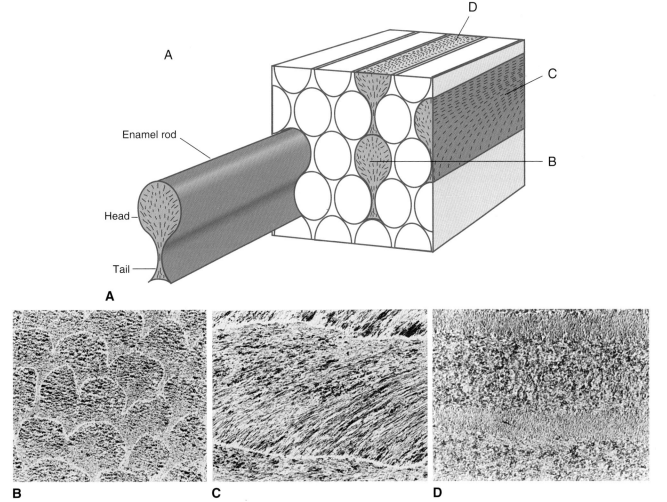

FIGURE 12-6 Enamel rod, the basic unit of enamel. **A:** Its relationship to the enamel of the tooth. **B:** Cross section of the enamel rod. **C** and **D:** Crystal orientation along the other two faces of an enamel block. (Transmission electron micrographs from Nanci A. *Ten Cate's Oral Histology*, ed 6. Mosby, St. Louis, 2003.)

The specific shape of each enamel rod is dictated by Tomes' process of the ameloblast. Generally, each enamel rod is cylindrical in longitudinal section. In most areas of enamel, the enamel rod is also 4 micrometers in diameter. There seems to be less of an emphasis on the classical model in cross section, with its keyhole or fish-scale shape, because there are so many variations in the structural arrangement of the enamel components.

In most of the enamel, the enamel rods are stacked in rows (see Figure 12-6). Surrounding the outer portion is the **interprismatic region,** or interrod enamels, as designated by some histologists. This interprismatic region appears different from the rod core on cross-sections because of its different crystalline orientation. Whether an organic rod sheath or lesser-mineralized interprismatic substance exists between the enamel rods remains controversial.

FURTHER MICROSCOPIC FEATURES OF MATURE ENAMEL

Mature enamel has certain microscopic features that must be identified to facilitate a subsequent discussion of the nature of enamel. The **dentinoenamel junction** (DEJ) between mature enamel and dentin appears scalloped on a cross section of a tooth (Figure 12-7). The convex side of the DEJ is toward the dentin, and the concave side is toward the enamel. This difference in the length of the enamel rods and corresponding dentinal tubules occurs during the apposition of the two tissues (see Chapter 6). Dental professionals must remember that the DEJ was formerly the basement membrane between the enamel organ and the dental papilla. In reality, the DEJ is simply a ridge between

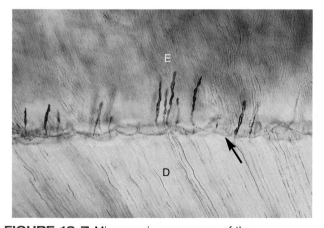

FIGURE 12-7 Microscopic appearance of the dentinoenamel junction (DEJ) *(arrow)* is scalloped, with the concave side of the DEJ toward the enamel *(E)*, and convex side toward the dentin *(D)*. (Courtesy of Dr. James McIntosh, PhD, Department of Biomedical Sciences, Baylor College of Dentistry, Dallas, TX.)

the two tissues that allows increased adherence between them, adding to the strength of the junction when the teeth are in function during mastication. Thus the DEJ is most pronounced in the coronal region, where occlusal forces are the greatest.

The **lines of Retzius** appear as incremental lines that stain brown in preparations of mature enamel (Figure 12-8). These lines are composed of bands or cross-striations on the enamel rods that, when combined in longitudinal sections, seem to traverse the enamel rods. On transverse sections of enamel, the lines of Retzius appear as concentric rings similar to the growth rings in a tree.

Associated with the lines of Retzius are the raised **imbrication lines** and grooves of **perikymata** noted on the nonmasticatory surfaces of some teeth in the oral cavity. The imbrication lines and perikymata are usually lost through wear, except on the protected cervical regions of some teeth, especially the permanent maxillary central incisors, canines, and first premolars.

The exact mechanism that produces these lines is still being debated. Some researchers hypothesize that the lines are a result of the diurnal, or 24-hour, metabolic rhythm of the ameloblasts, which consists of an active secretory work period followed by an inactive rest period. Thus each band on the enamel rod demonstrates the work/rest pattern of the ameloblasts that generally occurs over a span of a week.

The **neonatal line** is an accentuated incremental line of Retzius (Figure 12-9). The neonatal line marks the stress or trauma experienced by the ameloblasts during birth, again illustrating the sensitivity of the ameloblasts as they form enamel matrix. Microscopically, the darkened neonatal line marks the border between the enamel matrix formed before and after birth. As one would expect, the neonatal line is found in all primary teeth and in the larger cusps of the permanent first molars.

Enamel spindles are another microscopic feature of mature enamel and represent short dentinal tubules near the DEJ (Figure 12-10). Enamel spindles result from odontoblasts that crossed the basement membrane before it mineralized into the DEJ. Thus these dentinal tubules become trapped during the apposition of enamel matrix, and enamel becomes mineralized around them. Enamel spindles are especially noted beneath the cusps and incisal tips of the teeth. Clinical implications of enamel spindles are unknown at this time, and it is doubtful that these dentinal tubules contain live odontoblastic processes.

Enamel tufts are another microscopic feature and are noted as small, dark brushes with their bases near the DEJ (Figure 12-11). Enamel tufts are found in the inner one third of enamel and represent areas of less mineralization. They are an anomaly of crystallization and seem to have no clinical importance. Enamel tufts are best seen on transverse sections of enamel.

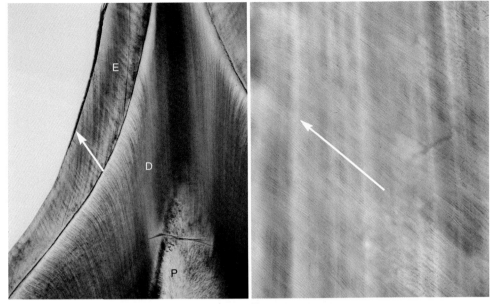

A

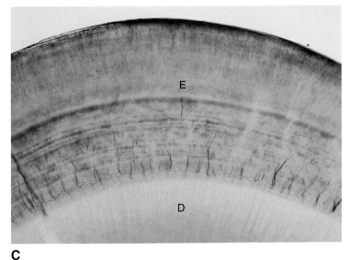

B

C

FIGURE 12-8 A microscopic view of the lines of Retzius that traverse the enamel rods in enamel. **A:** Long section of enamel (E) with its enamel rods (arrow) as it overlies dentin (D) and pulp (P) in the crown area. **B:** Close-up view of enamel rods (direction shown by arrow) so that the lines of Retzius are perpendicular to the rods. **C:** Cross section of enamel (E) as it overlies dentin (D) so that the lines of Retzius resemble the growth rings of a tree. (Courtesy of Dr. James McIntosh, PhD, Department of Biomedical Sciences, Baylor College of Dentistry, Dallas, TX.)

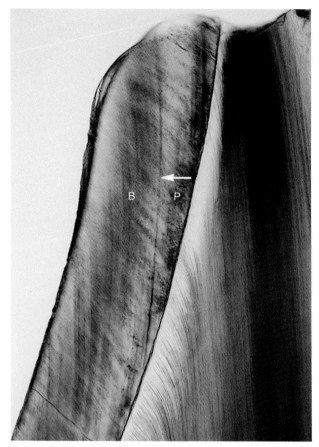

FIGURE 12-9 Microscopic view of the neonatal line *(arrow),* a pronounced line of Retzius, that corresponds to the birth of the individual. Thus it demarcates the enamel formed prenatally *(P)* and after birth *(B).* (Courtesy of Dr. James McIntosh, PhD, Department of Biomedical Sciences, Baylor College of Dentistry, Dallas, TX.)

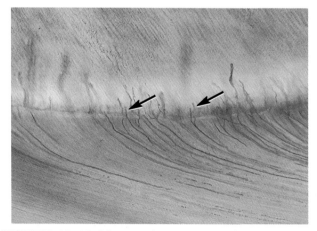

FIGURE 12-10 Microscopic appearance of enamel spindles *(arrows)* within the enamel and near the dentinoenamel junction. (Courtesy of Dr. James McIntosh, PhD, Department of Biomedical Sciences, Baylor College of Dentistry, Dallas, TX.)

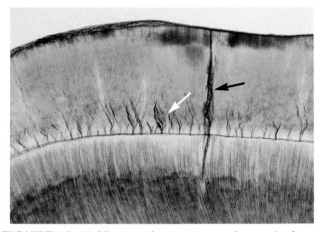

FIGURE 12-11 Microscopic appearance of enamel tufts *(white arrow)* and enamel lamella *(black arrow)* on this transverse section of enamel. (Courtesy of Dr. James McIntosh, PhD, Department of Biomedical Sciences, Baylor College of Dentistry, Dallas, TX.)

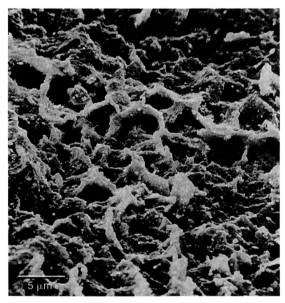

FIGURE 12-12 Photomicrograph showing the enamel rods after acid etching, which demineralizes the interprismatic region to allow the flow of the enamel sealant into the enamel for greater strength. (From Nanci A. *Ten Cate's Oral Histology,* ed 6. Mosby, St. Louis, 2003.)

Enamel lamellae are partially calcified vertical sheets of enamel matrix that extend from the DEJ near the tooth's cervix to the outer occlusal surface (see Figure 12-11). Enamel lamellae are narrower and longer than enamel tufts. This is another anomaly of crystallization that has unknown clinical importance. Enamel lamellae are best seen on transverse sections of enamel. Both enamel tufts and lamellae may be likened to geologic faults in mature enamel.

Clinical Considerations with the Microscopic Features of Enamel

Microscopic features must be taken into consideration during clinical treatment involving enamel. Enamel resembles a mild steel product in hardness, which also makes its brittle; therefore an underlying layer of more resistant dentin must be present to maintain its integrity. This property, along with the direction of the enamel rods, is taken into consideration during cavity preparation. The decay and adjacent portions of the enamel are removed in a way that allows all the enamel rods to remain supported by other rods and the underlying dentin. An isolated enamel rod is extremely brittle and breaks away easily. If enamel rods are undercut during cavity preparation, they may break, thus rendering the margin of restoration possibly leaky and thus defective. This brittleness of unsupported enamel also is noted during caries: The enamel breaks away easily, as the dentin is undermined beneath it.

In some cases, an acid etch is briefly used to remove some of the organic portions of the enamel crystals, enabling an enamel sealant to flow into the newly created gaps and thus offer more surface area for better adherence (Figure 12-12). This demineralization by acid etching is thus rendering seen grossly as the surface of enamel whitens. When placing these types of enamel sealants, dental professionals must be careful to protect the demineralized enamel surface from being contaminated and remineralized by saliva, thereby reducing sealant uptake. Acid etch is also used to prepare the enamel surface for other restorative procedures.

Whitening of the teeth to remove staining that has occurred as a result of lifestyle choices (e.g., ingestion of dark drinks and foods and use of tobacco) is of increased importance to the dental profession. Studies show that patients who have whitened their teeth take better care of them. Staining occurs in the interprismatic region internally on the enamel, which causes the tooth to appear darker or more yellow overall. In a perfect state, enamel is basically colorless, but it does reflect underlying tooth structure with its stains. Light reflection properties of the tooth are low. Oxygen radicals from the peroxide in the whitening agents come in contact with stains in the interprismatic spaces within the enamel layer. When this occurs, stains will be bleached. The teeth now appear lighter in color. Teeth not only appear whiter but also reflect light in increased amounts, which makes the teeth appear brighter as well.

CHAPTER 13

Dentin and Pulp

■ ■ ■

This chapter discusses the following topics:

- Dentin-pulp complex
- Dentin
  - Apposition of dentin matrix
  - Maturation of dentin
  - Components of mature dentin
  - Types of dentin
  - Microscopic features of mature dentin
  - Age changes in dentin
- Pulp
  - Anatomy of pulp
  - Microscopic features of pulp
  - Microscopic zones in pulp
  - Age-related changes in pulp
- Growth factors and dentin-pulp complex

■ ■ ■

After studying this chapter, the reader should be able to:

1. Define and pronounce the key terms in this chapter.
2. Discuss the dentin-pulp complex and describe the properties of dentin and pulp.
3. Discuss the apposition and maturation of dentin.
4. Outline the types of dentin.
5. Label the anatomical components of pulp.
6. Indicate and discuss the microscopic features of dentin and pulp.
7. Describe the age-related changes in pulp and dentin.
8. Integrate the knowledge of the histology with the clinical considerations involved in dentin and pulp.

■ ■ ■

Key Terms

Accessory canals
Apical foramen (ay-pi-kl for-ay-men)
Attrition (ah-trish-un)
Calcium hydroxyapatite
  (hy-drox-see-ap-ah-tite)
Caries
Cementum (see-men-tum)
Contour lines of Owen

Dentin: circumpulpal
  (serk-um-pul-pal), hypersensitivity
  (hi-per-sen-si-tiv-it-ee), intertubular
  (in-ter-tube-u-lar), mantle,
  peritubular, (pare-i-tube-u-lar),
  primary, secondary, tertiary
Dentinal fluid, tubules
Dentinogenesis (den-tin-oh-jen-i-sis)

Fibroblast (fi-bro-blast)
Gingival recession
  (re-sesh-un)
Globular dentin
Imbrication (im-bri-kay-shun) lines of
  von Ebner (eeb-ner)
Interglobular dentin
Neonatal line (ne-oh-nate-l)

Odontoblastic process
(oh-don-toe-**blast**-ik)
Odontoblasts (oh-**don**-toe-blasts)

Outer cells of the dental papilla
Predentin
Pulp: chamber, coronal, horns,

radicular (rah-dik-u-lar), stones
Pulpitis
Tomes' granular layer (tomes)

DENTIN-PULP COMPLEX

Unlike enamel, dentin and pulp cannot be viewed clinically if the teeth and associated periodontium are healthy. Dentin and pulp make up the inner portions of the tooth and are not exposed except when certain dental pathology exists. In addition, because of their shared embryological background, close proximity, and interdependence, dentin and pulp form a dentin-pulp complex. Thus this chapter discusses these two tissues together as one developmental and functioning unit.

Dental professionals must have an increased understanding of the histology of these two tissues. In the past, these two inner tissues were thought of as being analogous to a black box opened only by the dentist and thus hidden from the rest of the dental staff. With the advent of expanded responsibilities and increased preventive concerns for patients, all members of the dental team must be able to see into these interesting and important areas.

DENTIN

Mature dentin is a crystalline material that is less hard than enamel (see Table 6-2). Mature dentin is by weight 70 percent mineralized inorganic material, 20 percent organic material, and 10 percent water. This crystalline formation of mature dentin consists of mainly **calcium hydroxyapatite** with the chemical formula of $Ca_{10}(PO_4)_6(OH)_2$. This calcium hydroxyapatite is similar to that found in higher percentages in enamel and in lower percentages in bone and **cementum.** In addition, the crystals in dentin are platelike and smaller than those in enamel.

Small amounts of other minerals, such as carbonate and fluoride, are also present. Dentin is covered by enamel in the crown and cementum in the root and thus encloses the innermost pulp tissue. Thus dentin makes up the bulk of the tooth and protects the pulp.

Because of the translucency of overlying enamel, the dentin of the tooth gives the white enamel crown its underlying yellow hue. If the outer coverings of enamel and cementum are lost (discussed later), the exposed dentin is various shades of yellow-white and appears rougher in surface texture than enamel. Yet dentin is softer than enamel when instruments are

used, allowing removal with hand instruments even in a healthy state, unlike enamel.

On radiographs, the differences in the mineralization levels of different portions of the tooth can be noted. Enamel appears more radiopaque (lighter) than dentin, which appears more radiolucent (darker), and more radiopaque than pulp.

Clinical Considerations with Dentin

Attrition, which is the wearing away of a tooth surface through tooth-to-tooth contact, can also occur in dentin. Attrition is discussed in Chapter 12 in relation to enamel, demonstrated in Chapters 16 and 17 in relation to specific teeth, and in Chapter 20 in relation to oral habits. In contrast to hard enamel, this attrition can occur at a more rapid rate when dentin is exposed because its mineralized content is lower.

Coronal dentin can be exposed after attrition of the enamel and with certain enamel dysplasias. Coronal dentin can also become exposed when a patient asks to have the incisal edge filed with tooth-colored restorative materials on anteriors when trauma causes it to become chipped or worn. Root dentin can be exposed when the thin layer of cementum is lost as a result of **gingival recession** (Figure 13-1). Gingival recession, with its lower margin of the free gingival crest, is discussed in Chapter 10. Dentin that is lost externally is not fully replaced by the possible addition of secondary dentin inside the tooth along the outer pulpal wall (discussed later).

Another way that dentin is exposed and then lost is through **caries**, the demineralization and loss of portions of the tooth resulting from cariogenic bacteria (discussed later). Finally, cavity preparation by the dentist exposes and then removes carious dentin. Dentin demineralizes when the pH is less than 6.8.

Newly exposed dentin is already more yellow than the whiter enamel. When dentin remains exposed, over time it can also pick up food and tobacco stains, becoming more yellowish or even brown to black (see Figure 13-1). Dentin absorbs these stains because it is more porous than intact enamel. Dentin is porous from both its high organic content and the presence of dentinal tubules, acting as a sponge to contain these staining products. These stains are aesthetic concerns for some patients.

Removal of these stains by hand instrumentation or prophy jet device can remove even more dentin; thus ultrasonics, which remove no hard tooth products when used correctly, may be the correct choice for removal. Sensitivity can be curtailed with certain products or local anesthetia. Vital bleaching of the teeth may also be performed either at the office or in the home; bleaching at home must be done with appropriate supervision because it may lead to dentin hypersensitivity (discussed later).

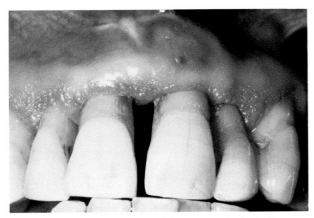

FIGURE 13-1 Clinical view of the areas of gingival recession. Note the difference in color between whiter enamel and darker dentin, which can also undergo staining when exposed.

Apposition of Dentin Matrix

Dentinogenesis is the process of dentin matrix or **predentin** formation that occurs during the apposition stage of tooth development. The exact time of the apposition stage varies according to the tooth that is undergoing development. Many factors can affect dentinogenesis (see Chapter 6).

Predentin is the initial material laid down by the **odontoblasts** (Figure 13-2). It is a mesenchymal product consisting of nonmineralized collagen fibers. Odontoblasts were originally the **outer cells of the dental papilla.** Dentin and pulp tissue thus have similar embryological backgrounds because both are derived from the dental papilla of the tooth germ. These odontoblasts are induced by the newly formed ameloblasts to produce predentin in layers, moving away from the dentinoenamel junction (DEJ). Unlike cartilage and bone, the odontoblast's cell body does not become entrapped in the product; rather, one long cytoplasmic extension remains behind in the dentin. Odontoblasts form approximately 4 micrometers of predentin daily.

Apposition of dentin, unlike enamel, occurs throughout the life of the tooth (discussed later). Although ameloblasts are lost after the eruption of the tooth and enamel production ceases, production of dentin continues because of the retention of the odontoblasts along the outer pulpal wall, inside the tooth.

Maturation of Dentin

Maturation of dentin or mineralization of predentin occurs soon after its apposition. The process of dentin maturation takes place in two steps or phases (Figure 13-3). Initially, the calcium hydroxyapatite crystals form as globules, or calcospherules, in the collagen

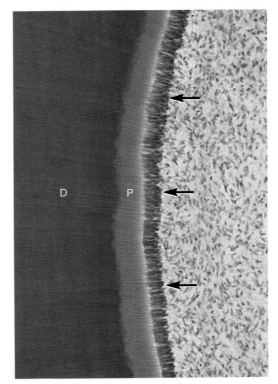

FIGURE 13-2 Microscopic view of odontoblasts *(arrows)* producing predentin *(P)* that will mature into dentin *(D)*. (Courtesy of Dr. James McIntosh, PhD, Department of Biomedical Sciences, Baylor College of Dentistry, Dallas, TX.)

fibers of the predentin, expanding and fusing together during the primary mineralization phase. This process is analogous to the wash of watercolor paint placed on wet paper for background as the blobs of color run into each other, although in dentin it is a three-dimensional process.

Later, new areas of mineralization occur as globules form in the partially mineralized predentin during the secondary mineralization phase. These new areas of crystal formation are more or less regularly layered on the initial crystals, and these also expand but fuse incompletely. This process is analogous to additional blobs of paint placed in specific areas over the painted background, but the colors of this additional layer do not run into each other to cover the page because the paper is no longer wet.

The incomplete fusion during the secondary mineralization phase results in differences noted in the microscopic features of the crystalline form of dentin. In areas where both primary and secondary mineralization have occurred with complete crystalline fusion, these appear as lighter rounded areas on dentin sections and are called **globular dentin** (Figure 13-4).

In contrast, the dark, arclike areas in dentin histological sections are called **interglobular dentin.** In these areas, only primary mineralization has occurred within the predentin, and the globules of dentin did not fuse completely. Thus interglobular dentin is

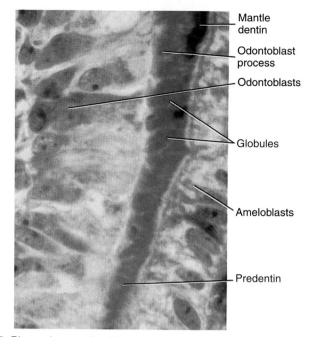

Mantle
dentin

Odontoblast
process

Odontoblasts

Globules

Ameloblasts

Predentin

FIGURE 13-3 Photomicrograph of the maturation of dentin showing the odontoblasts producing predentin, which contains odontoblastic processes. Note that the predentin matures by forming globules, which undergo mineralization or calcification into mature dentin (mantle). This area of dentin is adjacent to the dentinoenamel junction, with the ameloblasts on the opposite side. (From Nanci A. *Ten Cate's Oral Histology*, ed 6. Mosby, St. Louis, 2003.)

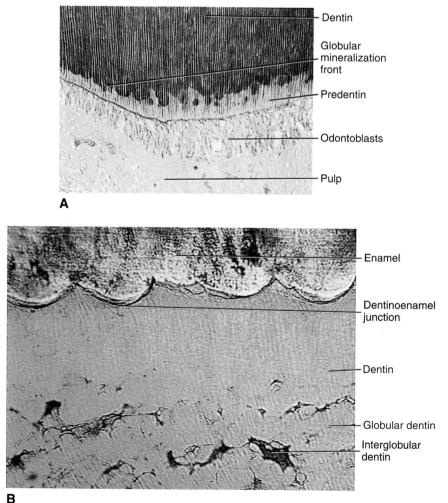

Dentin

Globular
mineralization
front

Predentin

Odontoblasts

Pulp

A

Enamel

Dentinoenamel
junction

Dentin

Globular dentin

Interglobular
dentin

B

FIGURE 13-4 Globular and interglobular dentin. **A:** Silver-stained section of dentin, demonstrating the globular mineralized front near the outer pulpal wall during primary mineralization. **B:** Ground section of mature dentin near the dentinoenamel junction, with highly mineralized or calcified globular dentin and less mineralized interglobular dentin after both primary and secondary mineralization. (From Nanci A. *Ten Cate's Oral Histology*, ed 6. Mosby, St. Louis, 2003.)

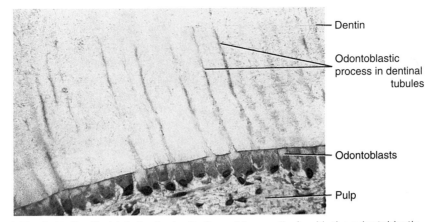

FIGURE 13-5 Dentinal tubules in dentin (top of the section), with the odontoblastic processes entering the tubules from the pulp tissue. The pulp tissue contains a layer of the cell bodies of odontoblasts to which the odontoblastic processes are still attached. (From Nanci A. *Ten Cate's Oral Histology*, ed 6. Mosby, St. Louis, 2003.)

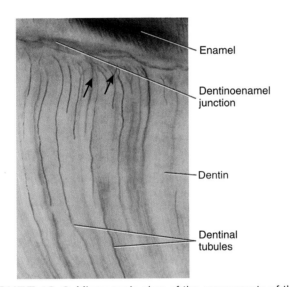

FIGURE 13-6 Microscopic view of the components of the dentinal tubule within the dentin, deep to the dentinoenamel junction and the enamel. The dentinal tubules contain odontoblastic processes *(arrows)* and dentinal fluid. (From Nanci A. *Ten Cate's Oral Histology*, ed 6. Mosby, St. Louis, 2003.)

slightly less mineralized than globular dentin. Interglobular dentin is especially evident in coronal dentin and near the DEJ and in certain dental anomalies (such as in dentin dysplasia; see Chapter 6).

Components of Mature Dentin

Within mature dentin, certain components, such as **dentinal tubules** and their contents, are noted (Figures 13-5 and 13-6). Dentinal tubules are long tubes in the dentin that extend from the DEJ in the crown area or dentinocemental junction (DCJ) in the root area to the outer wall of the pulp. After apposition of predentin

and maturation into dentin, the cell bodies of the odontoblasts remain in the pulp along its outer wall and inside the tooth (discussed later).

Like enamel, dentin is avascular. Nutrition for odontoblasts comes by way of the tubule from tissue fluid originally from the blood vessels located in the adjacent pulp tissue. Within the dentinal tubule is a space of variable size containing dentinal fluid, an odontoblastic process, and possibly an afferent axon.

The **dentinal fluid** in the tubule is presumably tissue fluid surrounding the cell membrane of the odontoblast, which is continuous from the cell body in the pulp. The **odontoblastic process** is a long cellular extension located within the dentinal tubule and still attached to the cell body of the odontoblast within the pulp. In a section of a tooth, odontoblastic processes within the dentinal tubule sometimes are not found at the periphery of dentin near the DEJ or DCJ. This absence may or may not be an artifact, given that cell structures are difficult to preserve in mineralized tissues.

Present evidence related to the controversy about the extent of the process within the tubule suggests that the process occupies the full length of the tubule from the DEJ or DCJ to the pulp during only the early stages of odontogenesis. In mature dentin, however, the process may or may not run the full length of the tubule to extend near the DEJ or DCJ.

A sensory or afferent axon is associated with part of the odontoblastic process in some dentinal tubules. This myelinated axon may not extend farther than the process and thus may not be found along the DEJ or DCJ. Yet the nerve cell body associated with the axon is located in the pulp along with the odontoblastic cell body. This axon is involved in the sensation of pain only (discussed later).

Primary curvature
of dentinal tubules

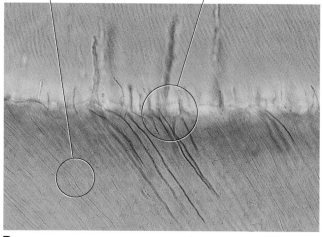

A

Secondary curvature
of dentinal tubules

Branching of
dentinal tubules

B

FIGURE 13-7 Two types of curvature of the dentinal tubules noted in dentin. **A:** Primary curvature. **B:** Secondary curvature, with branching noted near the dentinoenamel junction. (Courtesy of Dr. James McIntosh, PhD, Department of Biomedical Sciences, Baylor College of Dentistry, Dallas, TX.)

The direction of the tubule reflects the pathway of the odontoblast during apposition of predentin. There are two types of curvature established by the direction of the dental tubules: primary and secondary (Figure 13-7). The primary curvature of the dentinal tubules reflects the overall tubule course, which resembles a

large S-shaped curve. The secondary curvature of the tubule consists of small, delicate curves noted in the primary curvature, reflecting the smaller daily changes in odontoblast direction during apposition. Dentinal tubules are not interrupted by the interglobular areas of dentin but pass right through them. Tubules can branch at any point along the way from the DEJ or DCJ to the pulp. Dentinal tubules are crowded near the pulp because of the narrowing of this region (see Figure 13-5).

Clinical Considerations with Dentin Structure

The dentinal tubules serve as an entry for cariogenic microorganisms when caries extends from the enamel into the dentin (Figure 13-8). Microscopically, the microorganisms can be seen actually using the dentinal tubules as chutes toward the pulp because of their connection with the odontoblasts in the outer pulpal wall. When caries extends into the dentin from enamel (enamel caries is discussed in Chapter 12), the carious process moves more rapidly because of the increased organic composition of dentin as compared with enamel. In addition, because of the primary curvature of the dentinal tubules, the pulp may be affected at a more apical level than the level at which the external injury (such as caries) occurred. Cavity preparation takes this into account when carious dentin is removed.

When dentin is exposed as a result of caries, cavity preparation, recession, or attrition, the open dentinal tubules may be painful for the patient, causing **dentin hypersensitivity**. In some cases, the enamel and cementum do not meet, leaving the dentin exposed at the CEJ area (see Chapter 14). In addition, protective layers of cementum and dentin can be removed by aggressive scaling with hand instruments. Certain situations may trigger the short, sharp pain of dentin hypersensitivity, such as stimuli from thermal changes (cold water spray or ice), mechanical irritation (vibrations from instrumentation, handpieces, or ultrasonics), dehydration (stream of air or heat during cavity preparation), or chemical exposure (foods such as thick or hypertonic sweet, salty, or sour fluids; tooth-colored restorative materials; or vital bleaching agents). By contrast, the pain from other tooth-related situations are usually dull and chronic in nature.

However, dentin hypersensitivity is often diffuse, making localization difficult for the dental professional as well as the patient. This pain may wrongly be interpreted as a result of caries, pulpal or gingival infections, or soft tissue inflammation. Because of their chronic nature, attrition and recession may not be as painful as other forms of dentinal exposure because both are gradual and allow time for subtle changes to occur in the dentinal tubules to close them off from the stimulation (discussed later). Dentin hypersensitivity can occur with all teeth but is especially evident in premolars and canines, almost always on the facial or other cervical areas.

The latest theory of dentin hypersensitivity suggests that it is due to changes in the dentinal fluid associated with the processes, a type of hydrodynamic mechanism (Figure 13-9). This mechanism may be due to one or more of the following: evaporation and loss of dentinal fluid, movement of the fluid, and ionic changes in the fluid. These changes in the dentinal fluid are then transmitted to the afferent axon present in some tubules near the pulp, thus sending a painful message to the pulp and then on to the brain. That is possibly the reason that the previously mentioned painful situations are involved in dentin hypersensitivity: because they are involved in dentinal fluid movement within the tubule and because local anesthetics do not block sensation, as they would a fully innervated tissue, when they are placed on the surface of exposed dentin. However, in the future, more than one theory may explain surface dentinal pain.

Dentin hypersensitivity can be treated somewhat successfully with solutions applied either by professionals or within dentifrices. These desensitizing agents either temporarily block the exposed open ends of the dentinal tubules, similar to the way some staining products do, or interfere with nerve transmission in areas with dentin hypersensitivity. However, restorations sometimes are the only way to reduce hypersensitivity of the exposed dentinal surface in severe cases. Methods that will fully seal the dentinal tubules and thus prevent any dentin hypersensitivity are being studied.

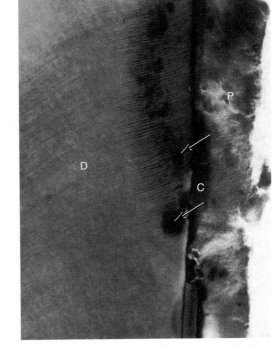

FIGURE 13-8 Photomicrograph of caries of dentin showing the cariogenic microorganisms entering the deeper portions of the dentin *(D)* by way of the dentinal tubules *(arrows)*. Note that the cementum *(C)* has already been invaded by the cariogenic microorganisms from the bacterial plaque biofilm *(P)* covering the root area. (From Perry DA, Beemsterboer PL, Taggart EJ. *Clinical Periodontology for Dental Hygienists,* ed 2. WB Saunders, Philadelphia, 2001.)

Types of Dentin

Dentin is not a uniform tissue in the tooth but differs from region to region (Table 13-1). Different types of dentin can be designated by their relationship to the dentinal tubules (Figure 13-10; see also Figure 13-5). Dentin that creates the wall of the dentinal tubule is called **peritubular dentin**. Peritubular dentin is highly mineralized after dentin maturation. The dentin that is found between the tubules is called **intertubular dentin**. Intertubular dentin is highly mineralized, but less so than peritubular dentin.

Dentin can also be categorized by its relationship to the DEJ and pulp (Figure 13-11). **Mantle dentin** is the first predentin that forms and matures within the tooth. Mantle dentin shows a difference in the direction of the mineralized collagen fibers compared with the rest of the dentin, with the fibers perpendicular to the DEJ. Mantle dentin also has more peritubular dentin than the inner portions of dentin and thus has higher levels of mineralization.

TABLE 13-1

Types of Dentin

Type	Location/Chronology	Description
Peritubular dentin	Wall of tubules	Highly calcified
Intertubular dentin	Between the tubules	Highly calcified
Mantle dentin	Outermost layer	First dentin formed
Circumpulpal dentin	Layer around outer pulpal wall	Dentin formed after mantle dentin
Primary dentin	Formed before completion of apical foramen	Formed more rapidly; is more mineralized than secondary
Secondary dentin	Formed after completion of apical foramen	Formed slower and is less mineralized than primary
Tertiary dentin	Formed as a result of injury	Irregular pattern of tubules

The layer of dentin around the outer pulpal wall is called **circumpulpal dentin**. All circumpulpal dentin is formed and matures after mantle dentin. The collagen fibers of circumpulpal dentin are mainly parallel to the DEJ compared with those of mantle dentin. The bulk of the dentin in a tooth is this type.

Dentin can also be categorized according to the time that it was formed within the tooth (Figure 13-12). **Primary dentin** is the dentin formed in a tooth before the completion of the apical foramen of the root, which is the opening in the root's pulp canal. Primary dentin is characterized by its regular pattern of tubules.

Secondary dentin is the dentin that is formed after the completion of the apical foramen and continues to form throughout the life of the tooth. Secondary dentin is formed more slowly than primary dentin and is less mineralized. Secondary dentin fills in along the outer pulpal wall. It is made by the odontoblastic layer that lines the dentin-pulp interface. Secondary dentin is noted for its regular pattern of tubules. Microscopically, a dark line shows the junction between the primary and secondary dentin that results from an abrupt change in the course of the odontoblasts during apposition. Certain medications placed during cavity preparation can promote the formation of secondary dentin and thus help protect the underlying pulp tissue.

Reparative, reactive, or **tertiary dentin** is dentin formed quickly in localized regions in response to a localized injury to the exposed dentin (see Figure 13-12). Tertiary dentin thus forms underneath the exposed dentin's tubules along the outer pulpal wall. The injury could be caries, cavity preparation, attri-tion, or recession. Odontoblasts in the area of the affected tubules might perish because of the injury, but neighboring undifferentiated mesenchymal cells of the pulp move and become odontoblasts. Tertiary dentin tries to seal off the injured area, thus the term

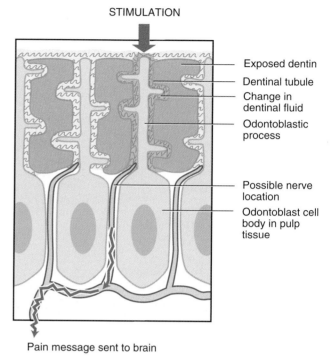

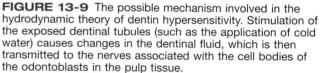

FIGURE 13-9 The possible mechanism involved in the hydrodynamic theory of dentin hypersensitivity. Stimulation of the exposed dentinal tubules (such as the application of cold water) causes changes in the dentinal fluid, which is then transmitted to the nerves associated with the cell bodies of the odontoblasts in the pulp tissue.

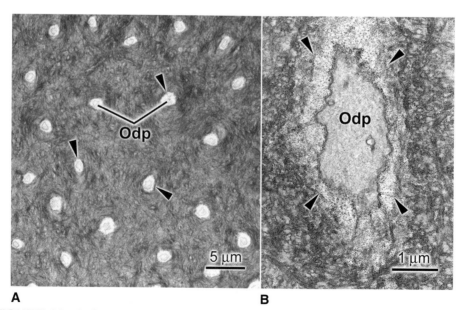

FIGURE 13-10 Cross section of dentinal tubules, composed of peritubular dentin *(arrows)* containing odontoblastic processes *(Odp)* and surrounded by intertubular dentin. **A:** Photomicrograph. **B:** Transmission electromicrograph. (From Nanci A. *Ten Cate's Oral Histology*, ed 6. Mosby, St. Louis, 2003.)

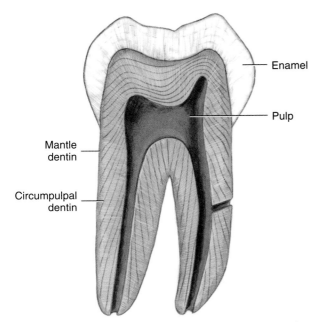

FIGURE 13-11 The two types of dentin in relation to the dentinoenamel junction and pulp: mantle dentin and circumpulpal dentin.

reparative dentin. The tubules in tertiary dentin assume a more irregular course than in secondary dentin.

A certain type of tertiary dentin, sclerotic dentin, is often found in association with the chronic injury of caries and also is noted to increase as the tooth ages. In this type of dentin, the odontoblastic processes die and leave the dentinal tubules vacant. The hollow dentinal tubules become retrofilled and occluded by a mineralized substance similar to peritubular dentin. This type of dentin may be involved in prolonging pulp vitality because it reduces the permeability of dentin. Clinically, the dentin in this type of arrested caries appears dark, smooth, and shiny.

Microscopic Features of Mature Dentin

When mature dentin is examined microscopically, certain features such as dentinal tubules and the types of dentin are noted. The dentinal process within the tubule is hard to discern microscopically. Other microscopic features are also noted and will be discussed further. These features can occur in both primary and secondary dentin.

The **imbrication lines of von Ebner** in dentin are incremental lines or bands that stain darkly and can be likened to the growth rings or incremental lines of Retzius noted in enamel (Figure 13-13). They show the incremental nature of dentin apposition and run at right angles to the dentinal tubules. With each daily 4-micrometer increment of dentin, the orientation of the deposited collagen fibers differs slightly. More severe changes occur every fifth day, giving rise at every 20 micrometers to an imbrication line.

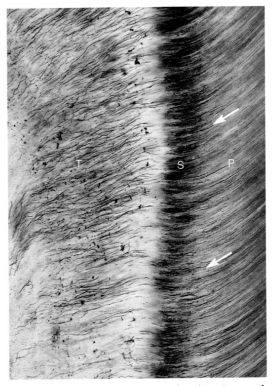

FIGURE 13-12 Microscopic view of various types of dentin in relation to the time they were formed: primary *(P)*, secondary *(S)*, and tertiary *(T)*. Note the dark line between the primary and secondary dentin *(arrows)* caused by an abrupt change in the course of the odontoblasts during apposition. Note also the more irregular course of dentinal tubules in tertiary dentin than in secondary dentin. (Courtesy of Dr. James McIntosh, PhD, Department of Biomedical Sciences, Baylor College of Dentistry, Dallas, TX.)

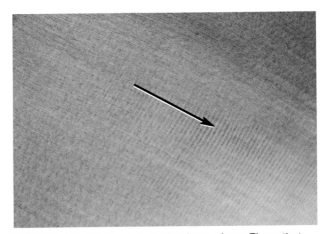

FIGURE 13-13 The imbrication lines of von Ebner that transverse the dentinal tubules (direction of dentinal tubules shown by *arrow*) in dentin. Note its regular pattern. (Courtesy of Dr. James McIntosh, PhD, Department of Biomedical Sciences, Baylor College of Dentistry, Dallas, TX.)

The **contour lines of Owen** are a number of adjoining parallel imbrication lines that are present in stained dentin. These contour lines demonstrate a disturbance in body metabolism that affects the odontoblasts by altering their formation efforts. They appear together

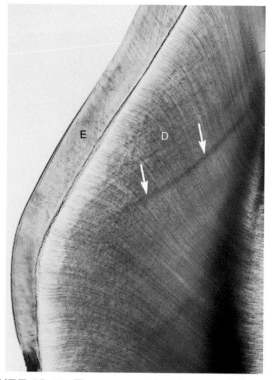

FIGURE 13-14 The pronounced contour line of Owen *(arrows)*, the neonatal line, and other parallel adjoining contour lines in dentin *(D)* underlying enamel *(E)*. (Courtesy of Dr. James McIntosh, PhD, Department of Biomedical Sciences, Baylor College of Dentistry, Dallas, TX.)

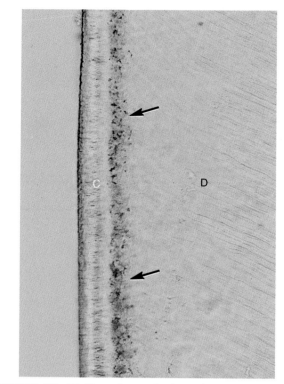

FIGURE 13-15 Tomes' granular layer *(arrows)* noted in dentin *(D)* near the dentinocemental junction underneath layers of cementum *(C)*. (Courtesy of Dr. James McIntosh, PhD, Department of Biomedical Sciences, Baylor College of Dentistry, Dallas, TX.)

as a series of dark bands. The most pronounced contour line is the **neonatal line** that occurs during the trauma of birth (Figure 13-14). Other contour lines occur with tetracycline staining of the teeth, in which the antibiotic becomes permanently and chemically bound to the dentin (see Chapter 3 for more information).

Tomes' granular layer is most often found in the peripheral portion of dentin beneath the root's cementum, adjacent to the DCJ (Figure 13-15). This area only looks granular because of its spotty microscopic appearance. The cause of the change in this region of dentin is unknown. It may be due to less calcified areas of dentin similar to interglobular dentin or loops of the terminal portions of branching dentinal tubules found near the DCJ similar to that of the DEJ.

Age Changes in Dentin

With increased age, the diameter of the dentinal tubule narrows because of deposition of peritubular dentin. This narrowing may be related to the decreased ability of pulp to react to various stimuli with age. With age, the passageways of the tubules to the pulp are not as wide open as in youth; thus the stimuli are not transmitted as rapidly and in as large amounts as they were

previously. Some studies show the complete obliteration of older tubules with mineralization of the associated odontoblastic processes.

Odontoblasts also undergo cytoplasmic changes, including a reduction in organelle content with age. As discussed previously, dentin becomes more exposed as a result of attrition and recession, which may or may not lead to dentin hypersensitivity.

PULP

The pulp is the innermost tissue of the tooth. Pulp appears as a less dense area on radiographs. The pulp of a tooth is a connective tissue with all the components of such a tissue (discussed later). Embryologically, the pulp forms from the central cells of the dental papilla. Thus pulp has a background similar to that of dentin because both are derived from the dental papilla of the tooth germ. During odontogenesis, when the dentin forms around the dental papilla, the innermost tissue is considered pulp.

One important consideration: The pulp is involved in the support, maintenance, and continued formation of dentin because the inner layer of the cell bodies of the odontoblasts remain along the outer pulpal wall (discussed later). Another function of the pulp is sensory because the cell bodies associated with the afferent axons in the dentinal tubules are located among this layer of odontoblasts. When the dentin or pulp is injured, the only sensation perceived by the brain is pain. Therefore changes in temperature, vibrations, and chemical changes that affect the dentin or pulp are perceived only as painful stimuli.

Pulp also has a nutritional function for the dentin because the dentin contains no blood supply of its own. Dentin depends on the pulp's vascular supply and associated tissue fluids for its nutrition. Nutrition is obtained by way of the tubules and their connection to the odontoblasts' cell bodies that line the outer pulpal wall.

Finally, the pulp has a protective function because it is involved in the formation of secondary or tertiary dentin, which increases the coverage of the pulp. In addition, if the pulp suffers any injury that also involves the odontoblasts, its undifferentiated mesenchymal cells can differentiate into fibroblasts, which then create fibers and intercellular substances, as well as odontoblasts, to create more dentin. The pulp also has white blood cells within its vascular system and tissues; these allow triggering of inflammatory and immune responses.

ANATOMY OF PULP

The mass of pulp is contained within the **pulp chamber** of the tooth (Figure 13-16). The shape of the pulp chamber corresponds to the shape of the tooth and is individualized for every tooth (see Chapters 16 and 17 for specific information). The pulp in the pulp chamber has two main divisions: the coronal pulp and the radicular pulp.

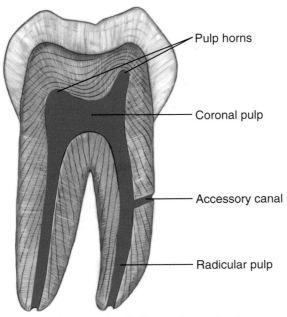

Pulp horns

Coronal pulp

Accessory canal

Radicular pulp

FIGURE 13-16 The anatomy of pulp.

The **coronal pulp** is located in the crown of the tooth. Smaller extensions of coronal pulp into the cusps of posterior teeth form the **pulp horns.** These pulp horns are especially prominent for the permanent dentition, under the buccal cusp of premolars and the mesiobuccal cusp of molars. To prevent exposure of the pulpal tissue, these regions must be taken into consideration during cavity preparation. Pulp horns are not found on anterior teeth.

The **radicular pulp**, or root pulp, is the portion of the pulp located in the root area of the tooth. It is also called the *pulp canal* by patients. The radicular pulp extends from the cervical portion of the tooth to the apex of the tooth. This portion of the pulp has openings from the pulp through the cementum into the surrounding periodontal ligament. These openings include the apical foramen and possibly accessory canals.

The **apical foramen** is the opening from the pulp at the apex of the tooth. This opening is surrounded by cementum and allows arteries, veins, lymphatics, and nerves to enter and exit the pulp from the periodontal ligament (PDL; Tables 13-2 and 13-3). Thus communication between the pulp and the PDL is possible because of the apical foramen. The apical foramen is the last portion of the tooth to form; it forms after the crown erupts into the oral cavity. In developing teeth, the foramen is large and centrally located. As the tooth matures, the foramen becomes smaller in diameter and is offset in position. The foramen may be located at the anatomical apex of the root but is usually located more slightly occlusally from the apex. If more than one foramen is present on the root, the largest one is designated as the apical foramen and the rest are considered accessory foramina.

Accessory canals may also be associated with the pulp and are extra openings from the pulp to the periodontal ligament (Figure 13-17; see also Figure 13-16). Accessory canals are also called *lateral canals* because

TABLE 13-2

Arterial Supply to the Teeth and Associated Periodontium

Teeth and Associated Periodontium	Major Branches of Maxillary Artery
Posterior maxillary and periodontium	Posterior superior alveolar artery
Anterior maxillary and periodontium	Infraorbital artery
Mandibular and periodontium	Inferior alveolar artery

(From Fehrenbach MJ, Herring SW. *Illustrated Anatomy of the Head and Neck*, ed. 2. WB Saunders, Philadelphia, 2002.)

TABLE 13-3

Nerve Supply to the Teeth and Associated Periodontium

Teeth and Associated Peridontium	Branches of Trigeminal Nerve
Maxillary anterior teeth, maxillary anterior facial periodontium	Anterior superior alveolar nerve from maxillary nerve
Maxillary anterior lingual peridontium	Nasopalatine nerve from maxillary nerve
Maxillary posterior teeth, maxillary posterior buccal periodontium	Middle superior alveolar and posterior superior alveolar nerve from maxillary nerve
Maxillary posterior lingual periodontium	Greater palatine nerve from maxillary nerve
Mandibular teeth and facial periodontium of the mandibular anterior teeth and premolars	Inferior alveolar nerve from mandibular nerve
Mandibular posterior buccal periodontium	Long buccal nerve from mandibular nerve
Mandibular lingual periodontium	Lingual nerve from mandibular nerve

(From Fehrenbach MJ, Herring SW. *Illustrated Anatomy of the Head and Neck*, ed. 2. WB Saunders, Philadelphia, 2002.)

they are usually located on the lateral portions of the roots of some teeth. Accessory canals form when Hertwig's epithelial root sheath encounters a blood vessel during root formation. Root structure then forms around the vessel, forming the accessory canal. Teeth have a variable number of these canals, which sometimes poses problems during endodontic therapy or root canal treatment (discussed later). Radiographs do not always indicate the number or position of these canals unless they are examined with instruments and radiopaque materials are used during this therapy.

Microscopic Features of Pulp

Because pulp is a connective tissue, it has all the components of such a tissue: intercellular substance, tissue fluid, cells, lymphatics, vascular system, nerves, and fibers (Figure 13-18). Intercellular substance and tissue fluid are discussed in Chapter 8.

As in all connective tissues, the **fibroblasts** are the largest group of cells in the pulp. Fibroblasts are also discussed in Chapter 8. The odontoblasts are the second largest group of cells in the pulp, but only their

Clinical Considerations with Pulp Tissue

When the pulp is injured by extensive caries, cavity preparation, or traumatic injury, it may undergo inflammation, or **pulpitis.** This inflammation initially remains localized within the confines of the dentin. The pressure from this confined pulpitis can result in extreme pain as the inflammatory edema presses on the afferent nerves contained in the pulp.

Pulpitis can later cause a pulpal infection in the form of a periapical abscess or cyst in the surrounding periodontium, spreading by way of the apical foramen. If the pulp dies from the infection, it must be removed. An inert radiopaque rubbery material (gutta-percha) is then placed within the pulp chamber, including the radicular pulp or root canal. This is called *endodontic therapy,* or *root canal treatment.*

Because the pulp is removed with this treatment, the tooth is no longer vital. An endodontically treated tooth may darken and become brittle and break during mastication. To prolong retention of the tooth, a full-coverage restorative

crown is sometimes placed on the natural crown to protect it from breaking and to improve its appearance. Internal or external nonvital bleaching may be necessary to reduce darkening. If an abscess or cyst formation develops in the periodontium as a result of pulpitis, surgery (apicoectomy) must be performed to remove the apical lesion.

Dental professionals must do their utmost to prevent injury to the pulp during restorative procedures. Such iatrogenic injury to the pulp can result from the heat or vibrations emitted by the handpiece during cavity preparation, causing physical damage. The pulp can also be injured by the restorative materials placed in the cavity preparation. Water-cooled handpieces with rapid rotation, which minimize the stress on the tooth, are now used successfully to reduce the incidence of pulpal damage. Liners are also currently placed over dentin before toxic restorative materials to prevent pulpal damage.

cell bodies are located in the pulp. The odontoblasts are located only along the outer pulpal wall.

In addition to fibroblasts and odontoblasts, the pulp contains undifferentiated mesenchymal cells. These cells are a rich resource for the dentin-pulp complex because they can transform into fibroblasts and odon-

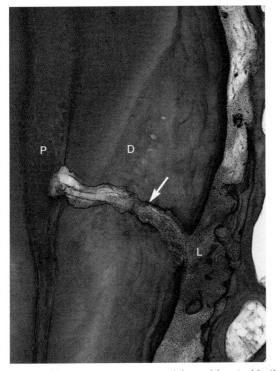

FIGURE 13-17 An accessory canal *(arrow)* located in the root. The root is composed of pulp *(P)* and dentin *(D)* covered by cementum. Note that the accessory canal is open to the periodontal ligament *(L).* (Courtesy of Dr. James McIntosh, PhD, Department of Biomedical Sciences, Baylor College of Dentistry, Dallas, TX.)

toblasts if either cell population is reduced after injury. The pulp also contains white blood cells in its tissue and vascular supply. White blood cell levels are normally low, unless the cells are ready to be triggered by an inflammatory or immune reaction. The red blood cells are located in the extensive vascular supply.

The fibers present in the pulp are mainly collagen fibers and some reticular fibers. The pulp contains no elastic fibers. Also present are an extensive vascular supply and rudimentary lymphatics.

Two types of nerves are associated with the pulp: myelinated nerves and unmyelinated. The myelinated nerves are the axons of sensory or afferent neurons that are located in the dentinal tubules in dentin. The associated nerve cell bodies are located between the odontoblasts' cell bodies in the odontoblastic layer of the pulp. The unmyelinated nerves are associated with the blood vessels.

Pulp stones, or denticles, are sometimes present in the pulp tissue (Figure 13-19). These are calcified masses of dentin complete with tubules and processes (true); in other cases, they are amorphous in structure (false). Pulp stones can be free, or unattached to the outer pulpal wall, or they can be attached to the dentin at the dentin-pulp interface. Pulp stones are formed during tooth development and also later as the pulp ages. They are quite common and may fill most of the pulp chamber. They are detected as radiopaque masses in radiographs. Stones pose a problem only during endodontic therapy.

Microscopic Zones in Pulp

Four zones are evident when pulp tissue is viewed microscopically: the odontoblastic layer, cell-free zone,

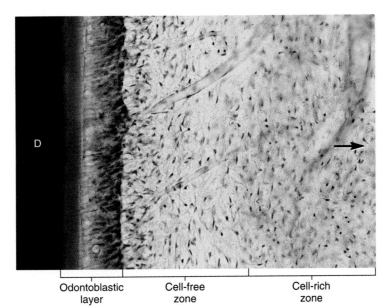

Odontoblastic layer   Cell-free zone   Cell-rich zone

FIGURE 13-18 Pulp tissue with its zones noted deep to the dentin *(D).* Note that the *arrow* points toward the inner zone of the pulpal core. (Courtesy of Dr. James McIntosh, PhD, Department of Biomedical Sciences, Baylor College of Dentistry, Dallas, TX.)

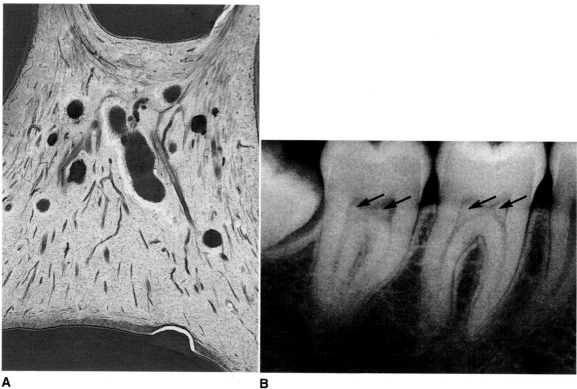

A   B

FIGURE 13-19 Pulp stones in a multirooted tooth. **A:** Microscopic appearance of pulp stones. **B:** Pulp stones *(arrows)*. (**A:** Courtesy of Dr. James McIntosh, PhD, Department of Biomedical Sciences, Baylor College of Dentistry, Dallas, TX.)

TABLE 13-4

Microscopic Zones in Pulp

Zones (From Outer to Inner Zones)	Description
Odontoblastic layer	This layer lines the outer pulpal wall and consists of the cell bodies of odontoblasts. Secondary dentin may form in this area from the apposition of these odontoblasts, causing the cell bodies to realign themselves. Cell bodies of the afferent axons from the dentinal tubules are located between cell bodies of the odontoblasts.
Cell-free zone	This zone contains fewer cells than the odontoblastic layer. The nerve and capillary plexus is located here.
Cell-rich zone	This zone contains an increased density of cells compared with the cell-free zone and also has a more extensive vascular system.
Pulpal core	This zone is located in the center of the pulp chamber, which, like the cell-rich zone, has many cells and an extensive vascular supply.

cell-rich zone, and pulpal core (Table 13-4; see also Figure 13-18). This chapter discusses these zones from the outermost zone closest to the dentin to the innermost zone of pulp.

The first zone of pulp closest to the dentin is called the *odontoblastic layer*. This zone lines the outer pulpal wall. It consists of a layer of the cell bodies of odontoblasts, whose odontoblastic processes are located in the dentinal tubules in the adjacent dentin. The odontoblasts are capable of forming secondary or tertiary dentin along the outer pulpal wall. If this occurs, the odontoblasts realign on the pulpal side next to this newly formed dentin. In addition, the cell bodies of the afferent axons from the dentinal tubules in dentin are located between the cell bodies of the odontoblasts.

The next zone is called the *cell-free zone*, but it is anything but empty. This zone was so named because it appears to be virtually free of cells at lower microscopic power. It is next to the odontoblastic layer, inward from the dentin. This cell-free zone consists of fewer cells than does the odontoblastic layer, but it is not entirely cell free. A nerve and capillary plexus is also located in this zone. No secondary or tertiary dentin is formed here initially, but newly formed dentin may encroach upon this zone.

The next zone after the cell-free zone is called the *cell-rich zone*, inward from dentin. The cell-rich zone, as its name implies, has an increased density of cells compared with the cell-free zone but does not contain as many cells as the odontoblastic layer. This zone also has a more extensive vascular system than does the cell-free zone.

The final zone of pulp is called the *pulpal core*, the innermost zone of pulp. The pulpal core is located in the center of the pulp chamber. This zone consists of many cells and an extensive vascular supply. Except for its location, it is very similar to the cell-rich zone.

Age-Related Changes in Pulp

With increased age, the pulp undergoes a decrease in intercellular substance, water, and cells as it fills with an increased amount of collagen fibers. This decrease in cells is especially evident in the number of undifferentiated mesenchymal cells. Thus the pulp becomes more fibrotic with increased age, leading to a reduction in the regenerative capacity of the pulp. Also, the overall pulp cavity can be made smaller by the addition of secondary or tertiary dentin, thus causing pulp recession.

GROWTH FACTORS AND DENTIN-PULP COMPLEX

The vitality of the dentin-pulp complex, both during health and after injury, depends on pulp cell activity and the signalling processes, which regulate the behavior of these cells. Research, particularly in recent years, has led to a better understanding of the molecular control of cellular behavior. Growth factors play a pivotal role in signalling the events of tissue formation and repair in the dentin-pulp complex. Harnessing these growth factors can provide exciting opportunities for biological approaches to dental tissue repair and the blueprint for tissue engineering of the tooth. These approaches offer significant potential for improved clinical management of dental disease and maintenance of tooth vitality.

CHAPTER 14

Periodontium: Cementum, Alveolar Bone, Periodontal Ligament

■ ■ ■

This chapter discusses the following topics:

- Periodontium
- Components of the periodontium
  - Cementum
- Alveolar bone
- Periodontal ligament

■ ■ ■

After studying this chapter, the reader should be able to:

1. Define and pronounce the key terms in this chapter.
2. Discuss the periodontium, and describe the properties of each of its tissues.
3. Discuss the development of the periodontium.
4. Outline the types of cementum and alveolar bone.
5. Label the fiber groups of the periodontal ligament and discuss their functions.
6. Demonstrate and discuss the microscopic features of the periodontium.
7. Describe the age-related changes in the periodontium.
8. Integrate the knowledge of the histology with the clinical considerations involving the periodontium, especially those changes associated with periodontal pathology.

■ ■ ■

Key Terms

Alveolar bone, crest (al-ve-o-lar)
Alevolar bone proper (al-ve-o-lar)
Alveolar crest group
Alveolodental ligament
  (al-ve-o-lo-**dent**-al)
Alveolus (plural, **alveoli**) (al-ve-o-lus,
  al-ve-o-lie)
Apical group
Arrest lines
Basal bone (bay-sal)
Calcium hydroxyapatite
  (hy-drox-see-**ap**-ah-tite)
Canaliculi (kan-ah-**lik**-u-lie)
Caries
Cemental spurs
Cementicles (see-**men**-ti-kuls)

Cementoblasts (see-men-toe-blasts)
Cementocytes
  (see-**men**-toe-sites)
Cementoenamel junction
Cementogenesis
  (see-men-toe-**jen**-i-sis)
Cementoid (see-**men**-toyd)
Cementum: acellular, cellular
  (see-**men**-tum)
Cortical bone
Dentinocemental junction
Edentulous (e-**den**-tu-lus)
Endochondral ossification
  (en-do-**kon**-dril os-i-fi-**kay**-shun)
Epithelial rests of Malassez
  (mal-ah-**say**)

Fibroblast (fi-bro-blast)
Gingival fiber group
Gingival recession
  (re-**sesh**-un)
Golden Proportions
Horizontal group
Hypercementosis
  (hi-per-see-men-**toe**-sis)
Interdental septum, ligament
  (in-ter-**den**-tal)
Interradicular group
Interradicular septum
  (in-ter-rah-**dik**-u-lar)
Intramembranous ossification
  (in-trah-**mem**-bran-us
  os-i-fi-**kay**-shun)

Lacuna (plural, **lacunae**) (lah-**ku**-nah, lah-**ku**-nay)
Lamina dura (lam-i-nah **dur**-ah)
Meckel's cartilage (**mek**-els **kar**-ti-lij)
Mesial drift (me-**ze**-il)
Oblique group

Odontoclast (oh-**don**-toe-klasts)
Osteoblasts
Osteoclasts
Periodontal ligament, space (pare-ee-o-**don**-tal)
Periodontium (per-e-o-**don**-she-um)
Principal fibers

Resorption (re-**sorp**-shun)
Reversal lines
Sharpey's fibers (shar-**peez**)
Trabecular bone (trah-**bek**-u-lar)
Vertical dimension of the face

PERIODONTIUM

The **periodontium** consists of the supporting soft and hard dental tissues between and including portions of the tooth and the alveolar bone (Figure 14-1). The periodontium serves to support the tooth in its relationship to the alveolar bone. Thus the periodontium includes the cementum, alveolar bone, and periodontal ligament, as well as individual components of these tissues. Some dental researchers include the gingiva in the category of the periodontium, but this tissue has only a minor role in the support of the tooth.

To understand the pathological changes that occur during the disease states involving the periodontium, dental professionals must appreciate the histology of the healthy, normal periodontium. Thus the underlying histological states of these tissues provide a clue to the clinical features within the periodontium, whether in a healthy or diseased state.

COMPONENTS OF THE PERIODONTIUM

Cementum

The **cementum** is the part of the periodontium that attaches the teeth to the alveolar bone by anchoring the periodontal ligament (Figure 14-2). In a healthy patient, the cementum is not visible because it usually covers the entire root, overlying Tomes' granular layer in dentin. Cementum is a hard tissue that is thickest at the tooth's apex and in the interradicular areas of multirooted teeth (50 to 200 micrometers) and thinnest at the **cementoenamel junction (CEJ)** at the cervix of the tooth (10 to 50 micrometers). Cementum has no innervation and is avascular, receiving its nutrition by way of its own cells from the surrounding periodontal ligament. Like dentin and pulp, cementum can form throughout the life of the tooth (see Chapter 6, Table 6-2 for more comparative information on cementum).

Mature cementum is by weight 65 percent mineralized or inorganic material, 23 percent organic material, and 12 percent water. This crystalline formation of mature cementum consists of mainly **calcium hydroxyapatite**, with the chemical formula of $Ca_{10}(PO_4)_6(OH)_2$. This calcium hydroxyapatite is similar to that found in higher percentages in enamel and dentin and most closely resembles the composition found in bone. Other forms of calcium are also present.

In certain situations when cementum is initially exposed, it is a dull pale yellow, lighter than dentin but darker than enamel's whitish shade (discussed later). When instruments are used, cementum feels grainy compared with the harder dentin and the even harder, smoother enamel surfaces. Because of its mineral level, cementum appears more radiolucent (darker) than enamel or dentin but more radiopaque (lighter) than pulp tissue when viewed by radiograph.

DEVELOPMENT OF CEMENTUM

Cementum, which develops from the dental sac, forms on the root after the disintegration of Hertwig's epithelial root sheath, as discussed in Chapter 6. This disintegration allows the undifferentiated cells of the dental sac to come into contact with the newly formed surface of root dentin, inducing these cells to become **cementoblasts**. The cementoblasts then disperse to cover the root dentin area and undergo **cementogenesis**, laying down **cementoid**. Unlike ameloblasts and odontoblasts, which leave no cellular bodies in their secreted

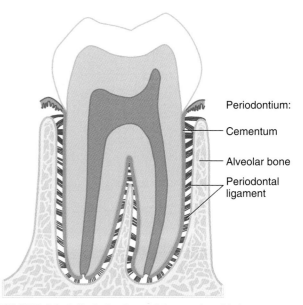

FIGURE 14-1 Periodontium of the tooth, with its components identified.

Periodontium:
— Cementum
— Alveolar bone
— Periodontal ligament

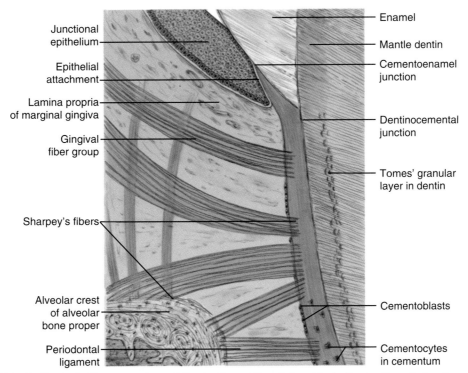

Junctional epithelium

Epithelial attachment

Lamina propria of marginal gingiva

Gingival fiber group

Sharpey's fibers

Alveolar crest of alveolar bone proper

Periodontal ligament

Enamel

Mantle dentin

Cementoenamel junction

Dentinocemental junction

Tomes' granular layer in dentin

Cementoblasts

Cementocytes in cementum

FIGURE 14-2 The cementum of the tooth and its relationship to the tooth and alveolar bone. Note Sharpey's fibers from the periodontal ligament into the cementum as well as Tomes' granular layer in the underlying dentin.

Clinical Considerations with Cementum

Cementum is exposed through **gingival recession** (Figure 14-3) (discussed also in Chapter 13 with regard to dentin). Because only a few layers of cementum cover the root, the exposed cementum is quickly worn off with mechanical friction, exposing the deeper dentin and leading to problems such as extrinsic staining and dentin hypersensitivity. Some initial studies are also showing that such morphology may result in an increased risk of cemental caries (discussed next).

The incidence of cemental caries increases in older adults as gingival recession occurs. Cemental **caries** is a chronic condition that forms a large, shallow lesion and slowly invades first the dentin and then the pulp tissue (Figure 14-4). Because dental pain is a late finding, many lesions are not detected early, resulting in restorative challenges and increased tooth loss. Xerostomia (dry mouth), poor manual dexterity for adequate oral care, and poor nutrition in older adults can complicate caries, and all these issues must be addressed during dental treatment of these patients. Increased controversy surrounds treatment of periodontal disease that involves the removal of the outer

layers of cementum during scaling of the roots. Bacterial plaque biofilm and the related hardened calculus are associated with the cemental surface of the root deep inside a periodontal pocket (Figures 14-5 and 14-6; see also Chapter 10). Some clinicians believe that bacterial toxins (endotoxins) have been absorbed into the outer portion of cementum from the adjacent bacterial plaque biofilm and that these outer layers of "toxic" cementum must be removed by manual scaling for the dentogingival tissues to heal and form a more occlusal epithelial attachment. Other clinicians believe that these toxins are loosely adherent to the cementum and that the cementum does not need to be scaled off to remove them. A more recent viewpoint is that ultrasonics can flush these toxins from the cementum without removing any of the hard tissue.

Research studies on cementum have not shown any conclusive differences between it and the toxic type of cementum, but clinicians subjectively report softer tissue textures and increased success with these types of treatment. More studies in this area are necessary as new treatments of periodontal disease are considered.

products, during the later stages of apposition, many of the cementoblasts become entrapped by the cementum they produce, becoming **cementocytes** (Figure 14-7).

When the cementoid reaches the full thickness needed, the cementoid surrounding the cemento-

cytes becomes calcified or matured and is then considered cementum. Because of the apposition of cementum over the dentin, the **dentinocemental junction (DCJ)** is formed. This interface is not as defined as that of the dentinoenamel junction, given

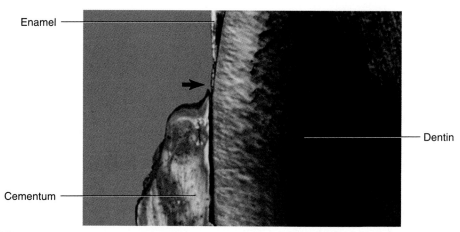

Enamel

Dentin

Cementum

FIGURE 14-3 Phase-contrast image of the cementoenamel junction. In some cases, cementum and enamel do not meet, leaving a region of exposed dentin (*arrow*) between them that may lead to tooth dentin hypersensitivity. (Courtesy P. Tambasco de Oliveira. From Nanci A. *Ten Cate's Oral Histology*, ed 6. Mosby, St. Louis, 2003.)

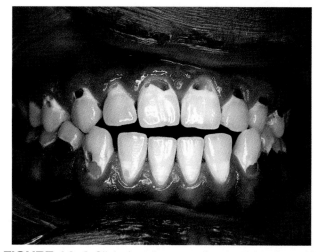

FIGURE 14-4 Clinical appearance of cemental caries, with some invasion into the adjacent dentin. Pulpal involvement is a late finding.

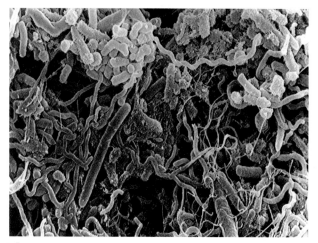

FIGURE 14-5 Scanning electron micrograph of subgingival bacterial plaque biofilm on the cemental root surface in a deep periodontal pocket. (Courtesy of Jan Cope, RDH, Director, Oregon Institute of Technology, Klamath Falls, OR.)

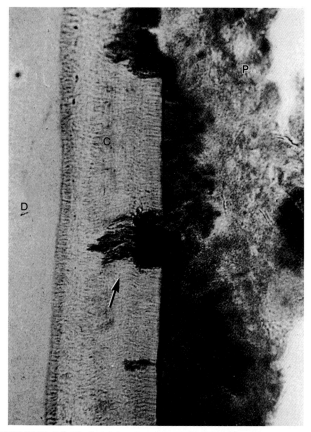

FIGURE 14-6 Calculus (*arrow*) embedded within the cementum (*C*) that overlies the dentin (*D*). Note that bacterial plaque biofilm (*P*) then overlies the calculus. Many times the calculus on the root is more mineralized than the cementum or even dentin. (From Newman MG, Takei HH, Carranza FA. *Clinical Periodontology*, ed 9. WB Saunders, Philadelphia, 2002.)

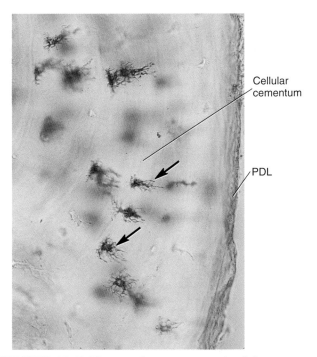

Cellular
cementum

PDL

FIGURE 14-7 Microscopic appearance of cellular cementum with its cementocytes (*arrows*). The cementocytes are within their lacunae, and their canaliculi are oriented toward the periodontal ligament (PDL) for nutrition. (Courtesy of Dr. James McIntosh, PhD, Department of Biomedical Sciences, Baylor College of Dentistry, Dallas, TX.)

that cementum and dentin are of common embryological background.

MICROSCOPIC APPEARANCE OF CEMENTUM

Cementum is composed of a mineralized fibrous matrix and cells (see Figures 14-2 and 14-11). The fibrous matrix consists of both Sharpey's fibers and intrinsic nonperiodontal fibers. **Sharpey's fibers** are a portion of the collagen fibers from the periodontal ligament that are each partially inserted into the outer part of the cementum at 90 degrees, or a right angle, to the cemental surface (as well as the alveolar bone on their other end). These fibers are organized to function as a ligament between the tooth and alveolar bone. The intrinsic nonperiodontal ligament fibers of the cementum are collagen fibers made by the cementoblasts and laid down in a nonorganized pattern, yet all these fibers run parallel to the DCJ.

The cells of cementum include the entrapped cementoblasts, the cementocytes (see Figure 14-7). Each cementocyte lies in its **lacuna** (plural, **lacunae**), similar to the pattern in bone. These lacunae also have canaliculi or canals. Unlike those in bone, however, these canals in cementum do not contain nerves, nor do they radiate outward. All the canals are oriented

toward the periodontal ligament and contain cementocytic processes that exist to diffuse nutrients from the ligament that is vascularized.

After the apposition of cementum in layers, the cementoblasts that do not become entrapped in cementum line up along the cemental surface in the periodontal ligament. These cementoblasts can form subsequent layers of cementum if the tooth is injured (discussed later).

Cementoenamel Junction

Three patterns may be present at the cementoenamel junction (CEJ). The classical view was that certain patterns dominated in certain oral cavities. New studies with the scanning electron microscope indicate that the CEJ may exhibit all of these patterns in an individual's oral cavity, and there is even considerable variation when one tooth is traced circumferentially (Figure 14-8; see also Figure 14-3). In some cases, the cementum may overlap the enamel at the CEJ. Novice clinicians may have difficulty discerning the CEJ from calculus around the cervix with this situation. However, compared with the usually spotty placement and roughness of calculus, cementum exhibits a uniform placement and roughness with an explorer.

Another situation at the CEJ is that the cementum and enamel may meet end to end, presenting no problems for the clinician or patient. Finally, another situation at the CEJ is that a gap may exist between the cementum and enamel, exposing dentin (see Figure 14-8). Thus patients may experience dentin hypersensitivity (see Chapter 13).

Cementum Repair

Similar to bone, cementum undergoes histological removal within the tissue as a result of trauma (Figure 14-9). This removal involves **resorption**, or the removal of cementum by the **odontoclast**, resulting in **reversal lines.** When stained, reversal lines appear as scalloped lines. Cementum is less readily resorbed than bone, an important consideration during orthodontic tooth movement (discussed later).

Repair of traumatic resorption involves apposition of cementum by cementoblasts in the adjacent periodontal ligament. Apposition of cementum is noted by its layers of growth, or **arrest lines,** which, when stained, look like smooth growth rings in a section of a tree. Reversal and arrest lines are prominent in cementum subjected to trauma from occlusal forces or to orthodontic tooth movement as well as during the shedding of primary teeth and eruption of the permanent tooth. However, unlike bone, cementum does not continually undergo remodeling or repair.

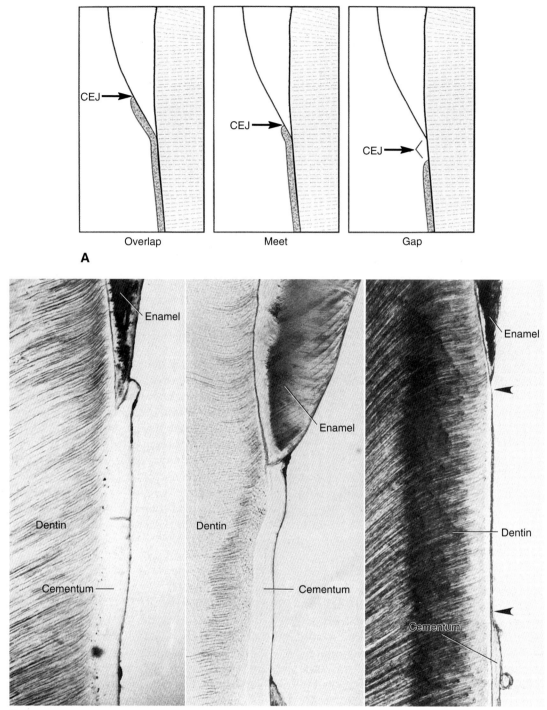

FIGURE 14-8 The three patterns that may be present at points along the cementoenamel junction (CEJ). One situation is that cementum may overlap enamel. Another situation is that they may meet end-to-end. Finally, there may be a gap between enamel and cementum, leaving dentin exposed. **A.** Diagram of patterns. **B.** Ground sections. (From Nanci A. *Ten Cate's Oral Histology*, ed 6. Mosby, St. Louis, 2003.)

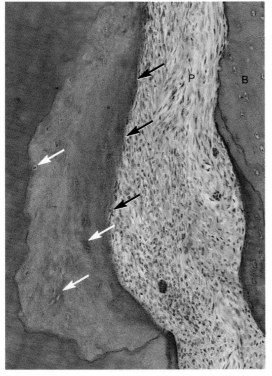

FIGURE 14-9 Reversal lines and arrest lines in cementum with embedded cementocytes (*white arrows*) that has undergone repair. On the surface of the cementum are the cementoblasts (*dark arrows*) with the surrounding periodontal ligament (*P*). Note that the alveolar bone (*B*) has similar lines as a result of bone remodeling. (Courtesy of Dr. James McIntosh, PhD, Department of Biomedical Sciences, Baylor College of Dentistry, Dallas, TX.)

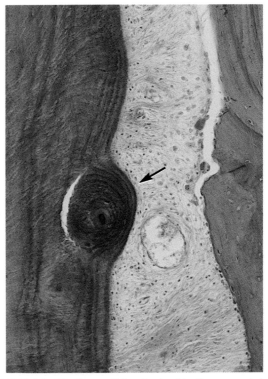

FIGURE 14-10 Cementicle attached to the cemental surface in the periodontal ligament (*arrow*). (Courtesy of Dr. James McIntosh, PhD, Department of Biomedical Sciences, Baylor College of Dentistry, Dallas, TX.)

 Clinical Considerations with Cementum

Cementicles are calcified bodies of cementum found either attached to the cemental root surface or lying free in the periodontal ligament (Figure 14-10). They form from the apposition of cementum around cellular debris in the periodontal ligament (PDL), possibly as a result of trauma to Sharpey's fibers. They become attached or fused from the continued apposition of cementum. Cementicles may be seen in radiographs and may interfere with periodontal treatment.

Cemental spurs can be found at or near the CEJ. These are symmetrical spheres of cementum attached to the cemental root surface, similar to enamel pearls. Cemental spurs result from irregular deposition of cementum on the root. They can present some clinical problems in differentiation from calculus, yet they are not easily removed and may also interfere with periodontal treatment.

TYPES OF CEMENTUM

Two basic types of cementum are formed by cemento-blasts: acellular and cellular (Figure 14-11 and Table

14-1). **Acellular cementum** consists of the first layers of cementum deposited at the DCJ and thus is also called *primary cementum.* It is formed at a slow rate and contains no embedded cementocytes. At least one layer of acellular cementum covers all of the root, and many layers cover the cervical one third near the CEJ (see Figure 14-3). The width of acellular cementum never changes.

The other type of cementum is **cellular cementum,** sometimes called *secondary cementum* (see Figures 14-6 and 14-11). Cellular cementum consists of the last layers of cementum deposited over the acellular cementum, mainly in the apical one third of the root. Cellular cementum is formed at a faster rate than acellular, and thus many embedded cementocytes are found within it. At its periphery are the cementoblasts in the periodontal ligament, which allow for the future production of more cellular cementum if needed. Thus the width of cellular cementum can change during the life of the tooth (discussed next), especially at the apex of the tooth. This type of cementum is especially common in interradicular areas. It is important to note that Sharpey's fibers in acellular cementum are fully mineralized; those in cellular cementum are generally mineralized only partially at their periphery.

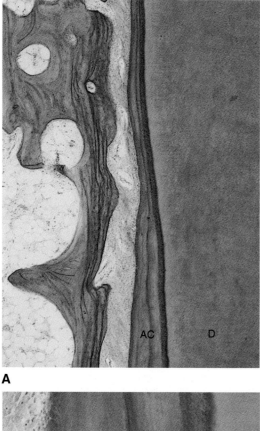

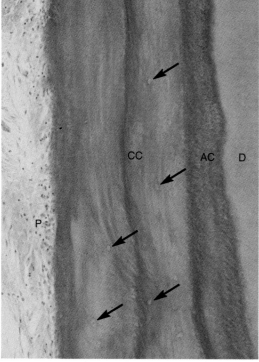

FIGURE 14-11 Two types of cementum on the root surface. **A:** Acellular cementum (*AC*) without cementocytes makes up the first layers of cementum deposited at the dentinocemental junction over the dentin (*D*). **B:** Layers of cellular cementum (*CC*) that contain embedded cementocytes (*arrows*) are the last layers of cementum deposited over the thin layer of acellular cementum (*AC*) adjacent to the dentin (*D*). The cells adjacent to the periodontal ligament (*P*) are cementoblasts. (Courtesy of Dr. James McIntosh, PhD, Department of Biomedical Sciences, Baylor College of Dentistry, Dallas, TX.)

TABLE 14-1

Comparison of Two Types of Cementum

Acellular	Cellular
First layer(s) deposited	Formed after acellular layer(s)
At least one layer over all of the root, with many layers near cervical one third	Layered over acellular, mainly in apical one third, especially interradicular region
Formed at a slower rate	Formed at a faster rate
No embedded cementocytes	Embedded cementocytes
Width constant over time	Layers sometimes added over time

Clinical Considerations for Cementum

Hypercementosis is the excessive production of cellular cementum, which mainly occurs at the apex of the tooth (Figure 14-12). This condition can result from trauma caused by occlusal forces and during certain pathological conditions, such as chronic periapical inflammation. It may also be a compensatory mechanism in response to attrition. It may be seen on radiographs as a radiopaque (light) mass at the root apex. Such deposits form bulbous enlargements on the roots that may interfere with dental extractions, should these become necessary.

Alveolar Bone

The **alveolar bone** is that part of the maxilla or mandible that supports and protects the teeth. The alveolar bone is also that part of the periodontium in which the cementum of the tooth is attached to it by way of the PDL (Figure 14-13). The alveolar bone is a hard, calcified tissue with all the components of other bone tissue (see Chapter 8). However, alveolar bone is more easily remodeled than cementum, thus allowing for orthodontic tooth movement (discussed later and in Chapter 6). When stained, the remodeled alveolar bone shows arrest lines and reversal lines, as does all bone tissue.

Like all bone, mature alveolar bone is by weight 60 percent mineralized or inorganic material, 25 percent organic material, and 15 percent water. This crystalline formation consists of mainly calcium hydroxyapatite with the chemical formula of $Ca_{10}(PO_4)_6(OH)_2$. This calcium hydroxyapatite is similar to that found in higher percentages in enamel and dentin and is most similar to that of cementum (see Table 6-2).

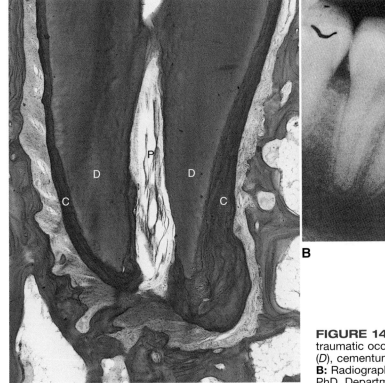

FIGURE 14-12 Hypercementosis at the root apex. This is due to traumatic occlusal forces of a tooth. **A:** Microscopic view with dentin (*D*), cementum (*C*), and radicular pulp tissue (*P*) noted in the root area. **B:** Radiographic presentation. (**A:** Courtesy of Dr. James McIntosh, PhD, Department of Biomedical Sciences, Baylor College of Dentistry, Dallas, TX.)

Clinical Considerations with Alveolar Bone

In orthodontic tooth movement, bone remodeling is forced (Figure 14-14). The bands, wires, or appliances put pressure on one side of the tooth and adjacent alveolar bone, creating a zone of compression in the PDL. This compression in the PDL leads to bone resorption. On the opposite side of the tooth and bone, a tension zone develops in the PDL and causes the deposition of new bone. Thus the tooth or teeth are slowly moved along the jaw bone to achieve a dentition that works in harmony (see Chapter 20). In this way, the width of the space between the alveoli and the root is kept about the same.

Mesial drift, or physiological drift, is a normal, natural movement phenomenon in which all the teeth move slightly toward the midline of the oral cavity over time (see Chapter 20). This can cause crowding late in life of a once-perfect dentition. It occurs quite slowly, depending mostly on the degree of wear of the contact points between adjacent teeth and on the number of missing teeth. Overall, amounts may total no more than 1 cm over a lifetime. However, this crowding may lead to poor oral hygiene. Occlusal drift or supereruption can also occur, especially with the posterior teeth (see Chapter 17). The exact mechanism that causes drifting of the dentition is still controversial; it may be an adjustment process to retain balance among the various portions of the masticatory apparatus or may just be related to the wear of the proximal and occlusal tooth surfaces.

ANATOMY OF THE JAW BONES

Each mature jaw bone, either the maxilla or mandible, is composed of two types of bone tissue with differing physiological functioning (discussed later; Figure 14-15). The portion that contains the roots of the teeth is called the alveolar bone, alveolar process, or alveolar ridge. The portion apical to the roots of the teeth is called the **basal bone,** which then forms the body of the maxilla or mandible. Both the alveolar bone and basal bone are covered by periosteum.

The alveolar bone is divided into the alveolar bone proper and the supporting alveolar bone. Microscopically, both the alveolar bone proper and the supporting alveolar bone have the same components: fibers, cells, intercellular substances, nerves, blood vessels, and lymphatics (see Chapter 8; see also Figure 14-13).

The **alveolar bone proper** is the lining of the tooth socket or **alveolus** (plural, **alveoli**) (see Figure 14-15). Although the alveolar bone proper is composed of compact bone, it may be called the *cribriform plate* because it contains numerous holes where Volkmann's canals pass from the alveolar bone into the PDL. The alveolar bone proper is also called *bundle bone* because Sharpey's fibers, a portion of the fibers of the PDL, are inserted here. Similar to those of the cemental surface, Sharpey's fibers in alveolar bone proper are each inserted at 90 degrees, or a right angle, but are fewer in number although thicker than those in cementum

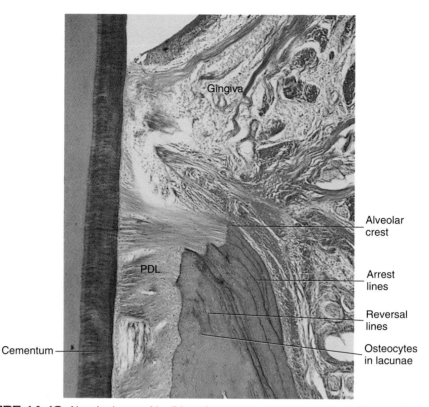

FIGURE 14-13 Alveolar bone with all its microscopic components, including arrest and reversal lines, is identified. Note that there has been a slight resorption of the alveolar crest owing to periodontal disease. (Courtesy of Dr. James McIntosh, PhD, Department of Biomedical Sciences, Baylor College of Dentistry, Dallas, TX.)

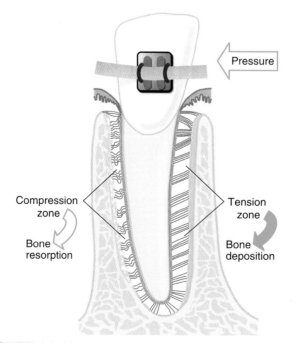

FIGURE 14-14 The process of orthodontic tooth movement.

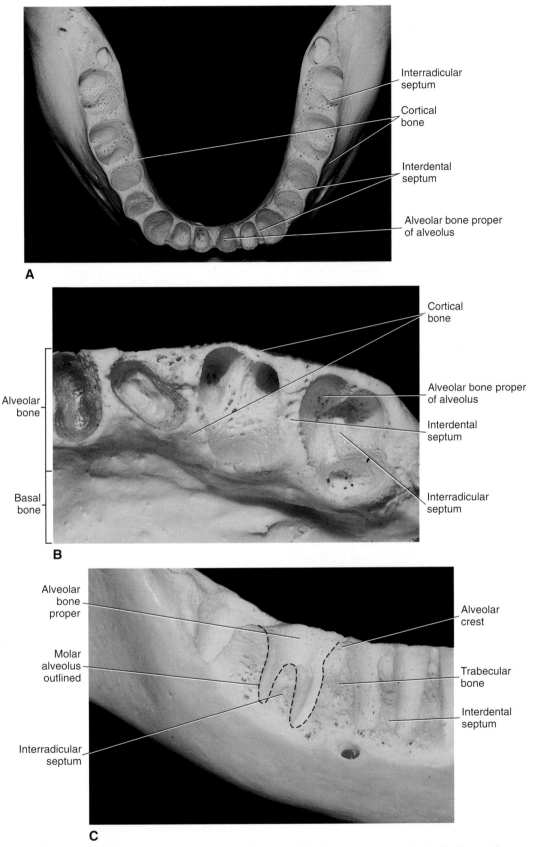

FIGURE 14-15 Anatomy of the alveolar bone. **A:** Mandibular arch of a skull with the teeth removed. **B:** Portion of the maxilla of a skull with the teeth removed. **C:** Cross section of the mandible with the teeth removed.

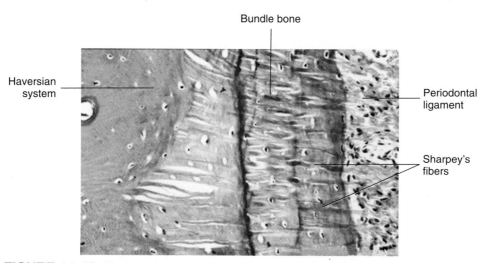

FIGURE 14-16 Microscopic view of the insertion of Sharpey's fibers from the periodontal ligament into the bundle bone or alveolar bone proper in the root area. Note the Haversian system within these plates of compact bone. (From Nanci A. *Ten Cate's Oral Histology*, ed 6. Mosby, St. Louis, 2003.)

(Figure 14-16). As in cellular cementum, Sharpey's fibers in bone are generally mineralized only partially at their periphery.

The alveolar bone proper consists of plates of compact bone that surround the tooth and assume the shape of the tooth. The alveolar bone proper varies in thickness from 0.1 to 0.5 millimeters. The lamina propria of the attached gingiva serves as a mucoperiosteum for the alveolar bone proper (see Chapter 9). A portion of the alveolar bone proper is seen on radiographs as the uniformly radiopaque (light) **lamina dura** (Figure 14-17). Integrity of the lamina dura is important when studying radiographs for pathological lesions.

The **alveolar crest** is the most cervical rim of the alveolar bone proper (Figure 14-18). In a healthy situation, the alveolar crest is slightly apical to the CEJ by approximately 1 to 2 mm. The alveolar crests of neighboring teeth are also uniform in height along the jaw bone.

A portion of the alveolar crest that is between neighboring teeth is seen on radiographs as a radiopaque (light) triangle at the most superior portion of the interdental bone (see Figure 14-17). It can be used for educating patients about bone loss levels in periodontal disease; however, it shows only the levels of alveolar bone proper interproximally. Bone loss can occur at any surface of the tooth and in varying amounts around the tooth.

The supporting alveolar bone consists of cortical and trabecular bone. The **cortical bone,** or cortical plates, consists of plates of compact bone on the facial and lingual surfaces of the alveolar bone (see Figure 14-15). These cortical plates are usually about 1.5 to 3 mm thick over posterior teeth, but the thickness is highly variable around anterior teeth. The cortical bone is not seen on periapical or bite-wing radiographs but only on occlusal radiographs as a uniformly

radiopaque (light) plate facial and lingual to the teeth (see Figure 14-17).

The **trabecular bone** consists of cancellous bone that is located between the alveolar bone proper and the plates of cortical bone (see Figure 14-15). Only the portions of trabecular bone between the teeth and between the roots are ever seen on any type of radiographs, and this trabecular bone appears less uniformly radiopaque or spongy than the uniformly radiopaque lamina dura of the alveolar bone proper.

The alveolar bone between two neighboring teeth is called the **interdental septum,** or interdental bone (Figure 14-19). It is easily seen on periapical and bite-wing radiographs (see Figure 14-17). The interdental septum consists of both the compact bone of the alveolar bone proper and cancellous bone of the trabecular bone. The alveolar bone between the roots of the same tooth is called the interradicular septum, or interradicular bone (Figure 14-20). The interradicular septum consists of both alveolar bone proper and trabecular bone. Only a portion of the interradicular septum is ever seen on periapical or bite-wing radiographs (see Figure 14-17).

DEVELOPMENT OF THE JAW BONES

Both the maxilla and mandible develop from tissues of the first branchial arch, or mandibular arch. The maxilla forms within the maxillary process, and the mandible forms within the fused mandibular processes of the mandibular arch. Both jaw bones start as small centers of **intramembranous ossification** located around the stomodeum. These centers then increase in diameter, growing into the mature jaw bones. (The histological development of bone tissue is discussed in Chapter 8.) Both jaw bones also have several skeletal units during their development, and these are related to the overall morphology, or form, of

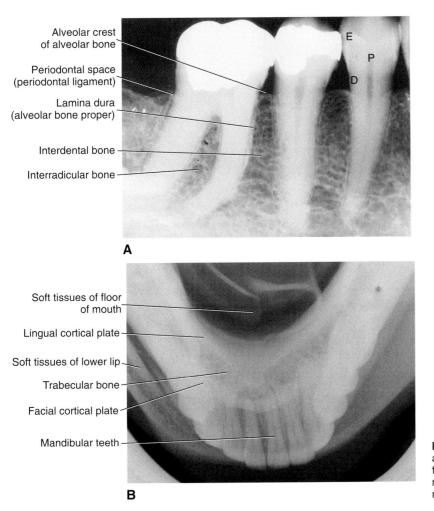

Alveolar crest
of alveolar bone

Periodontal space
(periodontal ligament)

Lamina dura
(alveolar bone proper)

Interdental bone

Interradicular bone

A

Soft tissues of floor
of mouth

Lingual cortical plate

Soft tissues of lower lip

Trabecular bone

Facial cortical plate

Mandibular teeth

B

FIGURE 14-17 Radiographs noting the anatomy of the alveolar bone and its associated tissues. **A:** Periapical radiograph of the mandible. **B:** Occlusal radiograph of the mandible.

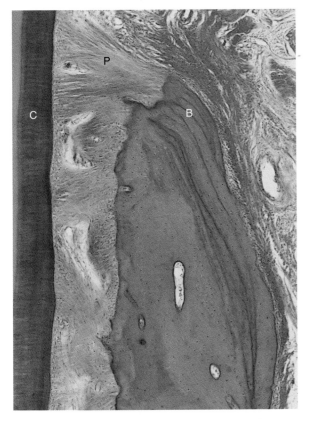

FIGURE 14-18 Photomicrograph of the alveolar crest of the alveolar bone proper (B) and its relationship to the root covered by cementum (C). Note that there is some resorption of the alveolar crest. The alveolar crest fibers of the periodontal ligament (P) are also present. (Courtesy of Dr. James McIntosh, PhD, Department of Biomedical Sciences, Baylor College of Dentistry, Dallas, TX.)

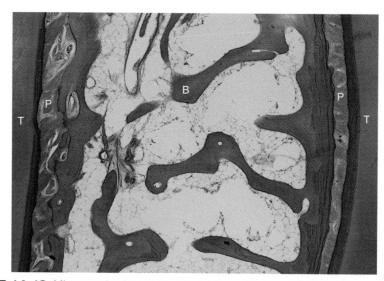

FIGURE 14-19 Microscopic view of interdental bone (*B*) found between the roots of two neighboring teeth (*T*) and surrounded on each side by the horizontal group of the periodontal ligament (*P*). (Courtesy of Dr. James McIntosh, PhD, Department of Biomedical Sciences, Baylor College of Dentistry, Dallas, TX.)

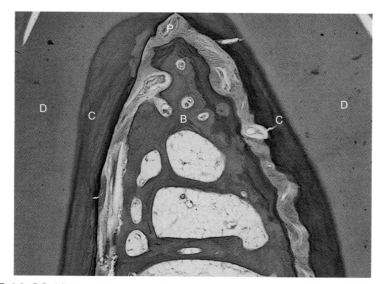

FIGURE 14-20 Microscopic view of interradicular bone between two roots (*B*) of a permanent mandibular molar and surrounded on each side by the interradicular group of the periodontal ligament (*P*). The tooth's roots are composed of dentin (*D*) and cementum (*C*). (Courtesy of Dr. James McIntosh, PhD, Department of Biomedical Sciences, Baylor College of Dentistry, Dallas, TX.)

Clinical Considerations with Alveolar Bone

The density of the alveolar bone in an area also determines the route that dental infection takes with abscess formation, as well as the efficacy of local infiltration during the use of local anesthesia. In addition, the differences in alveolar process density determine the easiest and most convenient areas of bony fracture used during tooth extraction.

After extraction of a tooth, the clot in the alveolus fills in with immature bone, which later is remodeled into mature secondary bone. However, with the loss of teeth, a patient becomes **edentulous**, either partially or completely, and the alveolar bone undergoes resorption (Figure 14-21). The underlying basal bone or body of the maxilla or mandible remains less affected, however, because it does not need the presence of teeth to remain viable.

Thus the alveolar bone depends on the functional stimulation from teeth during mastication and speech for preservation of its structure. Resorption of the alveolar bone can be complicated in postmenopausal women, who experience a shortage of estrogen, which normally helps maintain bone density and the loss of which may lead to the onset of osteoporosis. The placement of a denture, either partial or full, or a bridge can somewhat mimic the stimulation of the teeth in the alveolar bone. Over time, however, some amounts of bone are lost even with these types of tooth replacements.

The loss of alveolar bone, coupled with attrition of the teeth, causes a loss of height of the lower third of the **vertical dimension of the face** when the teeth are in maximum intercuspation (Figure 14-22; see Chapters 1 and 20 for more discussion). The extent of this loss is determined on the basis of clinical judgement using the **Golden Proportions.** This portion of the vertical dimension is important in determining the way in which the jaws and teeth function. In addition, a proper amount of height in the lower third of the face reduces the amount of facial wrinkles around the mouth as the skin ages, sags, and loses its resilience. With the loss of vertical dimension in the lower third, older patients can take on a cartoon "Popeye" facial appearance that is aesthetically displeasing and results in poor functioning of the teeth and jaws.

Ideally, an implant placed in an edentulous area preserves the integrity of the bone and serves as a permanent replacement for a lost tooth or teeth, preventing loss of vertical dimension (Figure 14-23). An implant has a core portion made of titanium that is surgically implanted in the alveolar bone of either jaw. The high success rate of these current implants has now been demonstrated.

The deeper part of this surgical portion of the implant has an open structure, allowing bone to bond to it, undergoing osseointegration of the implant to the surrounding alveolar bone. However, unlike teeth with a fibrous insertion of the PDL into the alveolar bone, an implant has no movement. An implant makes direct contact with the alveolar bone as well as with the surrounding connective tissue and superficial epithelium, which are called *periimplant tissues.* Research has shown that a sulcular epithelium that consists of the circular fibers of the PDL surrounds and is also attached to the superior portion of the implant by hemidesmosomes. After osseointegration and healing of the tissues, a prosthetic superstructure of a tooth or denture is then attached to the surgical portion of the implant.

Studies have shown that failure to obtain and maintain this cellular junction may lead to apical migration of the epithelium to the bone/implant interface, possible soft tissue encapsulation of the implant, and eventual implant failure resulting from mobility. Thus special devices are needed for professional and home care of an implant's superstructure to remove any deposits and prevent peri implant disease, especially because many patients with implants have a history of inadequate oral hygiene.

Now placement of an immediate load implant upon extraction of noninfected tooth or teeth is available. For this placement to be successful, adequate bone must exist and a sufficiently large implant must be placed; once placed, the implant must be able to resist occlusal forces. The temporary crown must be adjusted so that no forces are placed on it during function. Meeting these criteria allows osseointegration. After a period of 9 weeks a permanent crown can be placed, shortening treatment time by 4 to 6 months.

During chronic periodontal disease that has affected the periodontium (periodontitis), bone tissue is also lost (Figure 14-24). This bone loss may be due to the over-response of the immune system and the activation of certain osteoclast populations. This bone loss is first evident in the alveolar crest, which looks moth-eaten microscopically and radiographically (see Figure 14-13). The bone loss slowly continues down the alveolar bone; thus the tooth becomes increasingly mobile, increasing the possibility of tooth loss. Prevention of further loss of bone and thus control of the periodontal disease is paramount in the dental treatment plan for these patients and may include removal of deposits, use of antibiotics, and irrigation. Bone grafting, either from the oral cavity or from other sources, possibly with the use of guided tissue regeneration (GTR) membrane, may be included. Treatments similar to those for osteoporosis may be used in the future.

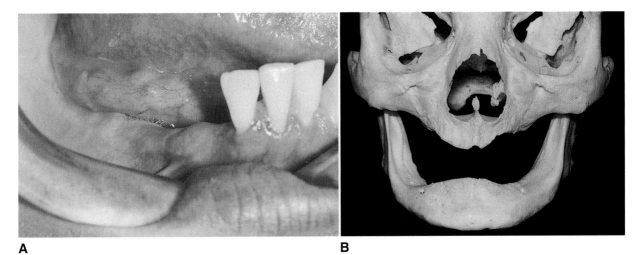

A   **B**

FIGURE 14-21 Edentulous state. **A:** Patient with alveolar bone loss of the posterior alveolar ridge of the mandible caused by loss of the posterior teeth. **B:** Skull that is completely edentulous, with bone loss of the alveolar ridges noted after tooth loss and only basal bone remains.

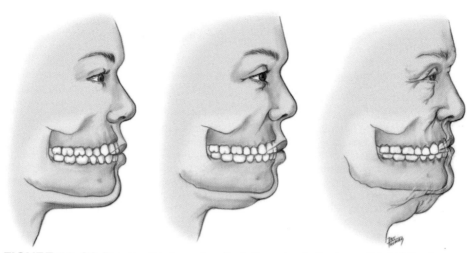

FIGURE 14-22 The possible loss of vertical dimension in the lower third of the face over the years (age 20, age 40, and age 60) as the alveolar bone is lost and the teeth undergo a reduction in height by slight attrition, the mechanical wear of the masticatory surface. Note the increase in wrinkles and lines around the mouth caused by these changes. This amount can be dramatically increased with tooth loss, severe periodontal disease, and increased levels of attrition.

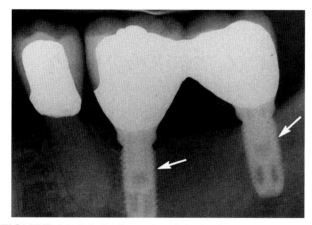

FIGURE 14-23 Radiographs of the implant areas in the mandible that have undergone osseointegration of the titanium device (*arrows*). (Courtesy of Dr. William Schmidt, DMD, MSD, Specialist in Prosthodontics and Implants, Seattle, WA.)

the bones. Each of these units is influenced in its growth pattern by some adjacent structure that acts on the developing bone.

Development of the Maxilla

The maxilla's primary center of intramembranous ossification for each half of the maxilla appears around the seventh week of prenatal development. It is located at the termination of the infraorbital nerve, just superior to the dental lamina of the primary maxillary canine tooth, in each maxillary process. Secondary ossification centers, the zygomatic, orbitonasal, nasopalatine, and intermaxillary, then appear and fuse rapidly with the primary centers. The two intermaxillary centers generate the alveolar ridge and primary palate region.

The subsequent growth of the maxilla can be subdivided into several skeletal units: the basal body unit, which develops beneath the infraorbital nerve, surrounding it to form the infraorbital canal; the orbital unit, which responds to the growth of the eyeball; the nasal unit, which depends on nasal septal cartilage for its growth; the alveolar unit, which forms in response to the maxillary teeth; and the pneumatic unit, which reflects maxillary sinus expansion. The primary bone initially formed in the maxilla is soon replaced by secondary bone as the face and oral cavity develop.

Development of the Mandible

During the sixth week of prenatal development, on each side of the embryo's mandibular arch, a primary ossification center appears in the angle formed by the division of the inferior alveolar nerve and its incisive and mental branches, on the lateral aspect of **Meckel's cartilage** or the first branchial arch cartilage (see Chapter 4).

In the seventh week, the first bone tissue in the body of the mandible forms. Bone formation spreads rapidly from the angle anterior to the midline. The anterior bone forms around Meckel's cartilage to produce a trough with medial and lateral plates that unite inferiorly around the incisive nerve. This trough extends to the midline on the embryo, where it comes into close approximation with a similar trough from the other side.

These two separate bilateral centers of ossification of the mandibular arch remain separated at the mandibular symphysis until shortly after birth. The trough turns into the mandibular canal as bone is formed over the incisive nerve joining the lateral and medial plates of initial bone.

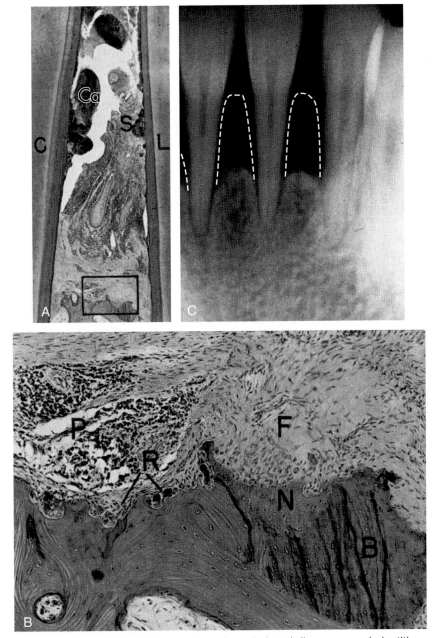

FIGURE 14-24 Bone loss caused by chronic periodontal disease or periodontitis. **A:** Microscopic view of periodontitis between a lateral incisor (*L*) and canine (*C*), showing calculus (*Ca*) and a periodontal pocket with suppuration (*S*). **B:** Close-up view of the rectangle showing bone resorption (*R*) from osteoclast activity beneath the inflammation in the periodontal ligament (*P*). Areas of fibrosis (*F*) are also noted. **C:** Radiograph of similar area showing severe bone loss (outline shows normal levels of alveolar bone). This bone loss initially involved the alveolar crest and moved apically as the periodontal disease progressed. (**A** and **B:** From Newman MG, Takei HH, Carranza FA. *Clinical Periodontology*, ed 9. WB Saunders, Philadelphia, 2002.)

Bone formation in the mandibular arch also spreads posteriorly toward the point where the mandibular nerve is divided into its lingual and inferior alveolar branches. This ossification initially forms a gutter, which later evolves into a canal that contains the inferior alveolar nerve.

The mandible subsequently develops as several skeletal units: a condylar unit that forms the articulation with the temporal bone; the body of the mandible,

which is the center of all growth of the mandible; the angular unit, which forms in response to the lateral pterygoid and masseter muscles; the coronoid unit, which forms in response to the temporalis muscle development; and the alveolar unit, which forms in response to the mandibular teeth.

Almost all of Meckel's cartilage disappears as the mandible develops. The primary bone formed along Meckel's cartilage is soon replaced by secondary bone.

Secondary cartilage appears between the tenth and fourteenth weeks of prenatal development to form the head of the condyle, part of the coronoid process, and the mental protuberance. Separate from Meckel's cartilage, the coronoid cartilage becomes incorporated into the expanding intramembranous bone of the ramus and disappears before birth. In the mental region, a similar situation occurs as the cartilage there disappears when the mandibular processes fuse.

The condylar cartilage appears initially as a cone-shaped structure and is the primordium of the condyle. Chondrocytes differentiate in the center and increase by interstitial and appositional growth. (Histology is discussed in Chapter 8.) By the middle of fetal life, most of the condylar cartilage is replaced with bone as a result of **endochondral ossification**, but its superior end persists into puberty. Thus the condylar cartilage acts as a growth center for the temporomandibular joint (see Chapter 19 for more information).

Developmental Disturbances with Alveolar Bone

The developmental dental anomaly called **anodontia**, in which tooth germs are congenitally absent, also affects the development of the alveolar processes (discussed further in Chapter 6). This occurrence can prevent the alveolar processes of either the maxilla or the mandible from developing. Proper development is impossible because the alveolar unit of each dental arch forms in response to the tooth germs in the area.

Periodontal Ligament

The **periodontal ligament (PDL)** is that part of the periodontium that provides for the attachment of the teeth to the surrounding alveolar bone by way of the cementum (see Figure 14-1). The PDL appears as the **periodontal space** of 0.4 to 1.5 mm on radiographs, a radiolucent area (dark) between the radiopaque (light) lamina dura of the alveolar bone proper and the radiopaque (light) cementum (see Figure 14-17).

The PDL is an organized fibrous connective tissue that also maintains the gingiva in proper relationship to the teeth. In addition, the PDL transmits occlusal forces from the teeth to the bone, allowing for a small amount of movement and acting as a shock absorber for the soft tissue structures around the teeth, such as the nerves and blood vessels (see Chapter 20 for more information).

Other functions of the PDL are discussed later. These other PDL functions include serving as the periosteum for the cementum and alveolar bone. Cells in the PDL also participate in the formation and resorption of the hard tissues of the periodontium. Additionally, the PDL has blood vessels that provide

nutrition for the cells of the ligament and surrounding cells of the cementum and alveolar bone.

Finally, the PDL and its nerve supply provide a most efficient proprioceptive mechanism, allowing us to feel even the most delicate forces applied to the teeth and any displacement of the teeth resulting from these forces (such as metal foil in candy wrappers). Unlike the soft connective tissue of the pulp, the PDL also transmits pain, touch, pressure and temperature sensations. Similar to the alveolar bone, the PDL develops from the dental sac of the tooth germ, as discussed in Chapter 6. Unlike other connective tissues of the periodontium, however, the PDL does not show the changes related to aging, although it can undergo drastic changes as a result of periodontal disease (discussed later).

Clinical Considerations with the Periodontal Ligament

Even after patients have endodontic therapy (root canal treatment) and the tooth becomes nonvital, they may feel discomfort when biting down or when the clinician taps the teeth to measure tooth percussion sensitivity. This discomfort is not due to sensations from the lost pulp tissue but from sensations within the PDL as it receives pressure from slight intrusive movements of the tooth during mastication. Many times the inflammation associated with pulpitis travels through the apical foramen to involve the periodontium, thus causing apical inflammation and destruction, and surgery may have to be performed to remove the apical lesion (apicoectomy).

COMPONENTS OF THE PERIODONTAL LIGAMENT

Because the PDL is a connective tissue, it has all the components of a connective tissue, such as intercellular substance, cells, and fibers (Figure 14-25; see also Chapter 8). The PDL also has a vascular supply, lymphatics, and nerve supply, which enter the apical foramen of the tooth to supply the pulp (see Chapter 13). Two types of nerves are found within the PDL. One type is afferent, or sensory, which is myelinated and transmits sensations that occur within the PDL; the other is autonomic sympathetic, which regulates the blood vessels.

Cells in the Periodontal Ligament

The PDL has all the cells that are in most connective tissues, such as blood cells and endothelial cells (Figure 14-26). Thus like all connective tissues, the **fibroblast** is the most common cell in the PDL. The PDL also has cells that are not in other connective tissues, such as a line of cementoblasts along the cemental surface. **Osteoblasts** are also present in the

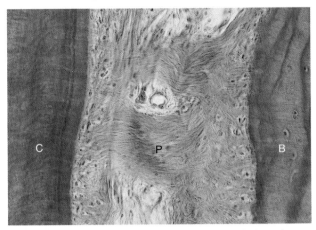

FIGURE 14-25 Microscopic view of the periodontal ligament (*P*), which is located between the alveolar bone (*B*) and cementum (*C*). (Courtesy of Dr. James McIntosh, PhD, Department of Biomedical Sciences, Baylor College of Dentistry, Dallas, TX.)

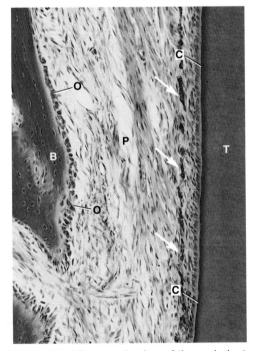

FIGURE 14-26 Microscopic view of the periodontal ligament (*P*), a connective tissue with many cells, including a layer of osteoblasts (*O*) on the alveolar bone proper (*B*) and layer of cementoblasts (*C*) on the cementum of the tooth (*T*). The periodontal ligament also includes the epithelial rests of Malassez (*white arrows*). (Courtesy of Dr. James McIntosh, PhD, Department of Biomedical Sciences, Baylor College of Dentistry, Dallas, TX.)

PDL at the periphery of the alveolar bone proper. In addition, the PDL has **osteoclasts** as well as odontoclasts. Each specific cell type can form either cementum or bone or even resorb these respective tissues, depending on the need of the tissues or the demands of the adjacent environment. Also present are undifferentiated mesenchymal cells, which can differentiate into any of these cells if any of these cell populations

are injured. Thus the PDL serves as a periosteum for the cementum and adjacent alveolar bone.

In addition, the **epithelial rests of Malassez** are present (see Figure 14-26). These groups of epithelial cells become located in the mature PDL after the disintegration of Hertwig's epithelial root sheath during the formation of the root (see Chapter 6).

Clinical Considerations for the Periodontal Ligament

The epithelial rests of Malassez can become cystic, usually forming nondiagnostic, radiolucent apical lesions that can be seen on radiographs. These groups of cells become cystic as a result of chronic periapical inflammation after pulpitis occurs. These cysts must be surgically removed and then observed for recurrence on follow-up visits.

Guided tissue regeneration (GTR) is being used in the treatment of alveolar bone loss and disorganization of the PDL caused by periodontal disease. This method to increase bone levels and strengthen the PDL uses a membrane of various materials that allows only osteoblasts and fibroblasts to produce either bone or PDL fibers at the diseased site. Guided tissue regeneration is becoming more successful because the membrane type being used results in less inflammation at the site.

FIBER GROUPS OF THE PERIODONTAL LIGAMENT

All the fibers in the PDL are collagen in structure. The PDL is wider near the apex and cervix of the tooth and narrower between these two end points. Most of the fibers are **principal fibers,** which are not individual fibers but are organized into groups or bundles according to their orientation to the mature tooth and related function; these bundles resemble spliced ropes. Each is approximately 5 micrometers in diameter. Researchers refer to these groups by various names, but this text uses the most common names known to dental professionals. Whether some nonorganized collagen fibers or secondary fibers of the PDL form an indifferent or intermediate plexus remains controversial.

During mastication and speech, certain forces are exerted on a tooth, such as rotational, tilting, extrusive, or intrusive. The principal fibers of the PDL distribute these forces, protecting its soft tissues and allowing some give when they occur, like a rubber band attached at both ends to two hard objects. The fibers can accomplish this task because the ends of each fiber are anchored within both cementum and the alveolar bone proper or in cementum alone from adjacent roots or teeth. The ends of the principal fibers that are within either cementum or alveolar bone proper are called Sharpey's fibers (see Figure 14-16). Sharpey's fibers are each partially inserted into these hard tissues of the periodontium at 90 degrees, or a right angle. Recent

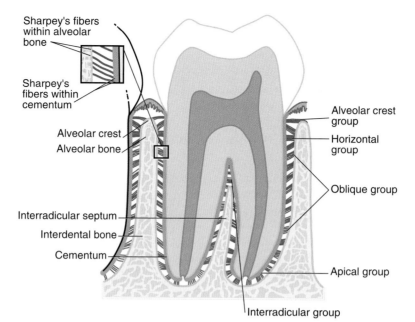

FIGURE 14-27 A sagittal section of the tooth and periodontal ligament. The fiber groups of the alveolodental ligament are identified: alveolar crest, horizontal, oblique, and apical as well as interradicular on multirooted teeth.

TABLE 14-2

Fiber Groups of the Alveolodental Ligament

Fiber Groups	Location	Function
Alveolar crest group	Originates in the alveolar crest of the alveolar bone proper and fans out to insert into the cervical cementum at various angles	To resist tilting, intrusive, extrusive, and rotational forces
Horizontal group	Originates in the alveolar bone proper apical to its alveolar crest and inserts into the cementum horizontally	To resist tilting forces and rotational forces
Oblique group	Originates in the alveolar bone proper and extends apically to insert more apically into the cementum in an oblique manner	To resist intrusive forces and rotational forces
Apical group	Radiates from the apical region of the cementum to insert into the surrounding alveolar bone proper	To resist extrusive forces and rotational forces
Interradicular group (only on multirooted teeth)	Inserted on the cementum of one root to the cementum of the other root(s) superficial to the interradicular septum	To resist intrusive, extrusive, tilting, and rotational forces

studies show that the fiber bundles go the length of the periodontal space and then branch along the two end points, increasing the strength of the ligament.

The main principal fiber group is the **alveolodental ligament**, which consists of five fiber groups: alveolar crest, horizontal, oblique, apical, and interradicular on multirooted teeth (Figure 14-27 and Table 14-2). If

viewed on sagittal section or from a facial or lingual view of the PDL, the fiber groups have different orientations from the cervix to the apex. If the alveolodental ligament is viewed on cross section, the fiber groups appear as spokes around the tooth (Figure 14-28). Thus the overall function of the alveolodental ligament is to resist rotational forces, or twisting of the

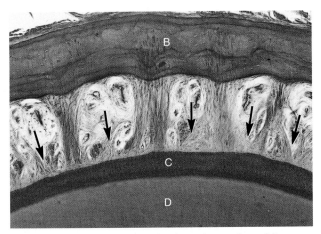

FIGURE 14-28 Microscopic view of a portion of the cross section of the tooth composed of cementum (*C*) and dentin (*D*) and highlighting the spokelike arrangement (*arrows*) of the alveolodental ligament, which originates in the alveolar bone proper (*B*) of the surrounding alveolus. (Courtesy of Dr. James McIntosh, PhD, Department of Biomedical Sciences, Baylor College of Dentistry, Dallas, TX.)

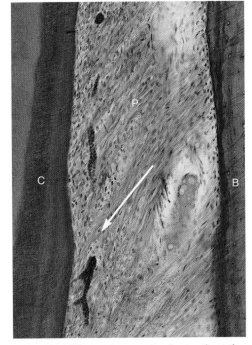

FIGURE 14-29 Photomicrograph of a tooth at the position of the oblique group of the periodontal ligament (*P*), which originates in the alveolar bone proper (*B*) and extends obliquely to insert more apically into the cementum (*C*; direction indicated by *arrow*). (Courtesy of Dr. James McIntosh, PhD, Department of Biomedical Sciences, Baylor College of Dentistry, Dallas, TX.)

tooth in its alveolus. Each of the five fiber groups also has its own function related to its orientation to the tooth.

The **alveolar crest group** of the alveolodental ligament originates in the alveolar crest of the alveolar bone proper and fans out to insert into the cervical cementum at various angles. The function of the alveolar crest group is to resist tilting, intrusive, extrusive, and rotational forces.

The **horizontal group** of the alveolodental ligament originates in the alveolar bone proper apical to its alveolar crest and inserts into the cementum horizontally. The function of the horizontal group is to resist tilting forces, which work to force the tooth to tip either mesially, distally, lingually, or facially, and to resist rotational forces.

The **oblique group** of the alveolodental ligament is the most numerous of the fiber groups and covers the apical two thirds of the root (Figure 14-29). This group originates in the alveolar bone proper and extends apically to insert more apically into the cementum in an oblique manner. The function of the oblique group is to resist intrusive forces, which try to push the tooth inward, as well as rotational forces.

The **apical group** of the alveolodental group radiates from the apical region of the cementum to insert into the surrounding alveolar bone proper. The function of the apical group is to resist extrusive forces, which try to pull the tooth outward, and rotational forces.

The **interradicular group** of the alveolodental group is found only on multirooted teeth. This group is inserted on the cementum of one root to the cementum of the other root (or roots) superficial to the interradicular septum and thus has no bony attach-

ment. This group works together with the alveolar crest and apical groups to resist intrusive, extrusive, tilting, and rotational forces.

Another principal fiber other than the alveolodental ligament is the **interdental ligament,** or transseptal ligament (Figures 14-30 and 14-31). This fiber group inserts mesiodistally or interdentally into the cervical cementum of neighboring teeth over the alveolar crest of the alveolar bone proper. Thus the fibers travel from cementum to cementum without any bony attachment. The function of the interdental ligament is to resist rotational forces and thus to hold the teeth in interproximal contact.

Some histologists also consider the **gingival fiber group** to be part of the principal fibers of the PDL (Figure 14-32). This is the name given to separate but adjacent fiber groups that are found within the lamina propria of the marginal gingiva. These fiber subgroups include the circular and gingival ligament as well as the alveologingival and dentoperiosteal fibers. They do not support the tooth in relationship to the jaws, resisting any forces of mastication or speech; rather, they support only the marginal gingival tissues to maintain their relationship to the tooth. Some textbooks contain extensive discussion of the different subgroups of the gingival fiber group, but simplification of the histology is useful here.

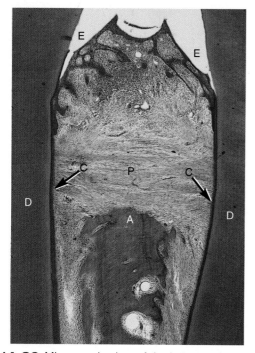

FIG. 14-30 Microscopic view of the interdental ligament of the periodontal ligament (*P*) between two neighboring teeth and superior to the alveolar crest (*A*). The teeth are composed of cementum (*C*), dentin (*D*), and an enamel space (*E*) owing to the fixation process. (Courtesy of Dr. James McIntosh, PhD, Department of Biomedical Sciences, Baylor College of Dentistry, Dallas, TX.)

The circular ligament is considered a fiber subgroup of the gingival fiber group. This fiber group is located in the lamina propria of the marginal gingiva. The circular ligament encircles the tooth, as shown on a cross section of a tooth. It reminds one of a sphincterlike "pulling of the purse strings" of the gingiva, which helps maintain gingival integrity.

The dentogingival ligament is another fiber subgroup of the gingival fiber group. This fiber group inserts in the cementum on the root, apical to the epithelial attachment, and extends into the lamina propria of the marginal gingiva. Thus the dentogingival ligament has only one mineralized attachment to the cementum. The dentogingival ligament works with the circular ligament to maintain gingival integrity, possibly of the marginal gingiva.

The alveologingival fibers are another subgroup of the gingival fiber group. These fibers extend from the alveolar crest of the alveolar bone proper and radiate coronally into the overlying lamina propria of the marginal gingiva. The alveologingival fibers possibly help to attach the gingiva to the alveolar bone because of their one mineralized attachment to bone. Another subgroup is the dentoperiosteal fibers, which course from the cementum, near the CEJ, across the alveolar crest. They possibly anchor the tooth to the bone and protect the deeper periodontal ligament.

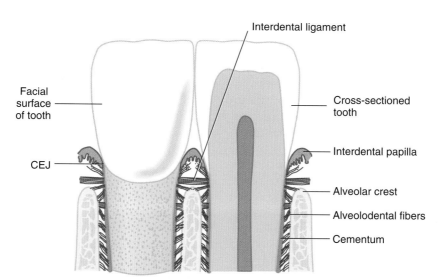

FIGURE 14-31 The interdental ligament, which inserts mesiodistally or interdentally into the cervical cementum of neighboring teeth over the alveolar crest of the alveolar bone proper. The function of the interdental ligament is to resist rotational forces and thus hold the teeth in interproximal contact.

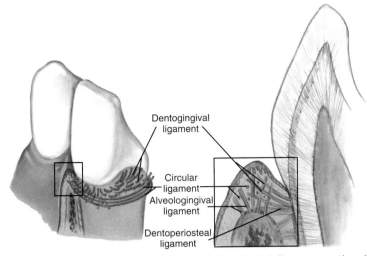

FIGURE 14-32 Some of the fiber subgroups of the gingival fiber group: the circular, dentogingival, alveologingival, and dentoperiosteal ligaments. Note that both of these are located in the lamina propria of the marginal gingiva and support only the gingival tissues to maintain their relationship to the tooth.

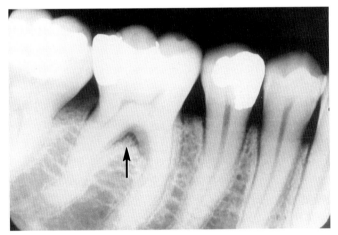

FIGURE 14-33 Occlusal trauma can be noted on radiographs with a widening of the radiolucent space between the radiopaque lamina dura of the alveolar bone proper and the radiopaque cementum. Thickening of the lamina dura in response is also possible.

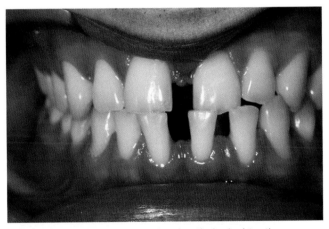

FIGURE 14-34 An example of pathological tooth migration caused by the weakened periodontium in which the occlusal forces need not be abnormal if the periodontal support is reduced by periodontal disease.

Clinical Considerations with the Periodontal Ligament

Occlusal trauma does not cause periodontal disease but can cause an acceleration of the progression of existing disease, and certain changes are noted in the PDL. When traumatic forces of occlusion are placed on a tooth, the PDL widens to take the extra forces. (Occlusal trauma is discussed further in Chapter 20.) Occlusal trauma can be viewed on radiographs as a widening of the radiolucent (dark) periodontal space between the radiopaque (light) lamina dura of the alveolar bone proper and the radiopaque (light) cementum (Figure 14-33). Clinically, occlusal trauma has the late manifestation of increased mobility of the tooth and possibly the presence of pathological tooth migration (Figure 14-34). This migration is due to the weakened periodontium, when even the occlusal forces need not be abnormal if the periodontal support is reduced.

Changes are also noted histologically in the PDL as a result of occlusal trauma: thrombosis, dilation, and edema of the blood supply; hyalinization of the collagen fibers; the presence of an inflammatory infiltrate; and nuclear changes in the osteoblasts, cementoblasts, and fibroblasts. No histological changes are noted in the gingival collagen fibers or in the junctional epithelium with occlusal trauma. Histological changes distinct from existing periodontal disease are reversible if the causes of trauma are eliminated.

The PDL also undergoes drastic changes with chronic periodontal disease that involves the deeper structures of the periodontium (periodontitis). The fiber groups of the PDL become disorganized, and their attachments to the alveolar bone proper or cementum by way of Sharpey's fibers are lost because of the resorption of these two hard dental tissues (see Figure 14-24). The first fiber group to be involved in changes caused by periodontal disease is the alveolar crest group of the alveolodental ligament.

The destruction of the PDL with periodontal disease then proceeds in an apical manner, affecting the horizontal, then oblique, and then apical and interradicular groups (if present), in that order. The teeth involved in advancement of periodontal disease become increasingly mobile, moving in ways that indicate the amount and type of fiber group lost.

The principal fiber group that remains the longest, despite the previous destruction of the alveolodental ligament, is the interdental ligament. The interdental ligament reattaches itself in a more apical manner as the periodontal disease proceeds apically, so that the teeth are at least held in interproximal contact. Thus when teeth are severely mobile interproximally, the prognosis is poor. Mobility and its amount and direction per tooth should be recorded in a patient's chart to achieve an overall diagnosis for a dentition with periodontal disease.

The interdental ligament is also responsible for the memory of tooth positioning within each dental arch. Therefore adequate time must be allowed to reattach the interdental ligament fully to its new position and thereby ensure the maintenance of the proper alignment established during orthodontic treatment. Retainers, removable and permanent, are used to maintain this desirable alignment.

UNIT IV

DENTAL ANATOMY

Overview of the Dentitions

After studying this chapter, the reader should be able to:

1. Define and pronounce the key terms of this chapter when discussing the teeth or portions of a tooth.
2. Describe the two dentitions of humans and their relationship to each other.
3. Define each dentition period and discuss the important clinical considerations for each dentition period.
4. Assign the correct universal designation for a tooth and the correct dentition period when examining a figure or a patient.
5. Integrate the knowledge of the dentitions into the dental treatment of patients.

Key Terms

Angle: line, point
Alveolar process (al-ve-o-lar)
Alveolus, alveoli (al-ve-o-lus, al-ve-o-lie)
Anatomical crown, root
Anterior teeth
Contact area
Crown
Cusp (kusp)
D-A-Q-T System
Dental anatomy
Dentition (den-tish-in): deciduous (de-sij-you-us), mixed, period, permanent, primary
Clinical crown, root

Contact area
Embrasures (em-bray-zhers)
Incisal (in-sigh-zl)
Height of contour
International Standards Organization Designation System
Interproximal (in-ter-prok-si-mal) space
Mandibular arch, teeth (man-dib-you-lar)
Masticatory surface (mass-ti-ka-tor-ee)
Maxillary arch, teeth (mak-sil-lare-e)
Occlusion (ah-kloo-zhun)

Palmer method
Posterior teeth
Quadrants (kwod-rints)
Ridges
Root, axis line, concavities
Sextants (sex-tants)
Surfaces: buccal (buk-al), distal (dis-tl), facial (fay-shal), labial (lay-be-al), lingual (ling-gwal), occlusal (ah-kloo-zl), mesial (me-ze-il), palatal (pal-ah-tal), proximal (prok-si-mal)
Thirds
Universal Tooth Designation System

THE DENTITIONS

The dentitions are initially discussed in this beginning of Unit IV. The term **dentition** is used to describe the natural teeth in the jawbones. As described in Chapter 6 in relation to tooth development, a person has two dentitions during a lifetime: primary and permanent. The first dentition present is the **primary dentition** (Figure 15-1). Pediatric patients and their supervising adults call these the *baby teeth.*

An older dental term for the primary dentition is the **deciduous dentition**. This term is derived from the concept that the primary dentition is exfoliated, or shed (just as deciduous trees shed their leaves), and replaced entirely by the **permanent dentition;** thus the permanent dentition is the second dentition to develop (Figure 15-2). The permanent dentition is also sometimes called the *secondary dentition,* or *adult teeth.*

By recent convention (or convenience), clinicians seem to prefer to mix and match their dental terms when referring to the two dentitions, as in *primary* and *permanent.* The permanent dentition is also collectively called the *succedaneous dentition* because many of these permanent teeth succeed primary predecessors or are succedaneous.

Still, dental personnel must remember that all the molars of the permanent dentition are nonsuccedaneous and are without any primary predecessors. Development of the primary dentition, eruption and shedding of the primary teeth, and development of the permanent dentition are discussed further in Chapter 6.

Tooth Types

The tooth types in both arches of the primary dentition, 20 teeth in all, include 8 incisors, 4 canines, and 8 molars (see Figure 15-1). The anatomy of the primary dentition is discussed further in Chapter 18.

The tooth types in both arches of the permanent dentition, 32 teeth in all, include 8 incisors, 4 canines, 8 premolars, and 12 molars (see Figure 15-2). Note that only the permanent dentition has premolars; the primary dentition has none. The anatomy of the permanent dentition is discussed further in Chapters 16 (anterior teeth) and 17 (posterior teeth).

Each tooth type has a specific form. This tooth form is related to the masticatory function of the tooth as well as to its role in speech and aesthetics. The form

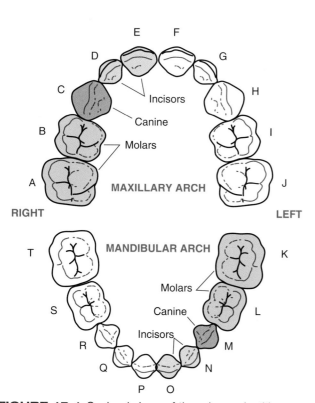

FIGURE 15-1 Occlusal views of the primary dentition during the primary dentition period. The types of teeth within it are identified.

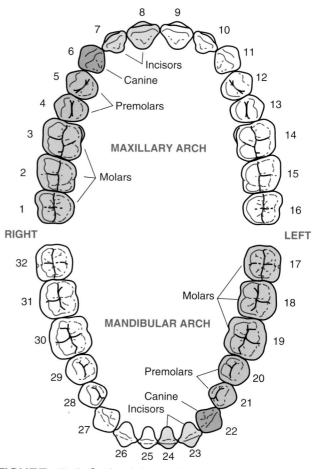

FIGURE 15-2 Occlusal views of the permanent dentition during the permanent period. The types of teeth within it are identified.

and function of each type are similar for both the primary and permanent dentitions.

The incisors function as instruments for biting and cutting food during mastication because of their triangular proximal form. The canines, because of their tapered shape and their prominent cusp, function to pierce or tear food during mastication.

The premolars, which are found only in the permanent dentition, function to assist the molars in grinding food during mastication because of their broad occlusal surface and their prominent cusps. The premolars also assist the canines in piercing and tearing food with their cusps. Finally, as the largest and strongest crowns, the molars function in grinding food during mastication, assisted by the premolars. This is due to the fact that molars have wide occlusal surfaces with prominent cusps.

 Clinical Considerations for Tooth Type

Variation of teeth within a particular tooth type is a given. This variation is of enduring interest to all clinicians. Because the specific shape of a tooth varies in each person and possibly within a dentition, a mold of the crown is made when integrating artificial caps or crowns within an individual dentition. The goal is to match as closely as possible the shape of the patient's teeth on the opposite side so the arch appears symmetrical and the caps or crowns fit the space provided. This mold is selected by comparing it with a mold guide of white plastic model crowns provided by various manufacturers.

The individual tooth form that functions most effectively can be lost as a result of caries, attrition, and trauma; change in form can affect mastication, especially in older patients, who may change to a soft but poor diet. Functional tooth form that has been lost can be approximated by restorative treatment in many cases. Restorations, crowns, bridges, partial or complete dentures, or implants may be used.

Tooth Designation

Both the primary and permanent teeth are designated by the National or **Universal Tooth Designation System** (Figure 15-3). This system is the most widely used in America today for designation of both dentitions because it is adaptable to electronic data transfer. This text uses the Universal System. With the Universal Tooth Designation System, the primary teeth are designated in a consecutive arrangement by using capital letters, *A* through *T,* starting with the maxillary right second molar, moving clockwise, and ending with the mandibular right second molar (see Figure 15-1).

The permanent teeth are designated by the Universal Tooth Designation System in consecutive arrange-

ment as the patient is observed from in front by using the digits *1* through *32,* starting with the maxillary right third molar, moving clockwise, and ending with the mandibular right third molar (see Figure 15-2). The clockwise convention is also used when charting restorations or periodontal conditions in the oral cavity for a patient.

However, the need for a system that can be used internationally, as well as by electronic data transfer, is recognized; thus the acceptance of the **International Standards Organization Designation System (ISO System)** by the World Health Organization (see Figure 15-3). With this system, the teeth are designated by using a two-digit code. The first digit of the code indicates the quadrant (see later discussion under general dental terms), and the second indicates the tooth in this quadrant. This is based on the Federation Dentitaire Internationale's (FDI) System.

Thus with the ISO System, the digits *1* through *4* are used for quadrants in a clockwise manner in the permanent dentition, and digits *5* through *8* are used in a clockwise manner for those quadrants of the primary dentition. For the second digit, which indicates the tooth, the digits *1* through *8* are used for the permanent teeth, and this designation is from the median line in a distal direction. The digits *1* through *5* are then used for the primary dentition, and this designation is also from the median line in a distal direction.

Another system commonly used in orthodontics is the **Palmer Method** (see Figure 15-3). It is very helpful for orthodontics because it allows discussion of the teeth that require treatment. In this system, the teeth are designated with a right-angle symbol indicating the quadrants with the tooth number inside, similar in numbering to the ISO System.

DENTITION PERIODS

Although there are two dentitions, three **dentition periods** occur throughout a person's lifetime because the two dentitions overlap (Table 15-1). Each patient should be assigned a dentition period to allow for the best dental treatment for that period. This specificity is especially important in the specialty of orthodontics, because growth during certain dentition periods is maximized to allow expansion of the jawbones and movement of the teeth. Appendix D of this text contains charts of developmental information on each permanent tooth.

Primary Dentition Period

The first dentition period is the **primary dentition period** (see Figure 15-1). This period begins with the

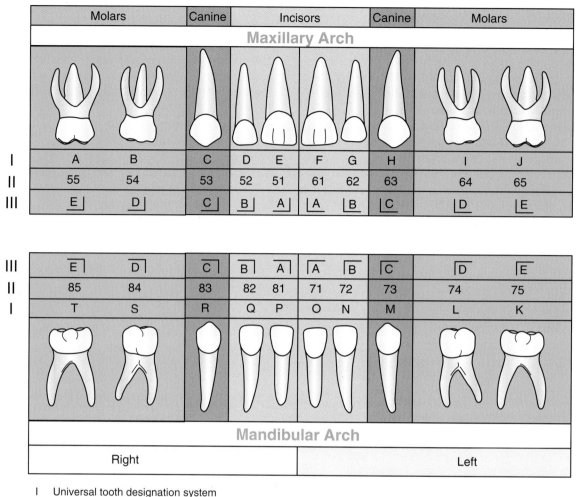

	Molars		Canine	Incisors				Canine	Molars	

Maxillary Arch

I	A	B	C	D	E	F	G	H	I	J
II	55	54	53	52	51	61	62	63	64	65
III	E⌋	D⌋	C⌋	B⌋	A⌋	⌊A	⌊B	⌊C	⌊D	⌊E

III	E⌋	D⌋	C⌋	B⌋	A⌋	⌊A	⌊B	⌊C	⌊D	⌊E
II	85	84	83	82	81	71	72	73	74	75
I	T	S	R	Q	P	O	N	M	L	K

Mandibular Arch

Right	Left

I   Universal tooth designation system

II   International Standards Organization designation system

III   Palmer Method

A

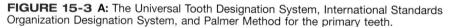

FIGURE 15-3 A: The Universal Tooth Designation System, International Standards Organization Designation System, and Palmer Method for the primary teeth.

eruption of the primary mandibular central incisors. Thus this period occurs between approximately 6 months and 6 years of age (see Chapter 6 for the chronological order of primary tooth eruption and Chapter 18 for their approximate ages). Only the primary teeth are present during this time. This period usually ends when the first permanent tooth erupts, a permanent mandibular first molar. The jawbones are beginning to grow during this period to accommodate the larger permanent teeth.

Mixed Dentition Period

The **mixed dentition period** follows the primary dentition period (Figure 15-4). This period occurs between approximately 6 and 12 years of age (see Chapter 6). Both primary and permanent teeth are present during this transitional stage. During this time, both shedding

of primary teeth and eruption of permanent teeth begin. Thus this period begins with eruption of the first permanent tooth, a permanent mandibular first molar. This period usually ends with shedding of the last primary tooth.

The color differences between the primary and permanent teeth become apparent during this period. The primary crowns are lighter in color than the darker permanent crowns owing to the fact that the permanent teeth have less opaque enamel and thus the yellow dentin is more visible. Also more evident is the difference in the crown size and root length between the smaller and shorter primary teeth and the larger and longer permanent teeth. The jawbones undergo their fastest and most noticeable growth during this period, consistent with the onset of puberty, to accommodate the larger teeth of the adult. Females shed their primary teeth and receive their permanent teeth slightly earlier than males, possibly reflecting the earlier overall physical maturation achieved.

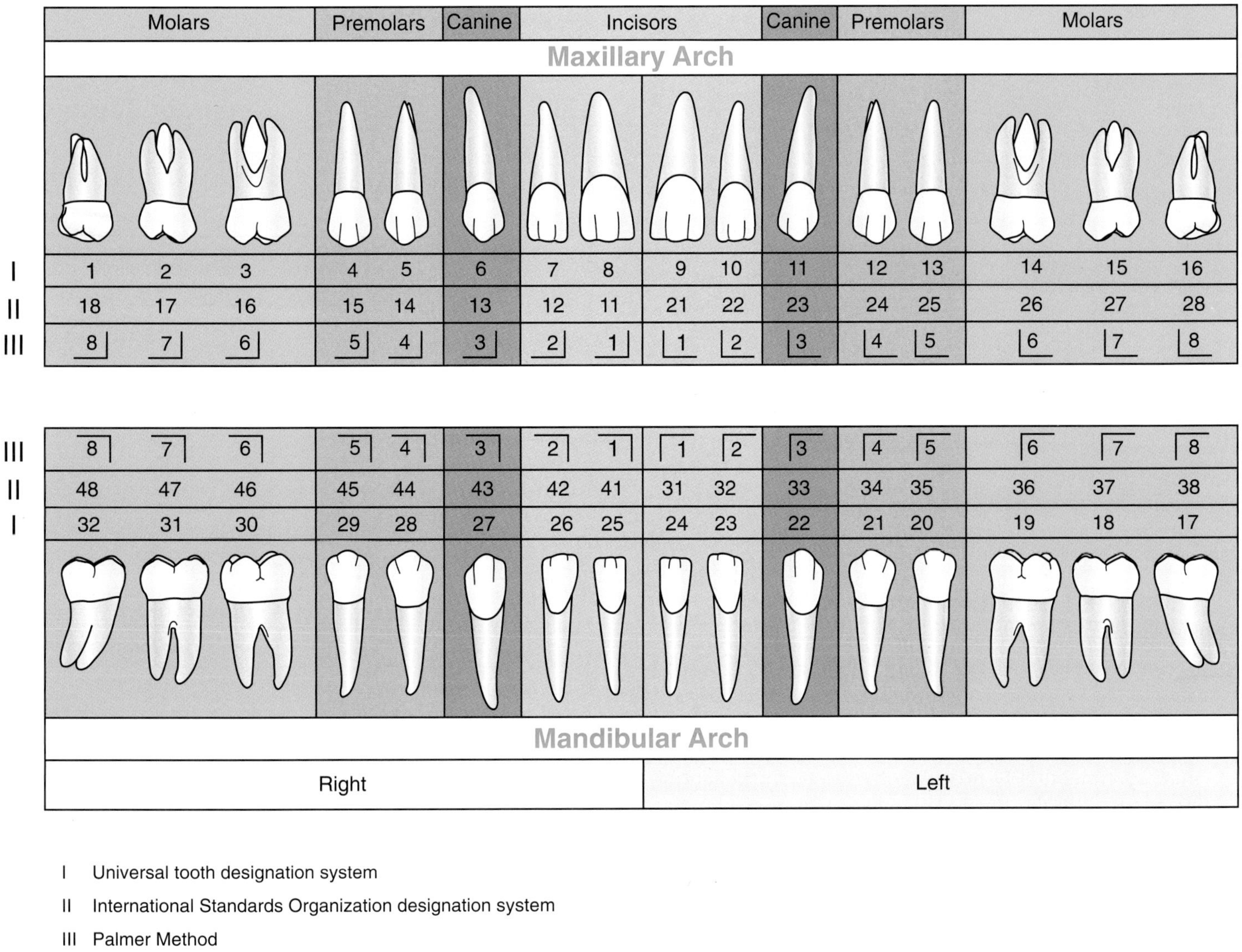

	Molars			Premolars		Canine	Incisors				Canine	Premolars		Molars		
								Maxillary Arch								

I	1	2	3	4	5	6	7	8	9	10	11	12	13	14	15	16
II	18	17	16	15	14	13	12	11	21	22	23	24	25	26	27	28
III	8⏌	7⏌	6⏌	5⏌	4⏌	3⏌	2⏌	1⏌	⌊1	⌊2	⌊3	⌊4	⌊5	⌊6	⌊7	⌊8

III	8⌐	7⌐	6⌐	5⌐	4⌐	3⌐	2⌐	1⌐	⌐1	⌐2	⌐3	⌐4	⌐5	⌐6	⌐7	⌐8
II	48	47	46	45	44	43	42	41	31	32	33	34	35	36	37	38
I	32	31	30	29	28	27	26	25	24	23	22	21	20	19	18	17

	Mandibular Arch	
Right		Left

I   Universal tooth designation system

II International Standards Organization designation system

III Palmer Method

B

FIGURE 15-3, cont'd B: The Universal Tooth Designation System, International Standards Organization Designation System, and Palmer Method for the permanent teeth.

TABLE 15-1

Dentition Periods and Clinical Considerations

	Primary Dentition Period	Mixed Dentition Period	Permanent Dentition Period
Approximate time span	6 months to 6 years	6 years to 12 years	After 12 years
Teeth marking start of period	Eruption of primary mandibular central incisor	Eruption of permanent mandibular first molar	Shedding of the last primary tooth
Dentition present	Primary	Primary and permanent	Usually permanent
Growth of jawbones	Beginning	Fastest and most noticeable	Slowest and least noticeable

Adapted from Ash MM. *Wheeler's Dental Anatomy, Physiology and Occlusions*, ed 8. WB Saunders, Philadelphia, 2002.

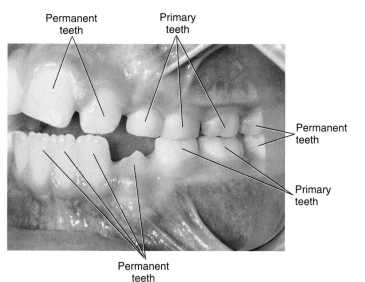

Permanent teeth

Primary teeth

Permanent teeth

Primary teeth

Permanent teeth

FIGURE 15-4 An example of the oral cavity during the mixed dentition period. The primary and permanent teeth are identified.

Permanent Dentition Period

The final dentition period is the **permanent dentition period** (see Figure 15-2). This period begins with shedding of the last primary tooth. Thus this period begins just after approximately 12 years of age and includes eruption of all the permanent teeth, except for teeth that are congenitally missing or impacted and cannot erupt (usually the third molars; see Chapter 6 for the chronological order of permanent tooth eruption and root completion and Table 15-2 for approximate ages as well as the tables in Appendix D of this text). The permanent teeth are usually the only teeth present during this period. Growth of the jawbones is not very noticeable as it slows and then eventually stops. Thus very little growth of the jaws occurs overall during this period, given that puberty has passed. Tooth types tend to erupt in pairs so that if any asymmetry exists, a radiograph of the area may be required. If you see a child who is unusually early or late in getting his or her teeth, inquire about family dental history.

TABLE 15-2

Approximate Eruption and Root Completion Ages for Permanent Teeth (in Years)

Maxillary Teeth	Eruption	Root Completion
Central incisor	7-8	10
Lateral incisor	8-9	11
Canine	11-12	13-15
First premolar	10-11	12-13
Second premolar	10-12	12-14
First molar	6-7	9-10
Second molar	12-13	14-16
Third molar	17-21	18-25
Mandibular Teeth	**Eruption**	**Root Completion**
Central incisor	6-7	9
Lateral incisor	7-8	10
Canine	9-1	12-14
First premolar	10-12	12-13
Second premolar	11-12	13-14
First molar	6-7	9-10
Second molar	11-13	14-15
Third molar	17-21	18-25

Adapted from Ash MM. *Wheeler's Dental Anatomy, Physiology and Occlusion*, ed 8. WB Saunders, Philadelphia, 2002. See also the ADA Oral Health Topics website at www.ada.org.

Clinical Considerations for the Mixed Dentition Period

The clinical considerations associated with the primary and permanent dentition periods are discussed later in each chapter devoted to them. The mixed dentition period has characteristic physiological and psychological effects. This dentition period is sometimes called the *ugly duckling stage* because of the different tooth colors, disproportionately sized teeth, and various clinical crown heights. In addition, temporary edentulous areas and crowding are noted. Additionally, in many cases, the surrounding gingiva responds to all these changes by becoming inflamed.

Oral hygiene is difficult for patients during the mixed dentition period because these changes may promote bacterial plaque biofilm retention. Supervising adults and child patients must be reminded to be especially diligent about oral hygiene care and reassured that this stage is only temporary. Preventive orthodontic care may also be initiated during this dentition period.

If gingival inflammation is only slight, with very little bacterial plaque biofilm formation, but bone loss around the newly erupted permanent first molars and lower anteriors is severe, early aggressive periodontitis (previously referred to as *juvenile periodontitis*) may be suspected. Early intervention in this serious periodontal disease can prevent further bone loss in the adult jaws.

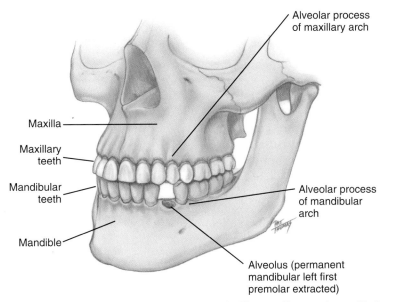

FIGURE 15-5 Oral cavity with the permanent teeth. The maxillary and mandibular arches and other structures are identified.

DENTAL ANATOMY TERMINOLOGY

Dental professionals must be able to understand and use dental anatomy terminology. Dental anatomy is the area of the dental sciences dealing with the morphology, or form, of the teeth, both crown and root. Restorative dentistry uses many dental anatomy terms when discussing treatment. Periodontal treatment of the teeth also necessitates using many of these terms, such as line angles, when probing around the teeth.

General Dental Terms

As noted earlier in Chapters 2 and 14, each tooth is surrounded and supported by the bone of the tooth socket, or **alveolus (plural, alveoli;** Figure 15-5). Each alveolus is located in the **alveolar process,** or tooth-bearing portion of each jawbone. Each alveolar process of the jawbones is also considered a dental arch, maxillary and mandibular.

The teeth in the **maxillary arch** of the upper jawbones, or maxillary arch, are the **maxillary teeth;** the teeth in the **mandibular arch** of the lower jawbone, or mandible, are the **mandibular teeth** (see Figure 15-5). Note that in this textbook the illustrations of teeth are oriented according to their position in the jaw of a person in anatomical position (see Appendix A). Thus maxillary teeth always show the root superior to the crown; mandibular teeth always show the root inferior to the crown.

Occlusion is the way that the teeth of the mandibular arch come into contact with those of the maxillary arch. The term **occlusion** is also used to describe the anatomical alignment of the teeth and their relation-

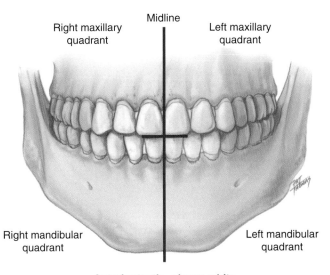

Anterior teeth - shown white
Posterior teeth - shown yellow

FIGURE 15-6 Oral cavity with the permanent teeth. The midline, quadrants, and anterior and posterior teeth are identified.

ship to the rest of the masticatory system (see Chapter 20 for more discussion).

Each dental arch has a midline, an imaginary vertical plane that divides the arch into two approximately equal halves, a right and a left (Figure 15-6). The midline is similar to the median, or midsagittal, plane of the body. The midline is an important consideration in the evaluation of a smile. Thus each dental arch can be further divided into two **quadrants,** with four quadrants in the entire oral cavity. Quadrants include the maxillary right quadrant, the maxillary left quadrant, the mandibular right quadrant, and the mandibular left quadrant. This designation is useful when planning a course of dental treatment for a patient over time.

Thus the correct sequence of words when describing a tooth is based on a **D-A-Q-T System:** *D* for dentition, *A* for arch, *Q* for quadrant, and *T* for tooth type. An example would be the permanent (*D*) mandibular (*A*) left (*Q*) first premolar (*T*).

Teeth can also be described according to their position in each dental arch in relationship to the midline (see Figure 15-6). The incisors and canines are considered **anterior teeth** because they are closer to the midline. In contrast, the molars (and premolars, if present) are considered posterior teeth because they are farther from the midline.

Some dental treatment plans also include the use of **sextants**, which divide each dental arch into three portions according to the relationship to the midline: the right posterior sextant, the anterior sextant, and the left posterior sextant. Thus the permanent maxillary right central incisor is in the maxillary anterior sextant. As a result of the mapping of nerve pathways, this information is quite useful in treatment plans that use local anesthesia for patient pain control.

To prevent miscommunication internationally, the ISO System also has designation of areas in the oral cavity (used also in their tooth designation system). These are designated by a two-digit number, and at least one of the two digits is zero (Table 15-3). An example of this system is that *00* designates the whole of the oral cavity, and *01* designates the maxillary area only.

Tooth Anatomy Terms

Each tooth consists of a crown and one or more roots (Figure 15-7). The crown has dentin covered by enamel, and each root has dentin covered by cementum. The inner portion of the dentin of both crown and root also covers the pulp cavity of the tooth. The pulp cavity has a pulp chamber, pulp canal (or canals) with

apex (or apices) and apical foramen (or foramina), and possibly pulp horn (or horns).

The enamel of the crown and cementum of the root usually meet close to the cementoenamel junction (CEJ), an external line at the neck or cervix of the tooth. The histology of the portions of a tooth is covered in Chapter 14, including a discussion of the various interfaces of the CEJ. At the CEJ, the cementum over the

TABLE 15-3

ISO System for Designation of Areas of Oral Cavity

Whole oral cavity	00
Maxillary area	01
Mandibular area	02
Upper right quadrant	10
Upper left quadrant	20
Lower left quadrant	30
Lower right quadrant	40
Upper right sextant	03
Upper anterior sextant	04
Upper left sextant	05
Lower left sextant	06
Lower anterior sextant	07
Lower right sextant	08

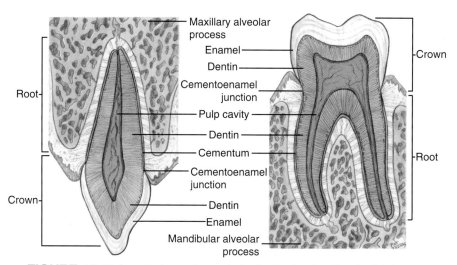

FIGURE 15-7 An anterior and a posterior tooth showing the dental tissues.

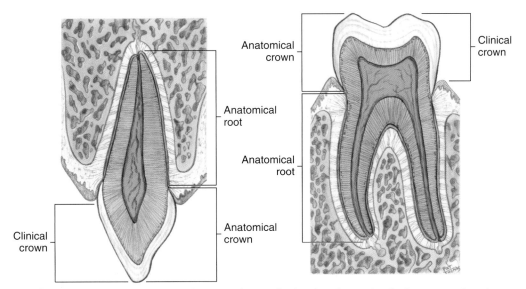

FIGURE 15-8 An anterior and a posterior tooth showing the anatomical crown and root as well as the clinical crown. The clinical root is not shown because this is a healthy peridontal situation without recession, which would expose a clinical root.

neck of each tooth may overlap the enamel, the enamel may meet the cementum edge to edge, or a small area of dentin may be exposed. The CEJ usually feels smooth or evenly grainy or has a slight groove when explored.

Portions of the crown and root of a tooth can also be defined in more specific ways (Figure 15-8). The **anatomical crown** is the portion covered by enamel. It remains mostly constant throughout the life of the tooth, except for attrition and other physical wear. The **clinical crown** is that portion of the anatomical crown that is visible and not covered by the gingiva. Its height is determined by the location of the gingival margin. The clinical crown of a tooth can change over time, especially as the gingiva recedes rootward. This text, when discussing the crown of a tooth, refers to the anatomical crown unless designated otherwise.

Similarly, the **anatomical root** is that portion of the root covered by cementum. The **clinical root** of a tooth is that portion of the anatomical root that is visible, subject to variability over time, again related to gingival recession. This text, when discussing the root of a tooth, refers to the anatomical root of a healthy tooth unless designated otherwise.

Teeth may have one or more roots, but all the roots of both dentitions have common traits. All roots are widest at the CEJ and taper toward the apex of the tooth. Roots have more bulk on the facial surface than on the lingual surface. The root tapers more dramatically on the lingual surface. Many surfaces of the roots have indentations, or **root concavities.** Some clinicians describe features of a tooth related to the **root axis line (RAL),** which is an imaginary line representing the long axis of a tooth, drawn in a way to bisect the root and the crown in the cervical area. The angulation

Clinical Considerations with Tooth Anatomy

Certain restorations may cover the entire crown area; these are called full restorative crowns (or "caps" by patients). A crown should ideally cover the entire prepared clinical crown, but enlarged gingival conditions or loss of crown structure may require a surgical periodontal procedure called *crown lengthening* to increase the amount of clinical crown and reduce the surrounding gingival tissues by removal.

Roots alone may also be retained after the crown of a root canal–treated tooth is removed if the periodontium is not adequate to support a prosthesis, such as a bridge or partial denture. The roots may have enough structure and gingival attachment to support a removable prosthesis, such as a complete or partial overdenture. Also, pins may be placed within the root and the crown to help with the buildup of restorative materials to support an individual crown restoration.

of the tooth and its roots is never strictly vertical within the alveolar bone (see Chapter 20 for more discussion).

Historically in dental education, the importance of clinical crown anatomy was emphasized, with limited emphasis on clinical root anatomy. Subsequently, dental professionals have seen an increased educational emphasis placed on detailed knowledge of root anatomy. This change in emphasis is due to a new recognition of the importance of precise periodontal root instrumentation to achieve oral health in cases of disease as well as preservation of the crown of the teeth by restorations. Initially, pocket analysis using a periodontal probe and a Nabor's probe (within furcation areas) yields the situational root morphology and deposit level. Once root morphology is understood and the patient's periodontal needs ascertained, the dental professional can also choose the correct instrument from the various ones available. In addition, the awareness of root morphology will prevent the destruction of the root by overinstrumentation.

Root concavities should be carefully considered during instrumentation appointments because treatment failures have been linked to deposits that have been left, either after therapy or oral hygiene; these deposits contribute to the continuation of the disease process. Studies show a significantly greater attachment loss for root surfaces with proximal root grooves compared with those that lack proximal root grooves. Whereas these concavities can act as predisposing factors in the periodontal disease process, the depressions also increase the attachment area, producing a root shape more resistant to damaging occlusal forces. Thus root contours present both harmful and protective effects that must be considered individually in the patient's periodontal prognosis.

Until recently, clinicians were not able to visualize the root surface unless surgery was performed. However, with the recent development of endoscopic technology with its small camera that can fit within a deepened sulcus, clinicians today are able to see the root surface in real time. When incorporated into clinical practice in the future, such devices may change the way many dental procedures are performed.

Tooth Orientational Terms

Each tooth has five surfaces: facial, lingual, masticatory, mesial, and distal. Thus each tooth is like a box with sides. Some of the surfaces of the tooth are identified by their orientational relationship to other orofacial structures (Figure 15-9). Tooth surfaces closest to the facial surface are considered **facial** surfaces. Those facial tooth surfaces close to the lips are also termed the **labial** surfaces. Those facial tooth surfaces close to the inner cheek are also considered the **buccal** surfaces. Therefore the anterior teeth have a labial surface, and posterior teeth have a buccal surface.

Those tooth surfaces closest to the tongue are termed the **lingual** surfaces. Those lingual surfaces closest to the palate on the maxillary arch are sometimes also termed the **palatal** surfaces. The **masticatory** surface is the chewing surface on the most superior surface of the crown. This is the **incisal** surface for anterior teeth and the **occlusal** surface for posterior teeth.

The masticatory surfaces of both anterior and posterior teeth have linear elevations, or **ridges,** which are named according to location. The masticatory surfaces of both canines and posterior teeth also have at least one major elevation, which is called a **cusp.**

Surfaces of both the crown and the root are also defined by their relationship to the midline (see Figure

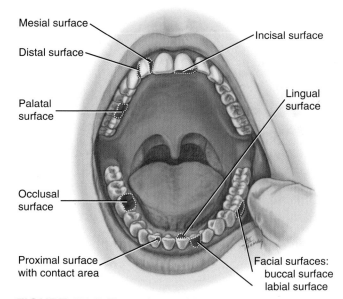

FIGURE 15-9 The surfaces of the teeth and their orientational relationship to other oral cavity structures, to the midline, and to other teeth are highlighted.

15-9). The surface closest to the midline is considered the **mesial** surface; the surface farthest away from the midline is considered the **distal** surface.

Together, both the mesial and the distal surfaces between adjacent teeth are considered the **proximal** surfaces. In other words, either surface of a tooth that is next to an adjacent tooth is referred to as a proximal surface, which may therefore be either the mesial or the distal surface. The area between adjacent tooth surfaces is called the **interproximal space**.

The area where the crowns of adjacent teeth in the same arch physically touch on each proximal surface is called the **contact area** (see Figure 15-9) or referred to by clinicians as the "contact." The contact areas on the mesial and distal are usually also considered the location of the height of contour on the proximal surfaces. The **height of contour,** or crest of curvature, is the greatest elevation of the tooth either incisocervically or occlusocervically on a specific surface of the crown (Figure 15-10). The facial and lingual surfaces of a tooth also have a height of contour that is easily seen when viewing the tooth's profile from the proximal.

It is noted when viewing teeth overall that the proximal CEJ curvature is greatest on the anterior and the least on the posterior teeth. However, this curvature is about the same on mesial and distal surfaces of the two teeth that face each other. In addition, on any given tooth, the height of curvature is greater on the mesial aspect of that tooth than it is on the distal.

When two teeth in the same arch come into contact, their curvatures next to the contact areas form spaces called **embrasures** (Figure 15-11). An embrasure is a triangular-shaped space between two teeth created by the sloping away of the mesial and distal surfaces and

ANTERIOR   POSTERIOR

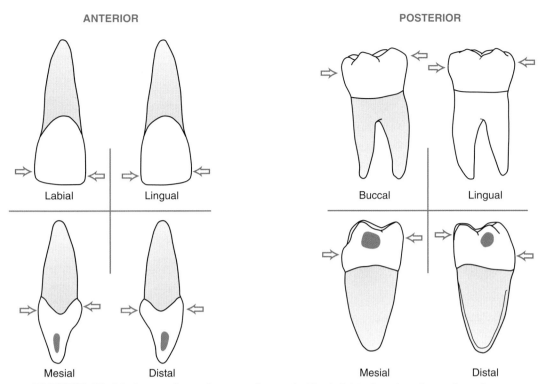

FIGURE 15-10 An anterior and a posterior tooth. The height of contour for each surface (with contact areas highlighted) is shown.

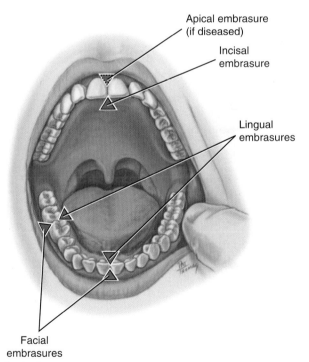

FIGURE 15-11 The embrasures (*red triangles*) formed between two teeth created by the sloping away of the mesial and distal surfaces, which may diverge facially, lingually, incisally/occlusally, or apically with loss of tissue. Note that posterior teeth have occlusal embrasures.

may diverge facially, lingually, occlusally, or apically with loss of tissue. These embrasures are continuous with the interproximal spaces between the teeth. There is an increasing angle of the occlusal embrasures

anterio-posteriorly. All these tooth contours, such as contact areas, heights of contour, and embrasures, are important in the function and health of the masticatory system (see Chapter 20 for more discussion). The form and alignment of the teeth serve to shelter the vulnerable gingivosulcular area from damage.

Each tooth can also be divided by imaginary lines to designate specific crown areas. A **line angle** is formed by the junction of two crown surfaces (Figure 15-12). The name of the line angle is derived by combining the names of those two surfaces. When combining terms such as *mesial* and *labial*, the *al* from the end of the first surface is dropped and an *o* is added and combined with the second surface, thus creating *mesiolabial*. If the first letter of the second word will result in doubling a vowel, such as *mesio-occlusal*, a hyphen is placed between the words, such as *mesio-occlusal*. An example of line angle would be the mesiolabial line angle, which is the junction of the mesial and labial surfaces.

Posterior teeth have *eight* line angles per tooth: mesiobuccal, distobuccal, mesiolingual, distolingual, mesio-occlusal, disto-occlusal, bucco-occlusal, and linguo-occlusal. Anterior teeth have only *six* line angles per tooth: mesiolabial, distolabial, mesiolingual, distolingual, labioincisal, and linguoincisal. Anterior teeth have fewer line angles because the mesial and distal incisal line angles are rounded; thus the mesioincisal and distoincisal line angles are practically nonexistent.

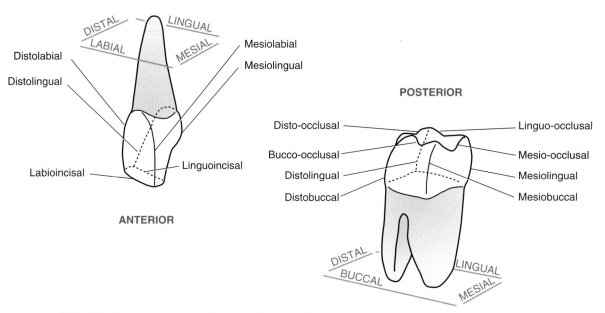

FIG. 15-12 An anterior and a posterior tooth. The designation of line angles of the crown is shown.

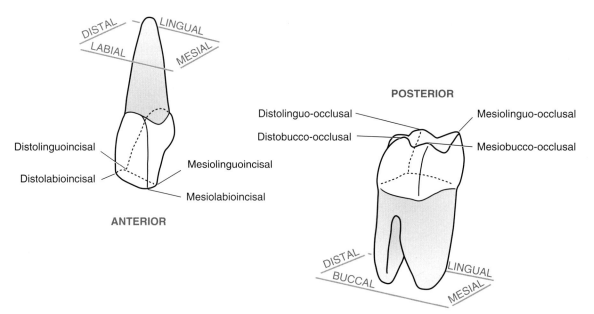

FIGURE 15-13 An anterior and a posterior tooth. The designation of point angles of the crown is shown.

A **point angle** is another way to determine a specific area of the crown (Figure 15-13). The junction of three crown surfaces, the point angle takes its name from those three surfaces. Each tooth has four point angles. Examples of point angles are mesiolabioincisal for an anterior tooth or mesiolabio-occlusal for a posterior tooth.

Finally, a crown surface can be divided both horizontally and vertically into three portions, or **thirds,** to designate specific tooth areas (Figure 15-14). An example is the middle third of the labial surface of a crown. The root can be divided into thirds only hori-

zontally. An example is the cervical third of the buccal surface of a root. The root is also divided vertically into halves by the root axis line, such that the halves are either labial-buccal-lingual or mesial-distal.

Note that in reference to line angles, point angles, thirds, or even a direction, there is an accepted sequencing of combined names of surfaces. The accepted sequence allows that the term *mesial* precedes *distal* and also that *mesial* and *distal* precede all other terms. The terms *labial, buccal,* and *lingual* follow *mesial* or *distal* but precede *incisal* or *occlusal* in any combination.

<table>
<tr><td>

Clinical Considerations for Tooth Surfaces

The tooth's angles, height of contour, and spaces define the "face" of a tooth when the design of a smile is considered because these features are what people see first when contemplating someone's smile. Altering placement and shape of these features changes the face of a tooth and its perceived size and the appearance of the smile. Note that the mesial part of the face and silhouette of a tooth is more angled vertically than the distal part of the face of a tooth.

After studying the surfaces of a tooth, dental professionals must be careful to note that access to proximal surfaces and interproximal space is more difficult than access to facial and lingual surfaces (although line angles can also present problems). This access problem occurs for the patient during oral care as well as for the clinician during instrumentation and restoration.

</td></tr>
</table>

CONSIDERATIONS FOR TOOTH STUDY

Many of the specific distinguishing features of a tooth can be seen only when the tooth is an extracted specimen. Extraction allows both the anatomical crown and the anatomical root to be viewed. Fewer features can be seen clinically when portions of the CEJ and root are covered by gingiva and only the clinical crown is visible. However, clinical views of the teeth are also important for observation of overall tooth arrangements and relationships. In Appendix C of this text are charts of the measurements of all the permanent teeth. Dental professionals should note that these are mean values of ideal teeth; real teeth vary in size among patients and do not always directly reflect jaw size.

Dental professionals should also note that most of the descriptions in this text are also of ideal teeth; although they are larger than life-size, they still use the same size relationships. These ideal teeth also have no wear or pathology, similar to plastic teeth. The features on most extracted specimens are sometimes harder to see and show signs of wear on both the crown and even the root apex, and the teeth may show caries and restorative treatment.

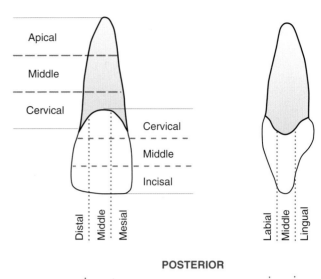
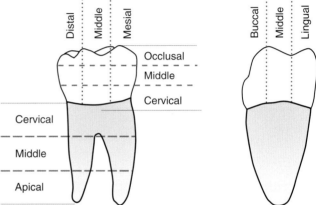

FIGURE 15-14 An anterior and a posterior tooth. The designation of crown and root thirds is shown.

However, extracted teeth provide a more realistic form of dental anatomy than plastic teeth; they have more clearly formed cusps, ridges, fossae, and pits. Variations of the ideal tooth form can thus be seen by students. Extracted teeth can also provide an opportunity for students to view relatively rare dental anomalies. Infection control procedures must be followed when handling extracted teeth (see *Workbook for Illustrated Dental Embryology, Histology, and Anatomy* for the detailed procedure).

CHAPTER 16

Permanent Anterior Teeth

■ ■ ■

This chapter discusses the following topics:

- Permanent anterior teeth
- Permanent incisors
  - Permanent maxillary incisors
  - Permanent mandibular incisors
- Permanent canines
  - Permanent maxillary canines #6 and #11
  - General features
  - Permanent mandibular canines #22 and #27

■ ■ ■

After studying this chapter, the reader should be able to:

1. Use the correct names and universal designation numbers of each permanent anterior tooth when examining a diagram and a patient.
2. Demonstrate the correct location of each permanent anterior tooth on a diagram and a patient.
3. Use and pronounce the key terms when discussing the permanent anterior teeth.
4. Describe the general and specific features of permanent anterior teeth and of each permanent anterior tooth type.
5. Discuss the important clinical considerations and developmental disturbances based on the anatomy of the permanent anterior teeth.
6. Integrate the knowledge of dental anatomy of the permanent anterior teeth into the dental treatment of patients.

■ ■ ■

Key Terms

Anodontia (an-ah-don-she-ah)
Attrition (ah-trish-un)
Avulsion (ah-vul-shin)
Canine eminence
   (kay-nine em-i-nins)
Canines (kay-nines)
Cementoenamel junction
Cingulum (sin-gu-lum)
Contact area
Crown
Cusp: slope, tip
Cuspid (kus-pidz)
Dens in dente

Dentigerous cyst (den-ti-jer-os)
Developmental depressions, groove,
   labial, pits
Diastema (di-ah-ste-mah)
Dilaceration (di-las-er-ay-shun)
Fossa (fos-ah) (plural, fossae, fos-ay)
Golden Proportions
Height of contour
Hutchinson's incisors (hutch-in-suns)
Imbrication lines (im-bri-kay-shun)
Impacted (im-pak-ted)
Incisal (in-sign-sl), angle, edge
Incisors (in-sigh-zers): central, lateral

Mamelons (mam-ah-lons)
Mesiodens (me-ze-oh-denz)
Peg lateral
Perikymata (per-ee-ki-mot-ah)
Ridge: incisal, labial, marginal
Root: accessory, concavities
Succedaneous (suk-seh-dane-ee-us)
Supernumerary
   (soo-per-nu-mer-air-ee)
Supplemental groove
Tubercles (too-ber-kls)

PERMANENT ANTERIOR TEETH

The permanent anterior teeth include the **incisors** and **canines** (Figure 16-1). All anterior teeth are composed of four developmental lobes: three labial lobes named *mesiolabial, middle labial,* and *distolabial,* and one lingual lobe (Figure 16-2). Two vertical **labial developmental depressions** outline the separations among the labial developmental lobes. These are called the *mesiolabial* and *distolabial developmental depressions.* All anterior teeth are **succedaneous** teeth replacing primary teeth of the same type. The development of the permanent teeth is discussed in Chapter 6.

The long **crown** of an anterior tooth has an **incisal** surface, which is its masticatory surface (Figure 16-3).

From the labial and lingual, the crown outline is trapezoidal, or four-sided, with only two parallel sides. The longer of the two parallel sides is toward the incisal.

The crown outline is triangular when viewed from the proximal, with the base of the triangle at the cervical and the apex at the **incisal edge** (Figure 16-4). These teeth are wider mesiodistally than labiolingually when compared with posterior teeth. For anterior teeth, the height of contour, or crest of curvature, for both the crown's labial and lingual surfaces is in the cervical third. Each contact area of anteriors are usually centered labiolingually on their proximal surfaces and have a smaller area than the contacts of posterior teeth. On each proximal surface, the **cementoenamel junction (CEJ)** curvature of all anterior teeth is greater than that of the posterior teeth.

The lingual surfaces of all anterior teeth have a **cingulum** (Figure 16-5). The cingulum is a raised, rounded area on the cervical third of the lingual surface in varying degrees of prominence or development on anterior teeth. The cingulum corresponds to the lingual developmental lobe. Ridges may also be present on the lingual surface. The lingual surface on anterior teeth is bordered mesially and distally on each side by a rounded raised border called a **marginal ridge**.

Some anterior teeth have a more complicated lingual surface with a **fossa** or even **fossae**, which are shallow, wide depressions (Figure 16-6). Some may also have **developmental pits,** which are located in the deepest part of each fossa. Other anterior teeth may have on their lingual surface a **developmental groove,** or primary groove, a sharp, deep, V-shaped linear depression that marks the junction among the developmental lobes.

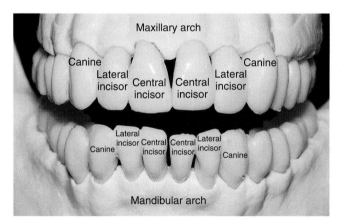

FIGURE 16-1 Frontal view of the skull. The permanent anterior teeth are identified and include the incisors and canines.

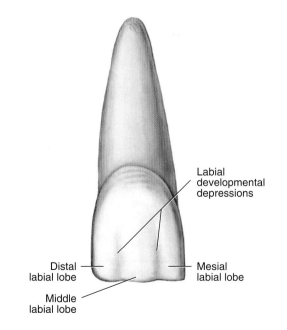

Labial View

FIGURE 16-2 An example of lobe development in a permanent anterior tooth.

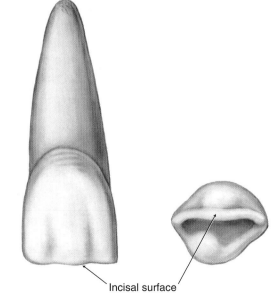

FIGURE 16-3 An example of an incisal surface on a permanent anterior tooth.

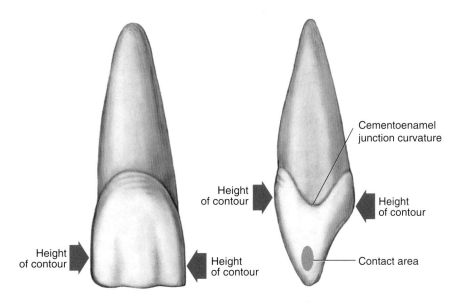

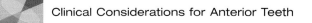

FIGURE 16-4 An example of a permanent anterior tooth with the contact area and height of contour identified.

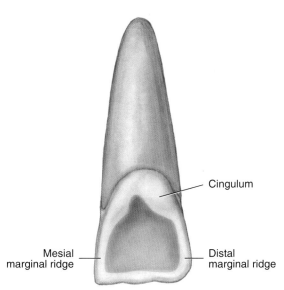

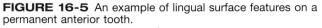

FIGURE 16-5 An example of lingual surface features on a permanent anterior tooth.

In addition, a **supplemental groove,** or secondary groove, may also be present on the lingual surface of anteriors. This is a shallower, more irregular linear depression. Supplemental grooves branch from the developmental grooves but are not always present in the same pattern on each different tooth type. In general, the more anterior the tooth, the fewer supplemental grooves are present and the smoother the lingual surface.

Anterior teeth usually have a single root, with some exceptions. The roots of maxillary anterior teeth have great lingual and slight distal inclination. The roots of mandibular anterior teeth vary in angulation from nearly vertical to great lingual inclination, with the canines possibly having a slight distal root inclination.

Clinical Considerations for Anterior Teeth

Patients may have difficulty in maintaining oral hygiene of anterior teeth because their arch position may allow the lips naturally to overhang the teeth. Thus patients may clean only the incisal two thirds of the crowns of anterior teeth with their toothbrushes, missing the associated cervical area and facial gingiva. This overhanging of the lips may also make instrumentation difficult.

Instrumentation may also be compromised in the area where the greater curvature of the CEJ is present interproximally on anterior teeth, where accessibility is limited and the teeth are in close proximity. The grooves on the lingual surface of anterior teeth may present areas for bacterial plaque biofilm retention if they extend to the root and are near the adjacent gingiva; for this reason, dental professionals may elect to reduce the grooves with a dental bur during a minor odontoplasty.

When the anterior teeth are restored, the **Golden Proportions** can be useful guidelines to balance the size of the teeth with one another. These guidelines designate that the ideal width of the maxillary lateral incisor as a factor of 1.0x, the width of the central incisors as 1.618x, and the width of the canines as 0.168x when observed in two dimensions from the facial aspect. Other formulas state that the maxillary central should be 60 percent wider than the lateral, and the lateral should be 60 percent wider than the canine from its midline to its mesial aspect. In addition, each incisor should also have an 8 : 10 width-to-length ratio.

In addition, consideration of smile design may involve the drawing of a line following the ideal outline formed by the incisal edges of the maxillary anterior teeth; this line should be 1 to 3 mm parallel or equidistant to the lower lip line. Some variation will occur with aging. Older individuals lose elasticity in the lips, which results in sagging, prominence of the mandibular teeth, and diminution of the maxillary teeth. People perceive straight smiles as more masculine and feminine smiles as more curved. In addition, if the lip line appears to be convex instead of concave compared with the lower lip line, people will perceive the smile as more youthful.

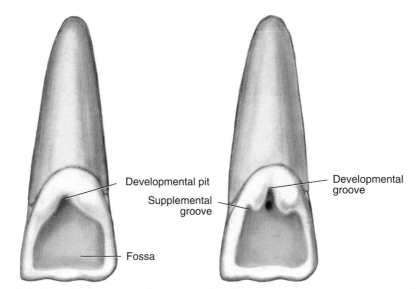

FIGURE 16-6 Additional examples of lingual surface features on a permanent anterior tooth.

PERMANENT INCISORS

General Features

The permanent incisors are the eight most anterior teeth of the permanent dentition, with four in each dental arch (Table 16-1). The two types of incisors are the **central incisors** and the **lateral incisors.** The central incisors are closest to the midline, and the lateral incisors are the second teeth from the midline. One of each type of incisor is present in each quadrant of each dental arch. Both types of incisors are mesial to the permanent canines when the permanent dentition is fully erupted. The permanent incisors are

---

Clinical Considerations for Incisors

The incisors function as instruments for biting and cutting food during mastication because of their incisal ridge, triangular proximal form, and arch position. They also support the lips and face and maintain vertical dimension. Additionally, they contribute to overall normal arch appearance. Finally, they are involved during the articulation of speech and assist in guiding jaw closure as the teeth come together.

Because of the anterior position of the permanent incisors, aesthetic concerns are important during restorative procedures. Restorative replacement of only a portion of the incisal edge of this tooth after traumatic fracture may also be difficult to maintain owing to this tooth's function in biting and cutting food.

The **mamelons** on the incisal ridge of incisors usually undergo **attrition**, the wearing away of a tooth surface caused by tooth-to-tooth contact, shortly after eruption as the tooth moves into occlusion (Figure 16-8 **A**; see also Figure 16-9 **C** and 16-18). Chapter 20 discusses attrition and occlusion in greater detail. The incisal ridge thus now appears flattened from its labial, lingual, or incisal views and becomes the **incisal edge.** Thus mamelons are usually most noticeable immediately after eruption; with attrition they become undetectable. Attrition can sometimes create a bow-shaped wear pattern on the incisal edge when viewed from the incisal.

With attrition, the maxillary incisors' incisal edges show lingual inclination and the mandibular incisors have a labial inclination to their incisal edges. Thus with this arrangement, the incisal edges of the maxillary and mandibular incisors are usually parallel to one another and mesh correctly during mastication. If mamelons are still present on the incisal ridge in an adult, it is because these teeth are not in occlusion, such as with an anterior open-bite relationship (see Figure 16-8 **B**, and see Chapter 20 for a discussion of open bite).

Thus mamelons occasionally do not wear down, especially when malalignment of the teeth and loss of tooth-to-tooth contact with occlusion exist. Most mature individuals do not like the appearance of mamelons and sometimes request to have them polished off; some patients even request placement of restorative materials to achieve a straight-appearing incisal edge. Part of the reason that the mamelons are so noticeable if present long after eruption is that these extensions are made of enamel, with no dentin layer underneath. This and their thinness contributes to their translucent appearance as opposed to the rest of the clinical crown, which is almost always more opaque than the mamelons. Given this translucent quality, mamelons often appear to be a different shade than the rest of the tooth and therefore are sometimes much more distinct.

TABLE 16-1

Anatomical Information on Permanent Incisors

	Maxillary Central Incisor	Maxillary Lateral Incisor	Mandibular Central Incisor	Mandibular Lateral Incisor
Universal number	#8 and #9	# 7 and #10	# 24 and #25	#23 and #26
General crown features	Incisal edge and incisal angles			
Specific crown features	Widest crown MD, greatest CEJ curve, and height of contour; distal offset cingulum, shallow lingual fossa, marginal ridges	Greatest crown variation, like a smaller maxillary central, prominent lingual surface; centered cingulum, pronounced marginal ridges	Smallest and simplest tooth, bilaterally symmetrical; small centered cingulum, subtle lingual fossa, and equal subtle marginal ridges	Like a larger mandibular central, not bilaterally symmetrical; appears twisted distally; small, distally placed cingulum; lingual fossa and moderate mesial marginal ridge longer than distal
Height of contour	Cervical third			
Mesial contact	Incisal third			
Distal contact	Junction of incisal and middle thirds	Middle third or junction with incisal third	Incisal third	Incisal third
Distinguishing right from left	Sharper MI angle, rounder DI angle, more pronounced mesial CEJ curvature			
General root features	Single-rooted			
Specific root features	Overall conical shape; no proximal root concavities		Bow shaped on cross section; root is longer than the crown; proximal root concavities give double-rooted appearance	
	Rounded apex; triangular in cross section	Root curves distally, with sharp apex; oval in cross section; same or longer than central but thinner		

CEJ = cementoenamel junction; DI = distoincisal; MD = mesiodistally; M = mesioincisal.

succedaneous and replace the primary incisors of the same type. On occasion, the permanent incisors seem to spread out as a result of spacing during initial eruption. With the eruption of the permanent canines, these spaces often close. When newly erupted, each incisor also has three mamelons, or rounded enamel extensions on the incisal ridge from the labial or lingual views (Figure 16-7). These mamelons are extensions from the three labial developmental lobes.

The incisors are also the only permanent teeth with two **incisal angles** formed from the incisal ridge (or incisal edge, as described later) and each proximal surface. Permanent incisors of both types are the only

permanent teeth with a nearly straight **incisal ridge,** which is a linear elevation on the masticatory or incisal surface when newly erupted—thus the name **incisors.**

The lingual surface has a cingulum that corresponds to the lingual developmental lobe, although its prominence or development differs for each type of incisor. These teeth also have a lingual fossa and marginal ridges on the lingual surface, again in differing developmental levels for each type of incisor. The height of contour for both labial and lingual surfaces of all incisors is at the cervical third, as is the case for all anterior teeth.

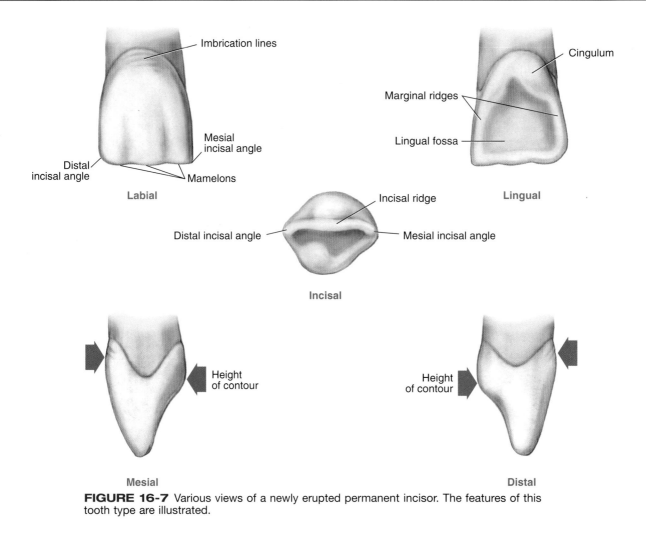

FIGURE 16-7 Various views of a newly erupted permanent incisor. The features of this tooth type are illustrated.

Developmental Disturbances of Incisors

The crown of a permanent incisor can be affected with **dens in dente** (discussed further in Chapter 6). This disturbance leaves the tooth with a deep lingual pit resulting from invagination of the enamel organ into the dental papilla. This pit may lead to pulpal exposure and pathology. Dens in dente may be hereditary and is more common with a maxillary lateral incisor.

The crowns of permanent incisors, similar to molars, can be affected in children with congenital syphilis. A pregnant woman infected with syphilis transmits the spirochete *Treponema pallidum,* a sexually transmitted organism, to her fetus via the placenta. This organism may cause localized enamel hypoplasia, which can result in **Hutchinson's incisors**. This disturbance occurs during tooth development. (Enamel hypoplasia is discussed in Chapter 6.)

A Hutchinson's incisor has a crown with a screwdriver shape from the labial view and is wider cervically and narrow incisally, with a notched incisal edge. Children may also have other developmental anomalies, such as blindness, deafness, and paralysis from congenital syphilis. Treatment of these teeth with restorative materials may improve their appearance.

A sharp, small, extra cusp or talon (claw) cusp occasionally appears as a projection from the cingulum of incisor teeth. These types of cusps can interfere with occlusion; however, grinding them down is a hazardous endeavor. Talon cusps often contain a prominent pulp horn, which is extremely susceptible to exposure in younger patients.

Permanent Maxillary Incisors

GENERAL FEATURES

The permanent maxillary incisors are the four most anterior teeth of the permanent maxillary arch. Each has a crown that is larger in all dimensions, especially mesiodistally, compared with a permanent mandibular incisor. In addition, the labial surfaces are more rounded from the incisal aspect, with the tooth tapering toward the lingual.

All lingual surface features, including the marginal ridges, lingual fossa, and cingulum, are more promi-

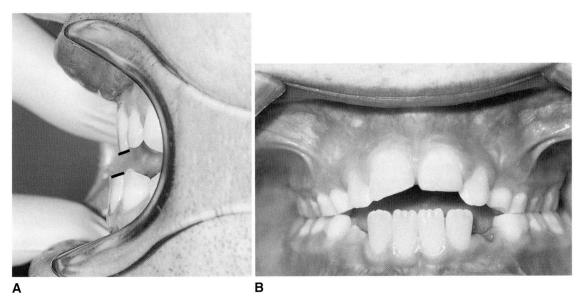

FIGURE 16-8 Examples of clinical appearance of the incisal edges on permanent incisors. **A:** Lateral view of permanent incisors altered by attrition on their incisal surfaces (see *dark lines* on incisal edges). **B:** Frontal view of mamelons present in a mixed dentition on the incisal edges of permanent incisors resulting from an open bite.

Clinical Considerations for Maxillary Incisors

If a permanent maxillary incisor has increased prominence of the lingual marginal ridges and a deeper lingual fossa, it may be considered a shovel-shaped incisor (Figure 16-9, *A*). It can also have an accentuated cingulum (Figure 16-9, *B*), with deepened grooves, and show incisal edge attrition (Figure 16-9, *C*).

Another lingual feature if present on the maxillary incisors, a lingual pit, is susceptible to caries development (Figure 16-10, *A-C*). The susceptibility of this developmental pit to caries is from both increased bacterial plaque biofilm retention and the weakness of the enamel forming the walls of the pit (see Chapter 12 for more information on enamel features). If the lingual pit is deep, a developmental disturbance of dens in dente must be considered and changes made in the patient's treatment plan (discussed earlier). Also present may be a vertically placed linguogingival groove (Figure 16-10, *D*), which originates in the lingual pit and extends cervically and slightly distally onto the cingulum. The linguogingival groove is also more common on maxillary laterals and may result in caries.

In addition, supragingival tooth deposits such as bacterial plaque biofilm and stain can collect in the prominent lingual surface concavities of maxillary incisors (see Figure 16-9, *D*). During instrumentation the proximal surfaces of these teeth are more accessible from the lingual than the facial approach because of the increased tapering of the tooth to the lingual. Dental professionals must be careful to check for deposits in any mesial and distal root concavities at the CEJ if this area is exposed as a result of recession.

Finally, many dental professionals believe that competency of the lips to maintain a lip seal when at rest can affect the position of the maxillary incisors (see Chapter 20 for further discussion). Competent lips allow these tooth tips to lie below the lower lip border, helping to maintain normal inclination. Incompetent lips that fail to provide a lip seal do not control this inclination and may even allow the maxillary incisors to lie in front of the lower lip, exaggerating already buccally inclined teeth. A tongue thrust is a complicating factor that may be associated with this problem. These dental professionals also believe that with overactive and tight lips, the maxillary incisors become lingually inclined.

---

nent on the maxillary incisors than on the mandibular incisors. Finally, the incisal edge is just labial to the long axis of the root from either proximal view.

Each root is short compared with those of other permanent maxillary teeth and usually is without root concavities. Bulbous and pronounced crowns may also create deep mesial and distal concavities at the CEJ.

The permanent central and lateral incisors of the maxillary arch resemble each other more than they resemble the similar type of incisors of the opposing arch. Generally, a maxillary central incisor is larger than a maxillary lateral incisor, but overall they have a similar form. Both types of maxillary incisors are wider mesiodistally than labiolingually.

PERMANENT MAXILLARY CENTRAL INCISORS #8 AND #9
Specific Overall Features (Figure 16-11)

The permanent maxillary central incisors erupt between 7 and 8 years of age (root completion occurs

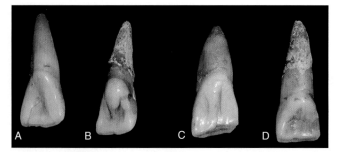

FIGURE 16-9 Various lingual views of a permanent maxillary incisors. **A:** Shovel shape. **B:** Accentuated cingulum, with deepened grooves. **C:** Attrition on incisal surface and showing lingual inclination. **D:** Stain in the lingual fossa.

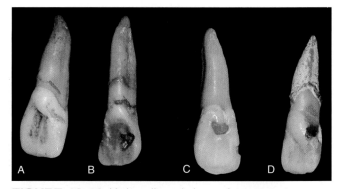

FIGURE 16-10 Various lingual views of permanent maxillary incisors. **A:** Lingual pit. **B:** Lingual pit with caries. **C:** Lingual pit caries repaired. **D:** Linguogingival groove, resulting in caries.

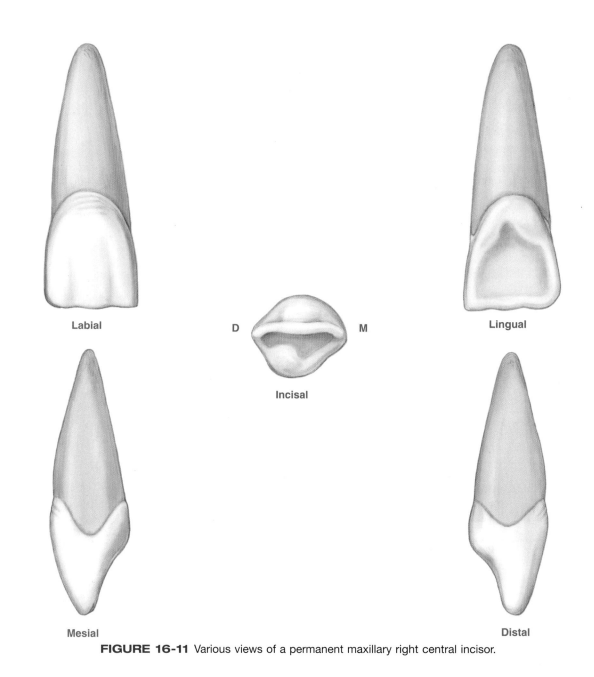

Labial

D   M

Incisal

Lingual

Mesial

Distal

FIGURE 16-11 Various views of a permanent maxillary right central incisor.

at age 10). Thus these teeth usually erupt after the mandibular central incisors. Many children want these two teeth to come in fast to fill their wide arch space when they shed their four primary maxillary incisors, as in the old song "All I Want for Christmas Is My Two Front Teeth."

The maxillary central incisors are the most prominent teeth in the permanent dentition because of both their large size and their anterior arch position. In consideration of smile design, the central incisors should be dominant with perspective in such a way that each tooth posteriorly appears to get smaller. In addition, the maxillary centrals are the largest of all the incisors. The two maxillary central incisors usually share a mesial contact area. The outline of the crown of a permanent maxillary central incisor from the labial or lingual view is trapezoidal, four-sided with two parallel sides. It has the widest crown mesiodistally of any permanent anterior tooth.

The maxillary central incisor has a single conical **root,** smooth and slightly straight, usually with a rounded apex. Thus the root is thick in the cervical third and narrows through the middle to the blunt apex. The root is one and one-half times the length of the crown. The root of this central incisor is also about the same length or shorter but wider than the lateral of the same arch. Bulbous crowns may create deep mesial and distal concavities at CEJ. The pulp cavity of a maxillary central incisor mirrors the shape of the tooth (Figure 16-12). There is only one root canal, which is rather large. The pulp chamber has three sharp elongations, the mesial, distal, and central pulp horns. These pulp horns correspond to the three labial developmental lobes of the tooth. The central pulp horn is usually shorter than the other two and more rounded. The root is oval in cervical cross section, being slightly wider on the labial surface and narrower at the lingual.

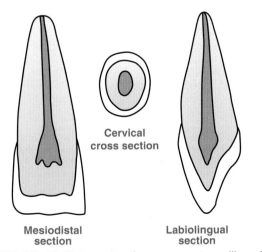

Cervical
cross section

Mesiodistal
section

Labiolingual
section

FIGURE 16-12 Pulp cavity of a permanent maxillary right central incisor.

Labial View Features

The crown of a maxillary central incisor is narrowest at the cervical third and becomes wider toward the incisal edge on the labial surface (see Figure 16-11). The incisal ridge is nearly straight. Two labial developmental depressions may extend the length of the crown from the cervical to the incisal, showing the division of the surface into three labial developmental lobes. The crown usually has **imbrication lines,** or slight ridges, that run mesiodistally in the cervical third. Between them are the grooved **perikymata.** The CEJ on the labial surface has more curvature to the distal.

From the labial view, both incisal angles can be seen on the maxillary central incisor. The overall mesial outline is slightly rounded, with a sharp mesioincisal angle. The overall distal outline is even more rounded, with a rounded distoincisal angle. The difference in sharpness of the central's mesioincisal and distoincisal angle *helps to distinguish the right maxillary central incisor from the left.*

The mesial contact with the other maxillary central is in the incisal third (see Figure 16-7). The distal contact with the maxillary lateral is at the junction of the incisal and middle third, located farther cervically than the mesial contact.

Lingual View Features

The lingual surface of the crown of a maxillary central incisor is narrower overall than the labial surface (Figure 16-13). The CEJ on the lingual surface usually has more curvature to the distal. The single cingulum is wide, well-developed, and located slightly off center toward the distal.

From the lingual view, the mesial marginal ridge is longer than the distal marginal ridge. The single lingual fossa is wide yet shallow and is located immediately incisal to the cingulum. The lingual fossa varies in depth and diameter. Outlining the incisal border of the lingual fossa, the raised linguoincisal edge is on the same level as the bordering marginal ridges.

On the lingual surface, a horizontally placed lingual groove may be present (although it is more common on maxillary laterals), separating the cingulum from the lingual fossa. The lingual groove may make the cingulum appear scalloped.

A lingual pit may also be present at the incisal border of the cingulum in the lingual groove on the maxillary central incisor. Also present may be a vertically placed linguogingival groove, which originates in the lingual pit and extends cervically and slightly distally onto the cingulum.

Proximal View Features

The CEJ curvature on the mesial surface is deep incisally and has the greatest depth of curvature of any

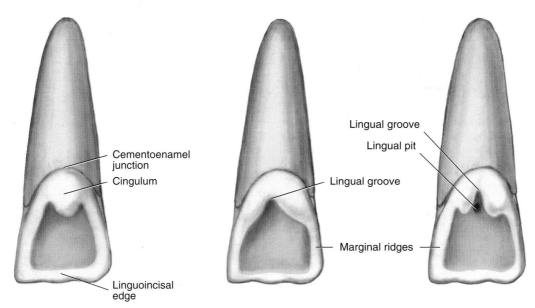

FIGURE 16-13 Variations of form of the lingual surface of the permanent maxillary right central incisor (with the lingual fossae highlighted).

tooth surface in the permanent dentition, which *helps to distinguish the right maxillary central incisor from the left* (see Figure 16-11). The height of contour for both the labial and lingual surfaces is also greater on this tooth than on any tooth in the permanent dentition and is located at the cervical third, as in all incisors.

The incisal edge is located slightly labial to the long axis of the tooth. The incisal outline is also sloped toward the lingual from its longest and most labial portion. The distal view is similar to the mesial, although the curvature of the CEJ is less on the distal than on the mesial surface.

Incisal View Features

Overall, the shape of the crown of a maxillary central incisor from the incisal view is triangular, with the labial outline broadly rounded. This is a useful view for observing the slight distal placement of the cingulum. On the lingual surface of the incisal view, the mesial marginal ridge again appears longer than the distal marginal ridge. Note that the incisal edge lies just labial to the long axis of the root.

 Clinical Considerations with Maxillary Central Incisors

The incisal edge or even the entire permanent maxillary central incisor is especially at risk for traumatic fracture or tooth displacement because of the tooth's most anterior and labial position (especially of its incisal edge) and its early eruption into the oral cavity. Because of these two factors and without full root completion, the entire tooth in a child may undergo **avulsion**, which is complete displacement of the tooth from the socket resulting from extensive trauma to the area. Even if the tooth is only fractured, pulpal pathology may occur in the tooth and result in the need for endodontic therapy or loss of tooth vitality as the pulp dies.

An open contact, or **diastema**, can also exist between the permanent maxillary central incisors, which can be a wide and unattractive space. Both the cause and treatment of this type of diastema are controversial. Treatment may involve surgery to reduce the impact of a tight maxillary labial frenum, with or without orthodontic treatment. "Winged" incisors may be present, but they are not a disturbance of development but rather a special case of rotation of the maxillary central incisors; it is usually described as a distinctive bilateral rotation to the mesial.

Developmental Disturbances with Maxillary Central Incisors

One common location for a supernumerary tooth is between the two permanent maxillary central incisors (see Chapter 6 for more discussion). This is called a **mesiodens**. It is due to the presence of an extra tooth germ resulting from an abnormal initiation process during tooth development, a **supernumerary tooth**. The presence of this extra tooth may affect spacing in the maxillary arch whether it is erupted or not.

The tooth may also have a dwarfed root, which results in a lack of periodontal support for the tooth and may affect the prognosis of the tooth if it is involved in periodontal disease.

PERMANENT MAXILLARY LATERAL INCISORS #7 AND #10
Specific Overall Features (Figure 16-14)

The permanent maxillary lateral incisors erupt between 8 and 9 years of age (root completion occurs

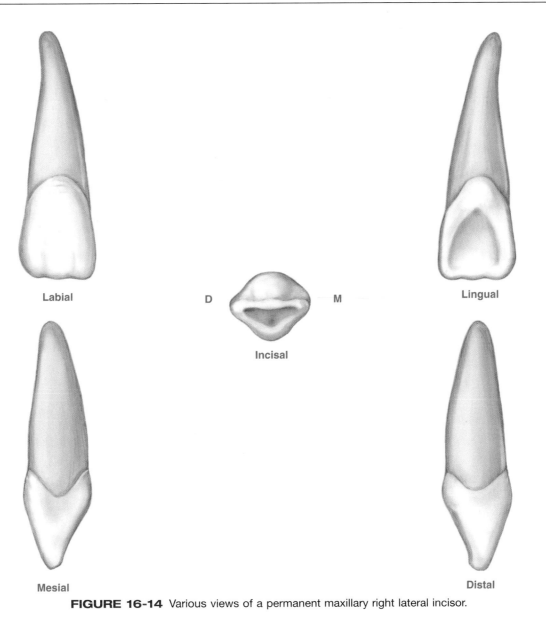

Labial

Lingual

D   M

Incisal

Mesial

Distal

FIGURE 16-14 Various views of a permanent maxillary right lateral incisor.

at age 11). Thus these teeth usually erupt after the maxillary central incisors.

The crown of a maxillary lateral incisor has the greatest degree of variation in form of any permanent tooth, except for the permanent third molars. A maxillary lateral usually resembles a maxillary central incisor in all views of the tooth but has a smaller and slightly more rounded crown.

A maxillary lateral incisor has a single conical root that is relatively smooth and straight but may curve slightly to the distal. Its crown is one to one and one-half times shorter than the length of the root. The root of the lateral incisor is also about the same length as or longer than the central but is thinner, particularly mesiodistally, and is also wider labiolingually. This tooth is frequently confused with a small permanent mandibular canine, but the root usually has no depressions on the proximal surface, as is common on a

mandibular canine. A linguogingival groove may be present on the root (and possibly on the crown). The apex of the root is not rounded like the central but is sharp.

The pulp cavity of the maxillary lateral incisor is very simple in form, with a single pulp canal and a pulp chamber (Figure 16-15). The pulp chamber does not have three sharp pulp horns as it does in a maxillary central incisor. Instead, the pulp chamber of a maxillary lateral incisor usually has one rounded form or two less-sharp pulp horns, a mesial and distal pulp horn. The shape of the root on cross section is oval.

LABIAL VIEW FEATURES

The labial developmental depressions and imbrication lines on the labial surface are less common on a maxillary lateral than on a central incisor (see Figure

16-14). The crown is smaller than that of a central incisor and less symmetrical.

Generally, it resembles a central in its mesial outline, with the mesial contact with the maxillary central at the incisal third or at the junction of the incisal and the middle third, farther cervically than the central. The distal outline is always more rounded than the central and has a more cervical distal contact area with the maxillary canine, at the middle third or at the junction of the incisal and the middle third.

From the labial view, both incisal angles are more rounded on a maxillary lateral than on a central incisor. Although similar to a central incisor, a maxillary lateral has different incisal angles from the labial. The lateral's mesioincisal angle is sharper than the distoincisal angle, which *helps to distinguish the right maxillary lateral incisor from the left.*

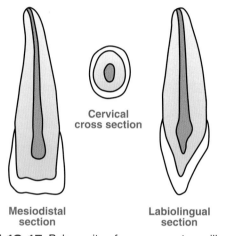

Cervical
cross section

Mesiodistal
section

Labiolingual
section

FIGURE 16-15 Pulp cavity of a permanent maxillary right lateral incisor.

LINGUAL VIEW FEATURES

The lingual surface of the **crown** of a maxillary lateral incisor is narrower than the labial surface, as is the case with a central (Figure 16-16). A maxillary lateral has a prominent yet centered and more narrow cingulum than does a central incisor, with a deeper lingual fossa. The marginal ridges are pronounced: The longer mesial marginal ridge is nearly straight, and the shorter distal marginal ridge is quite straight. The linguoincisal ridge is also well-developed.

On the lingual surface, a horizontal lingual groove that separates the cingulum from the lingual fossa is more common on a maxillary lateral incisor and better developed than on a central. Also, a lingual pit is more common on a lateral than on a central and is located on the incisal surface of the cingulum, along the lingual groove.

Also present on the lingual surface of a maxillary lateral incisor may be a vertical linguogingival groove that originates in the lingual pit and extends cervically and slightly distally onto the cingulum. The linguogingival groove may extend onto the root surface. The linguogingival groove is also more common on this tooth than on a maxillary central. Rarely, the root has a deep distolingual marginal groove, a developmental groove that starts on the distal marginal ridge on the lingual surface and extends onto the root.

PROXIMAL VIEW FEATURES

The crown of a maxillary lateral incisor is triangular on a mesial view, as are all anterior teeth (see Figure 16-14). The CEJ curvature is similar to that of a central, although it is not as deeply curved on a lateral. Also similar to a central, a lateral's CEJ is more curved on the mesial surface than the distal of this tooth, which

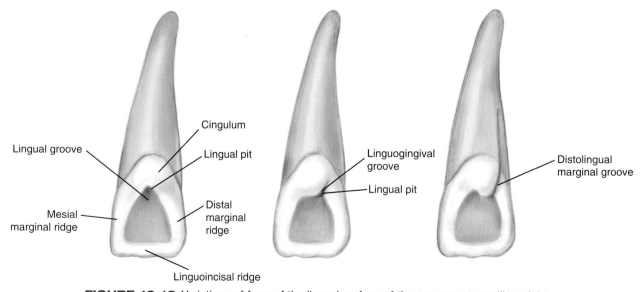

Lingual groove

Cingulum

Lingual pit

Mesial
marginal ridge

Distal
marginal
ridge

Linguoincisal ridge

Linguogingival
groove

Lingual pit

Distolingual
marginal groove

FIGURE 16-16 Variations of form of the lingual surface of the permanent maxillary right lateral incisor (with the lingual fossae highlighted).

helps to distinguish the right maxillary lateral incisor from the left. The incisal edge is usually labial to the long axis of the tooth. The distal view is similar to that of the mesial, although the CEJ is not as deeply curved.

INCISAL VIEW FEATURES

The outline of the crown of a maxillary lateral incisor is more rounded or oval from the incisal view, not triangular as is a central. The crown's mesiodistal measurement is somewhat wider than the labiolingual measurement. Thus the labial surface is more rounded than that of a central.

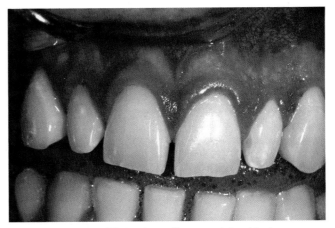

FIGURE 16-17 Bilateral maxillary peg lateral incisor showing examples of partial microdontia.

Clinical Considerations with Maxillary Lateral Incisors

Because of the variations in form and the possibility of developmental disturbances (see the next section), permanent maxillary lateral incisors present challenges during preventive, restorative, and orthodontic procedures. Unattractive open contacts may be seen in the dental arch in this area because of these variations in form as well as asymmetrical tooth size and position across the maxillary arch.

The linguogingival groove can be considered a clinically adverse factor because deposits can accumulate in the nichelike groove. This condition tracks the periodontal destruction apically as the groove advances, resulting in the formation of a deeply localized periodontal lesion. Studies have found deeper mean probing pocket depth and a greater degree of severe gingivitis in the groove region. Careful, repeated pocket depth probing is essential to monitor these high-risk areas in a patient.

Developmental Disturbances with Maxillary Lateral Incisors

A permanent maxillary lateral incisor is one of the most common teeth of the permanent dentition to exhibit partial microdontia (all disturbances are discussed further in Chapter 6). This disturbance leads to a smaller lateral incisor crown, or **peg lateral**, either unilaterally or bilaterally (Figure 16-17). This disturbance occurs in the process of proliferation during tooth development. It may be hereditary or may result from other factors. Treatment to improve appearance may include restorative materials.

The permanent maxillary lateral incisors are also more commonly involved in partial **anodontia** and thus may be congenitally missing. This disturbance results from an absence of the appropriate individual tooth germ (or germs) in the area, either unilaterally or bilaterally in about 1 or 2 percent of the population, from a failure in the initiation process during tooth development. Partial anodontia may present aesthetic problems for patients and can result in problems in occlusion. Thus missing teeth may require prosthetic replacement or implant.

Finally, a permanent maxillary lateral incisor may have one or more **tubercles**, or accessory cusps, on the cingulum. **Dilaceration** of the crown or root, showing angular distortion, may occur, making extraction and endodontic treatment difficult.

Permanent Mandibular Incisors

GENERAL FEATURES

The permanent mandibular incisors are the smallest teeth of the permanent dentition and the most symmetrical. More uniformity in form is seen among these teeth than among any other of the permanent dentition. The central and lateral incisors of the mandibular arch resemble each other more than do the similar types of incisors of the maxillary arch.

Generally, a mandibular lateral incisor is slightly larger than a central, exactly the opposite of the situation in the maxillary arch. The incisal ridge usually also wears from attrition mainly on the labial surface to become the incisal edge. The incisal edge is just lingual to the long axis of the root. Each mandibular incisor has a crown that is wider labiolingually than mesiodistally, this being unlike the maxillary incisors. Both mandibular incisors also have smoother and less complex lingual surface features than the maxillary incisors, including a cingulum, lingual fossa, and marginal ridges.

Proximal root concavities are also present on both types of mandibular incisors and, if deep enough, give the teeth a double-rooted appearance. The root of a mandibular incisor is elliptical, an elongated oval on cervical cross section. Thus the root is extremely narrow on the labial and lingual surfaces and wide on both proximal surfaces. The root is longer than the crown for both incisors (see Figures 16-19 and 16-21).

Clinical Considerations with Mandibular Incisors

Although the concavity of the lingual surface of all mandibular incisors is smoother than that of maxillary incisors, supragingival tooth deposits such as bacterial plaque biofilm, calculus, and stain tend to collect in the concavity. This buildup of deposits is aided by the mandibular incisors' position in the oral cavity near the duct openings of the submandibular and sublingual salivary glands in the floor of the mouth. Saliva, with its mineral content, is released from these glands and causes the bacterial plaque biofilm to mineralize more quickly into calculus.

With attrition, the wearing away of a tooth surface caused by tooth-to-tooth contact, the incisal edge can change on the mandibular incisors (discussed further in Chapter 20). Thus these incisors may lose their symmetrical form, exposing the inner dentin (Figure 16-18). With severe attrition, the incisal edge also becomes a concavity lined with exposed dentin. This porous dentin becomes intrinsically stained and unattractive. This area may also be affected by dentin hypersensitivity (see Chapter 13).

Instrumentation may be more difficult in this area because many patients have overlapping mandibular incisors owing to inadequate mandibular arch size and other occlusal factors. This crowding increases with age because of normal physiological mesial drift. If the incisors tip incisally back toward the tongue, instrumentation is also extremely difficult. Use of a mouth mirror is essential in all these cases.

Prolonged instrumentation with metal scalers can narrow even further the already narrow labial and lingual root surfaces of the permanent mandibular incisors. The crowns of the teeth can thus be placed in jeopardy during mastication because of unsupported cervical enamel. Finally, the proximal surface of the roots is difficult to explore with instruments because of the limited interproximal space and the oval root shape. The presence of proximal root concavities may also increase the difficulty of root instrumentation.

PERMANENT MANDIBULAR CENTRAL INCISORS #24 AND #25

Specific Overall Features (Figure 16-19)

The permanent mandibular central incisors erupt between 6 and 7 years of age (root completion occurs at age 9). Thus these teeth usually erupt before the maxillary central incisors.

The mandibular central incisors are the smallest and simplest teeth of the permanent dentition; thus they are smaller than the lateral incisors of the same arch.

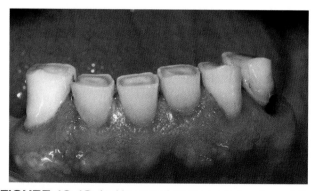

FIGURE 16-18 Attrition noted on the incisal surface of the permanent mandibular incisors, as well as canines.

The two mandibular centrals usually share a mesial contact area.

This tooth has a simple root, which is widest labiolingually and then mesiodistally. The root has pronounced proximal root concavities, which vary in both length and depth. A shallow depression extends longitudinally along the midportion of root. Dental professionals must remember that root proximation with a contralateral tooth may cause access difficulty.

The pulp cavity for this tooth is quite simple because it has a single pulp canal and three pulp horns (Figure 16-20). The root is a narrow oval in cross section.

Labial View Features

The crown of a mandibular central incisor is quite symmetrical from the labial view, having a fan shape (see Figure 16-19). The imbrication lines and developmental depressions usually are not present or are extremely faint. The mesial contact with the other mandibular central is at the incisal third. The distal contact with the lateral incisor is also at the incisal third.

From the labial view, both the incisal angles, the mesioincisal angle and distoincisal angle, are sharp or only slightly rounded; the mesioincisal angle is slightly sharper than the distoincisal angle, which *helps to distinguish the right mandibular central incisor from the left*. Nevertheless, distinguishing between the right and left central incisors is often difficult. The mesial and distal outlines are nearly straight from the CEJ to the relatively straight incisal edge.

Lingual View Features

The crown of a mandibular central incisor is narrower on the lingual surface than the labial. The outline of the crown of a mandibular central incisor is the most symmetrical of all incisors, either maxillary or mandibular. Overall, the lingual surface is smooth and has a small, centered cingulum.

On the lingual surface, the single lingual fossa is barely noticeable; therefore the mesial marginal ridge and distal marginal ridge are barely noticeable as well. Because the cingulum is centered, the faint mesial and distal marginal ridges have the same length.

Proximal View Features

The CEJ curvature is higher incisally on the mesial than on the distal surface, which *helps to distinguish the right mandibular central incisor from the left*. The incisal edge is usually straight but can be rounded and is lingual to the long axis of the root. The distal view is similar to the mesial view of the tooth, except that the CEJ curves less incisally on the distal than on the mesial surface.

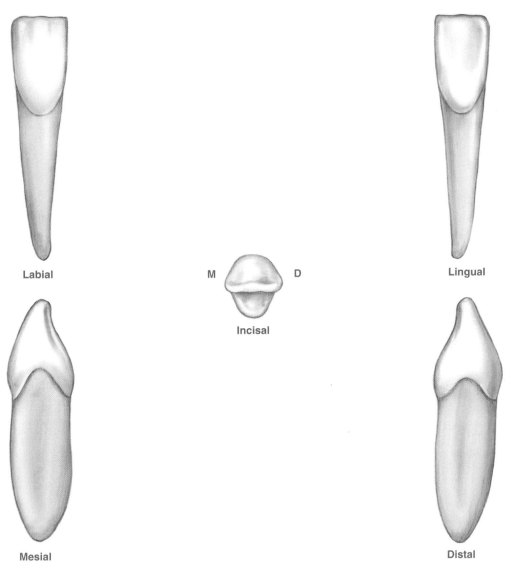

Labial

M   D

Incisal

Lingual

Mesial

Distal

FIGURE 16-19 Various views of a permanent mandibular right central incisor.

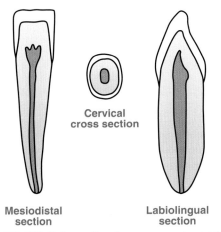

Cervical
cross section

Mesiodistal
section

Labiolingual
section

FIGURE 16-20 Pulp cavity of a permanent mandibular right central incisor.

Incisal View Features

This tooth has a nearly symmetrical crown outline on the incisal view. The incisal edge is usually at a right angle, or perpendicular, to the labiolingual axis of the crown of the tooth and overall is just lingual to the long axis of the root. The labiolingual measurement is also wider than the mesiodistal measurement on incisal view. Again, on the lingual surface, the faint mesial marginal ridge and distal marginal ridge are the same length.

    Developmental Disturbances with Mandibular Central Incisors

Developmental disturbances are rarely noted in the permanent mandibular central incisors. One rare exception is that the teeth may have an **accessory root** or bifurcated root, with the two branches having labial and lingual orientations.

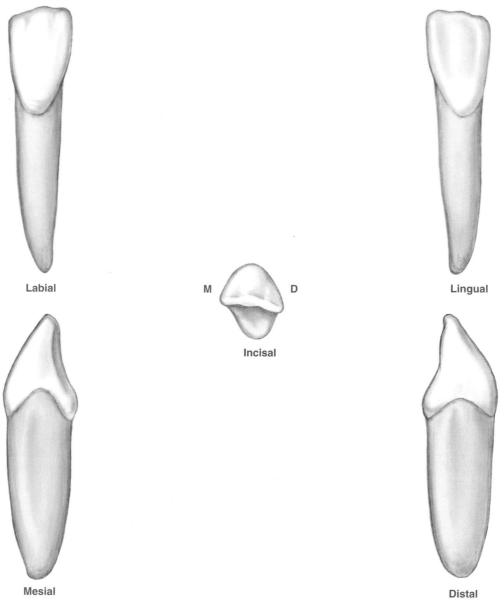

Labial   M   D   Lingual

Incisal

Mesial   Distal

FIGURE 16-21 Various views of a permanent mandibular right lateral incisor.

PERMANENT MANDIBULAR LATERAL INCISORS #23 AND #26

Specific Overall Features (Figure 16-21)

The permanent mandibular lateral incisors erupt between 7 and 8 years of age (root completion occurs at age 10). Thus these teeth usually erupt after the mandibular central incisors.

A mandibular lateral is slightly larger overall than a central incisor. There is also more variation in form than with the central. The crown of a permanent mandibular lateral incisor is also slightly larger than that of a central, but it resembles a central in most other ways. From both the labial and lingual views, the crown of mandibular lateral appears tilted or twisted distally in comparison with the long axis of the tooth (this gives the impression that the tooth haas been bent at the CEJ).

The single root of a mandibular lateral is usually straight, slightly longer and wider than that of a central. The root, like that of a mandibular central, has pronounced proximal root concavities, especially on the distal surface. These vary in both length and depth. The pulp cavity for this tooth is quite simple because it has a single pulp canal and three pulp horns (Figure 16-22).

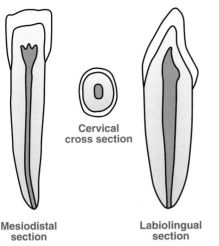

Cervical
cross section

Mesiodistal   Labiolingual
section   section

FIGURE 16-22 Pulp cavity of a permanent mandibular right lateral incisor.

Labial View Features

The crown of a mandibular lateral incisor is not as symmetrical as that of a central and appears tilted or twisted distally on the root from the labial view (see Figure 16-21). The tooth is not symmetrical because the distal outline is slightly more rounded and shorter compared with the slightly flatter and longer mesial outline. The incisal angles are different: The mesioincisal angle of the incisal edge is sharper than the distoincisal angle, which *helps to distinguish the right mandibular lateral incisor from the left.* The labial developmental depressions are deeper than on the central incisors.

From the labial view, the mesial contact with a mandibular central incisor is in the incisal third. The distal contact with a mandibular canine is in the incisal third but is located more cervically than the mesial contact.

Lingual View Features

The crown of a mandibular lateral incisor lacks bilateral symmetry and appears tilted or twisted distally on the root from the lingual view. Overall, the lingual surface has more prominent features compared with the lingual surface of a central incisor. The small single **cingulum** lies just distal to the long axis of the root.

On the lingual surface, both the mesial marginal ridge and distal marginal ridge are more developed than on a central, although the mesial marginal ridge is longer than the distal marginal ridge. A single lingual fossa is also present. A lingual pit is rarely present on a lateral but more often than on a central.

Proximal View Features

The greater height of the CEJ curvature on the mesial than the distal surface *helps to distinguish the right*

mandibular lateral incisor from the left. Also from the mesial view, more of the lingual surface is visible because of the distal tilt or twist of the incisal edge. The distal view is similar to the mesial view of the tooth, but the CEJ is curved less on the distal than the mesial surface.

Incisal View Features

A more rounded appearance is noted both labially and lingually from the incisal view of a mandibular lateral incisor as compared with that of a mandibular central. The entire incisal edge is not straight mesiodistally, as it is in a central; instead, the incisal edge curves toward the lingual in its distal portion. Also, the incisal angles are different: The distoincisal angle is visibly more lingual than the mesioincisal angle, and the cingulum appears displaced toward the distal. Again, on the lingual surface, the mesial marginal ridge is longer than the distal marginal ridge.

 Developmental Disturbances with Mandibular Lateral Incisors

Developmental disturbances are rare in a permanent mandibular lateral incisor, as in a central. One rare exception is that the tooth may have an accessory root or bifurcated root, with the two branches having labial and lingual orientation.

PERMANENT CANINES
General Features

The permanent canines are the four anterior teeth located at the corners of each quadrant for each dental arch (Table 16-2). Thus a permanent canine is the third tooth from the midline in each quadrant, distal to the incisors and mesial to the posterior teeth. Patients commonly call the canines their "eye teeth." An older dental term for canines was **cuspids** because they were the only teeth in the permanent dentition with one cusp. They get their present dental name of *canines* from the Latin word for dog because they resemble dogs' teeth. Patients often complain of the slightly deeper yellow color of their canines compared with their incisor teeth, a normal color in the dentition that is actually placed in dentures to mimic a natural look.

Both the maxillary and mandibular canines resemble one another. The crown of each is about the same size and, when viewed from the proximal, appears triangular, like all anterior teeth. When viewed from the labial or lingual, however, the canine crown outline appears pentagonal, with five sides, similar to the premolars. Canines are also wider labiolingually than the incisors, even wider than maxillary central incisors.

TABLE 16-2

Anatomical Information on Permanent Canines

	Maxillary Canine	Mandibular Canine
Universal number	#6 and #11	#22 and #27
General crown features	Single cusp, with tip and slopes, labial ridge, marginal ridges and lingual ridge, cingulum, and lingual fossae; longest tooth in each arch or dentition	
Specific crown features	Prominent lingual anatomy, sharp cusp tip	Smoother lingual anatomy, less sharp cusp tip
Height of contour	Labial: cervical third Lingual: middle third	
Mesial contact	Junction of incisal third and middle thirds	Incisal third
Distal contact	Middle third	Junction of incisal and middle thirds
Distinguishing right from left	Shorter mesial cusp slope, more cervical contact on distal, more pronounced mesial CEJ curvature	
	Shorter distal outline on labial view with depression between the distal contanct and CEJ	Shorter and rounder distal outline on labial view, with a shorter mesial slope than distal
General root features	Long, thick single root; ovoid on cross section; proximal root concavities	
Specific root features	Blunt root apex	Developmental depressions on mesial and distal giving tooth double-rooted appearance; pointed apex

CEJ = cementoenamel junction.

Similar to the other anterior teeth, each of the canines has an incisal edge (Figure 16-23). Different from the incisors is the **cusp tip,** which is in line with the long axis of the root for both maxillary and mandibular canines when first erupted. Because of the presence of the cusp tip, the incisal edge of canines is divided into two **cusp slopes** or ridges, rather than being nearly straight across like the incisors.

The mesial cusp slope is usually shorter than the distal cusp slope for both the maxillary and mandibular canines when they first erupt. The mesial cusp slope of a maxillary canine occludes with the distal cusp slope of a mandibular canine. The length of these cusp slopes and position of the cusp tip can change with attrition (discussed later).

The canines are the only teeth in the permanent dentition with a vertical and centrally placed **labial ridge**. This labial ridge is a result of greater development of the middle labial developmental lobe in comparison with the mesial and distal labial developmental lobes. Mamelons are not normally present on the incisal edge as they are on incisors, but a small notch may be seen on either cusp slope. The height of contour on labial and lingual surfaces is in the cervical third for the canines, similar to all anterior teeth.

Each canine also has a cingulum and marginal ridges on its lingual surface, like the incisors (Figure 16-24). The cingulum corresponds to the lingual developmental lobe, as in the incisors, but is larger than on any incisor. As with the incisors, however, the canine crown is narrower on the lingual surface than on the labial surface, with the crown tapering lingually.

In addition, canines have a vertical, centrally placed lingual ridge that extends from the cusp tip to the cingulum. The lingual ridge creates two separate and shallow lingual fossae between it and the bordering marginal ridges. These lingual fossae are more pronounced on the maxillary canines than on the mandibular.

The permanent canines are the longest teeth in the dentition. Each has a particularly long, thick root. The root is usually one and one-half times the length of the crown. This long and large root is externally manifested by the vertically oriented and labially placed bony ridge called the **canine eminence** of the alveolar bone, especially in the maxillary arch. Proximal root concavities are located on both proximal root surfaces. The root is ovoid or egg shaped on cervical cross section (see Figures 16-27 and 16-30).

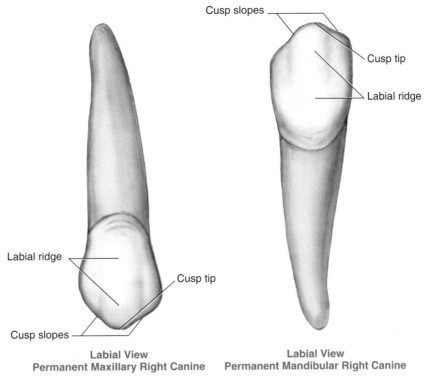

Cusp slopes

Cusp tip

Labial ridge

Labial ridge

Cusp tip

Cusp slopes

Labial View
Permanent Maxillary Right Canine

Labial View
Permanent Mandibular Right Canine

FIGURE 16-23 Labial views of newly erupted permanent canines and their features.

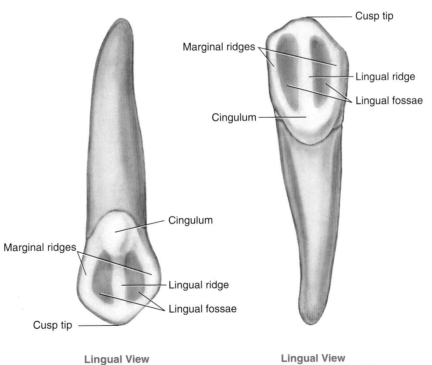

Cusp tip

Marginal ridges

Lingual ridge

Lingual fossae

Cingulum

Cingulum

Marginal ridges

Lingual ridge

Lingual fossae

Cusp tip

Lingual View
Permanent Maxillary Right Canine

Lingual View
Permanent Mandibular Right Canine

FIGURE 16-24 Lingual views of permanent canines and their features (lingual fossae highlighted).

Clinical Considerations with Canines

Because of their tapered shape and prominent cusp, the permanent canines function to pierce or tear food during mastication. Canines, because of their arch position, serve as a major support of facial muscles and keep the overall vertical dimension of the face intact.

Without their presence, normal facial contours cannot be maintained and a loss of height occurs in the lower third of vertical dimension. Dentists consider the canines the cornerstones of the dental arch because of their arch position, tooth form, and function.

The canines also support the incisors and premolars in their functions during mastication and speech. During occlusal movement, they act as guideposts (see Chapter 20 for more information). In this respect, they serve as a protective functional device for a type of lower jaw movement called *lateral deviation*. Finally, canines can help relieve any excessive horizontal forces imposed on posterior teeth.

The permanent canines are the most stable teeth in the dentition, one reason being their long root length, which offers an increased amount of periodontal tissue support. In addition, the proximal root concavities help furnish increased periodontal anchorage for these teeth. Thus these teeth have a significantly reduced risk of loss as a result of periodontal disease or traumatic injury and are usually the last teeth lost in a failing dentition. The canines often serve as the stabilizing anchors for replacements of lost teeth in prosthetic procedures, such as the placement of partial dentures. These teeth are also important cosmetically because each one holds the commissure (corner of lip) out, reducing the appearance of lip lines or wrinkles.

Caries usually does not occur with canines, another factor that makes them an extremely stable tooth in the dentition. Canines seldom have carious lesions because the crown portion usually has a form that promotes self-cleansing and does not retain bacterial plaque biofilm or other deposits.

However, changes can occur in the length of each canine cusp slope and in the movement of the position of the usually centered cusp tip. In older individuals, the lengths of the cusp slopes are often altered by attrition, the wearing away of a tooth surface caused by tooth-to-tooth contact (Figure 16-25; see Chapter 20 for more discussion). With wear, each cusp tip of the maxillary canines is moved to the distal of center, with mesial displacement of the cusp tip for the mandibular canine. This wear also lengthens the mesial cusp slope, shortens the distal slope for the maxillary canines, and shortens the mesial cusp slope and lengthens the distal slope for the mandibular canines. The wear pattern on a canine from the incisal view can appear either diamond shaped or triangular.

It is also noted that proximal surfaces of the canines are more accessible from the lingual than the facial approach during instrumentation. This is because of the convergence of the proximal surfaces toward the lingual.

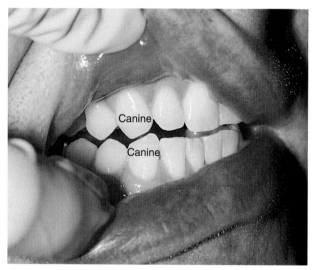

FIGURE 16-25 Lateral view of permanent canines altered on their incisal surfaces by attrition. The cusp tip of maxillary canines is moved to the distal of center, with mesial displacement of the cusp tip for the mandibular canine. This also lengthens the mesial cusp slope and shortens the distal one for the maxillary canines and shortens the mesial cusp slope and lengthens the distal one for the mandibular canines.

Permanent Maxillary Canines #6 and #11

SPECIFIC OVERALL FEATURES (FIGURE 16-26)

The permanent maxillary canines erupt between 11 and 12 years of age (root completion occurs between the ages of 13 and 15). Thus these teeth usually erupt after the mandibular canines, after the maxillary incisors, and possibly after the maxillary premolars.

The crown of a maxillary canine is similar in length or even shorter than that of a maxillary central incisor. Labiolingually, the crown is considerably wider than that of a central incisor, but a canine crown is noticeably narrower mesiodistally. The cingulum on the lingual surface is more developed and larger than that of a central incisor of the same arch, making the tooth stronger during mastication.

A maxillary canine does somewhat resemble a mandibular canine. However, the cusp is more developed and larger and the cusp tip is sharper on a maxillary tooth. In addition, the entire lingual surface features of the maxillary canine are more prominent, including the lingual ridge and marginal ridges.

Finally, an entire maxillary canine is as long as a mandibular canine, but the crown is as long as or

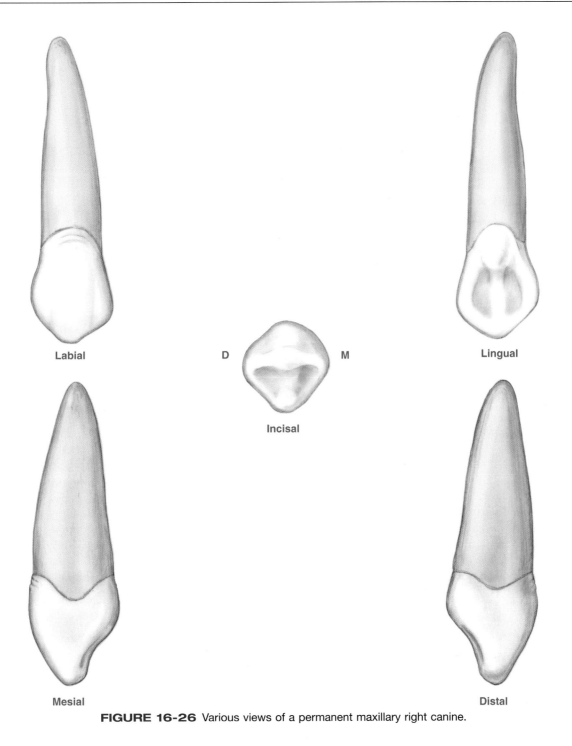

Labial

D M

Incisal

Lingual

Mesial

Distal

FIGURE 16-26 Various views of a permanent maxillary right canine.

slightly shorter than that of a mandibular canine. The long root is single and has a blunt apex; it is the longest root in the maxillary arch. Developmental depressions are evident on both proximal surfaces of the root but are especially pronounced on the distal surface owing to the distal prominence of crown at CEJ. Moderate to deep proximal concavities are also possible. The pulp cavity of a maxillary canine consists of a single pulp canal and a large pulp chamber (Figure 16-27). The pulp chamber usually has only one pulp horn.

LABIAL VIEW FEATURES

The mesial half of the crown of a maxillary canine resembles a portion of an incisor, and the distal half resembles a portion of a premolar, showing the transition from the incisors to the premolars in the maxillary arch (see Figure 16-26). Normally, imbrication lines and perikymata are present in the cervical third of the surface, especially in newly erupted teeth.

Two faint and vertical mesial and distal labial developmental depressions extend from the cervical

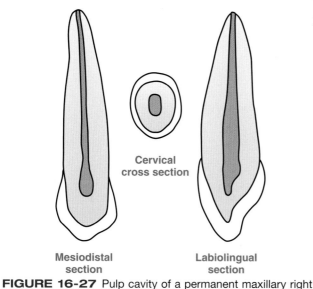

FIGURE 16-27 Pulp cavity of a permanent maxillary right canine.

Mesiodistal section

Labiolingual section

Cervical cross section

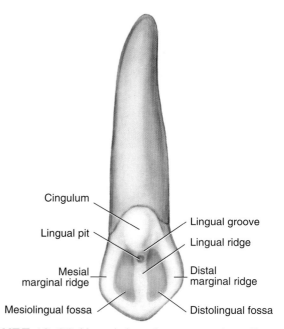

Cingulum

Lingual pit

Mesial marginal ridge

Mesiolingual fossa

Lingual groove

Lingual ridge

Distal marginal ridge

Distolingual fossa

FIGURE 16-28 Lingual view of a permanent maxillary right canine and features (lingual fossae highlighted).

to the incisal and separate the three labial developmental lobes. These depressions are located on either side of the vertical, centrally placed labial ridge. This ridge is most noticeable in the incisal portion of the labial surface.

The mesial outline of the labial surface of the maxillary canine is usually rounded from the mesial contact area to the CEJ, but overall it is straighter than the distal outline. The distal outline is shorter than the mesial outline and usually has a depression between the distal contact area and the CEJ, which *helps to distinguish the right maxillary canine from the left*. From the labial view, the mesial and distal contacts are on two different levels, which *helps to distinguish the right maxillary canine from the left*. The mesial contact with the lateral incisor is at the junction of the incisal and middle thirds. The distal contact with the first premolar is more cervical, at the middle third.

As previously discussed, the single cusp is round and the mesial cusp slope of a maxillary canine is shorter than the distal cusp slope when first erupted, which *helps to distinguish the right maxillary canine from the left*. The **CEJ** on the labial surface is evenly curved toward the root.

LINGUAL VIEW FEATURES

The mesial, distal, and incisal lingual outlines of a maxillary canine are similar to those on the labial view of the tooth (Figure 16-28). The overall dimension of the lingual surface is less than that of the labial surface, however, because the mesial and distal surfaces converge slightly toward the lingual. The cingulum is large and usually smooth and is centered mesiodistally on the lingual surface.

The lingual surface also has a prominent mesial marginal ridge and distal marginal ridge. A vertical, centrally placed lingual ridge is also present from the cingulum to the cusp tip, separating two lingual fossae, the shallow but visible mesiolingual fossa and distolingual fossa. On a maxillary canine, the cingulum and the incisal half of the lingual surface are sometimes separated by a shallow lingual groove. This groove may contain a lingual pit near its center. The lingual pit may also be present without the lingual groove.

PROXIMAL VIEW FEATURES

The CEJ curves higher incisally on the mesial than on the distal surface, which *helps to distinguish the right maxillary canine from the left* (see Figure 16-26). The cusp tip is toward the labial. The distal view of the tooth is similar to the mesial view, but the CEJ curvature is less on the distal than on the mesial surface.

INCISAL VIEW FEATURES

Again, the labiolingual width of a maxillary canine is large in comparison with that of any other anterior tooth, making it an extremely strong tooth during mastication. Additionally, the crown outline is asymmetrical. The mesial portion of the crown has greater labiolingual bulk. The distal portion of the crown appears thinner than the mesial and gives the impression of being stretched to make contact with the first premolar.

More specifically, the mesial half of the labial outline is quite rounded, and the distal half is frequently concave. The distal half of the lingual outline is also frequently concave because the distal fossa is deeper and thus more pronounced. The mesial marginal ridge is longer than the distal marginal ridge. The cusp slopes seem to form a nearly straight line.

Clinical Considerations with Maxillary Canines

Because the permanent maxillary canines erupt after the maxillary incisors and possibly the maxillary premolars, their arch space often is partially closed and they may erupt labially or lingually to the surrounding teeth. The maxillary canines may also fail to erupt fully, remaining **impacted** within the alveolar bone. An impacted tooth is an unerupted or partially erupted tooth that is positioned against another tooth, bone, or even soft tissue in a way that makes complete eruption unlikely. As a result, surgical exposure and follow-up orthodontic treatment may be needed. This problem may be prevented by careful evaluation of patients with mixed dentition and institution of preventive orthodontic care. In addition, the distal prominence of the crown is at the CEJ and may cause instrumentation difficulties during work on the distal root surface.

Developmental Disturbances with Maxillary Canines

The cingulums on the maxillary canines may exhibit tubercles, or extra cusps (discussed further in Chapter 6) that are located near the most incisal level of the cingulum. A lingual pit is often associated with the presence of tubercles.

In a separate developmental disturbance, the root of maxillary canines may undergo distorted angulations or dilaceration, and there may be several curvatures along its length. With root curvature in the apical third, the root is usually curved distally. Finally, developmental cyst formation may occur within the dental tissues of an impacted crown of a maxillary canine, resulting in a **dentigerous cyst**.

Permanent Mandibular Canines #22 and #27

SPECIFIC OVERALL FEATURES (FIGURE 16-29)

The permanent mandibular canines erupt between 9 and 10 years of age (root completion occurs between the age of 12 and 14). Thus these teeth usually erupt before the maxillary canines and after most of the incisors have erupted.

A mandibular canine closely resembles a maxillary canine. Although the entire tooth is usually as long, a mandibular canine is narrower labiolingually and mesiodistally than a maxillary canine. The crown of this tooth can be as long or even longer than that of a maxillary canine.

The single cusp is not as well developed, and the two cusp ridges are thinner labiolingually than those of a maxillary canine. The single cusp tip usually is not as sharp. In addition, the cusp tip is on a line with the long axis of the root, but it is sometimes positioned lingually, similar to the mandibular incisors.

The lingual surface of the crown of a mandibular canine is smoother than that of a maxillary canine and has a less developed cingulum and two marginal ridges. Thus the lingual surface of this crown more closely resembles the form of the lingual surface of the adjacent mandibular lateral incisors, despite the added feature of a lingual ridge.

The single root of a mandibular canine may be as long as that of a maxillary canine but is usually somewhat shorter, although it still has the longest mandibular root. The root has a slight mesial inclination. The mesial developmental depression on the root is more pronounced and often deeper compared with that of a maxillary canine. A distal developmental depression similar to the mesial one is also apparent. These proximal concavities may extend the full length of the root. These depressions may be extremely pronounced, to the point of creating a facial and lingual component in the apical third and giving the tooth a double-rooted appearance. The root apex is also more pointed on this tooth than on a maxillary canine.

The pulp cavity of a mandibular canine resembles that of a maxillary canine in that they both usually have a single pulp canal and a large pulp chamber (Figure 16-30). There is also only one pulp horn. The major difference is that a mandibular canine may have two separate pulp canals. If the tooth has two canals, one is placed labially and the other lingually. The canals may join at the apex or have separate apical foramina.

LABIAL VIEW FEATURES

The labial surface on a mandibular canine is not as rounded as that on a maxillary canine, especially in the incisal two thirds of the tooth (see Figure 16-29). In contrast, however, a mandibular canine is generally more rounded than a mandibular incisor.

Imbrication lines are not normally present on the labial surface, unlike a maxillary canine. Two faint and vertically placed mesial and distal labial developmental depressions separate the three labial lobes, similar to the maxillary canine and incisors. These depressions are located on either side of the vertical, centrally placed labial ridge, which is not as prominent as that of a maxillary canine.

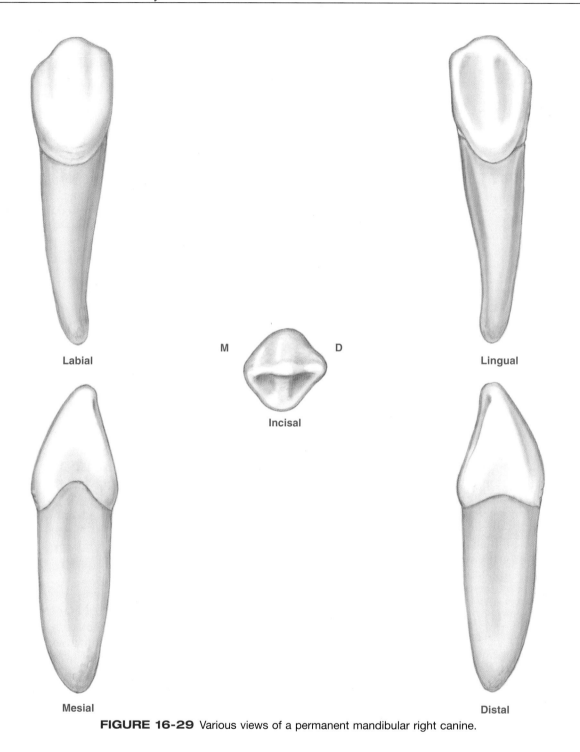

Labial

Lingual

M   D

Incisal

Mesial

Distal

FIGURE 16-29 Various views of a permanent mandibular right canine.

From the labial view, the mesial outline is almost a straight line from the mesial contact to the CEJ, straighter than on a maxillary canine. The distal outline is shorter and rounder than the mesial outline, similar to that of a maxillary canine. This feature *helps to distinguish the right mandibular canine from the left.*

From the labial view, similar to a maxillary canine, the mesial and distal contacts are on different levels, which *helps to distinguish the right mandibular canine from the left.* The mesial contact with the lateral incisor is in the incisal third. The distal contact with the first premolar is at the junction of the incisal and middle thirds, a more cervical location than that on the mesial side.

As discussed before, the cusp slopes are different: The mesial cusp slope of a mandibular canine is shorter than the distal cusp slope when first erupted from the labial view, which *helps to distinguish the right mandibular canine from the left.* With attrition, the central cusp tip moves to the mesial, shortening the already

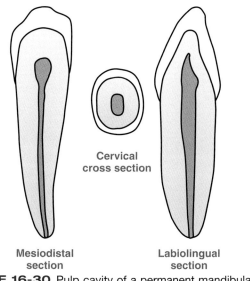

Cervical cross section

Mesiodistal section **Labiolingual section**

FIGURE 16-30 Pulp cavity of a permanent mandibular right canine.

short mesial cusp slope and further lengthening the distal cusp slope. The CEJ is evenly curved toward the root.

LINGUAL VIEW FEATURES

The lingual surface is relatively smooth, except for the faintly demarcated features of a lingual ridge, mesial marginal ridge, distal marginal ridge, and two lingual fossae, the distolingual fossa and mesiolingual fossa. The less developed cingulum on a mandibular canine is not centered as on a maxillary canine but lies distal to the long axis of the root. In addition, the cingulum also does not extend as far incisally as it does in the maxillary canines. Rarely are there any lingual pits or lingual grooves on this surface.

PROXIMAL VIEW FEATURES

A mandibular canine is again similar to a maxillary canine from a mesial view, with a similar triangular shape and pointed cusp on the crown. Again, the less developed cingulum and thinner marginal ridges are seen. The cusp tip is more lingually inclined without incisal wear, unlike the labially placed cusp tip on a maxillary canine.

The CEJ curvature on the mesial surface is more toward the incisal when compared to the same surface of a maxillary canine. Also, the CEJ curve is more toward the incisal on the mesial surface than the distal on this same tooth, which *helps to distinguish the right mandibular canine from the left.* The distal view is similar to the mesial aspect. The one exception is that the CEJ is curved less on the distal than on the mesial surface.

INCISAL VIEW FEATURES

A mandibular canine from this view is similar to a maxillary canine, but it is slightly more symmetrical compared with the maxillary tooth. Also, the crown is wider labiolingually than mesiodistally and is offset toward the mesial. The less developed cingulum is offset toward the distal. This placement still gives the tooth only a slight asymmetrical appearance from this view, less than a maxillary canine.

The mesial marginal ridge is longer than the distal marginal ridge. The labial outline is also more rounded mesiodistally than that of the mandibular incisors because of the pronounced labial ridge.

Developmental Disturbances with Mandibular Canines

Dilaceration (see Chapter 6 for more discussion) of the root can also occur with a mandibular canine, similar to a maxillary canine. Another developmental disturbance is an accessory root or bifurcated root in the apical third, with labial and lingual branches. This tooth is the anterior tooth most likely to have a bifurcated root, although this still is rare.

CHAPTER 17

Permanent Posterior Teeth

After studying this chapter, the reader should be able to:

1. Use the correct names and universal designation numbers of each permanent posterior tooth when examining a diagram and a patient.
2. Demonstrate the correct location of each permanent posterior tooth on a diagram and a patient.
3. Define and pronounce the key terms when discussing the permanent posterior teeth.
4. Describe the general and specific features of posterior teeth and each posterior tooth type of the permanent dentition.
5. Discuss the important clinical considerations and developmental disturbances based on the anatomy of the permanent posterior teeth.
6. Integrate the knowledge of dental anatomy of the permanent posterior teeth into the dental treatment of patients.

Key Terms

Andontia (an-ah-**don**-she-ah)
Bicuspid (bi-**kus**-pid)
Bifurcated (bi-fer-**kay**-ted)
Cementoenamel junction
Contact area
Crown
Cusp: planes, ridges, tip
Cusp of Carabelli (kare-ah-**bell**-ee), groove
Dentigerous cyst (den-**ti**-jer-os)
Dilaceration (di-las-er-**ay**-shun)
Enamel pearl

Fluting
Fossa (**fos**-ah) (plural, fossae, fos-ay): central, triangular
Furcation (fer-**kay**-shin), crotches
Groove: central, developmental, marginal, supplemental, triangular
Inclined cuspal planes
Impacted (im-**pak**-ted)
Molars (**mo**-lers), first, mulberry, (mull-bare-ee), peg third, second, third
Multirooted
Nonsuccadaneous (non-suk-seh-

dane-ee-us)
Oblique ridge
Occlusal (ah-**kloo**-zl): developmental pits, surface, table
Premolars (pre-**mo**-lers): first, second
Ridge, buccal, cervical, oblique (obleek), marginal, transverse (trans-**vers**), triangular
Root: accessory, concavities, fusion, trunk
Trifurcated (try-fer-**kay**-ted)
Tubercles (**too**-ber-kls)

PERMANENT POSTERIOR TEETH

The permanent posterior teeth include the **premolars** and **molars** (Figure 17-1). The **crown** of each posterior tooth has an **occlusal surface** as its masticatory surface, bordered by the raised **marginal ridges**, which are located on the distal and mesial (Figure 17-2). The occlusal surface also has two or more **cusps**. Some anatomists liken a cusp to a gothic pyramid, with four **cusp ridges** descending from each **cusp tip.** Between these cusp ridges are sloping areas, or **inclined cuspal planes.** These planes are named by combining the names of the two cusp ridges between which they lie.

Each cusp usually has four inclined **cuspal planes.** Some inclined planes are functional and thus involved in the occlusion of the teeth (see Chapter 20 for more discussion).

The occlusal surface is bordered by the marginal ridges, creating an inner **occlusal table** (Figure 17-3). There are also **triangular ridges** that are cusp ridges that descend from the cusp tips toward the central portion of the occlusal table (Figure 17-4). They are so named because the slopes of each side of the ridge are inclined in a way that resembles two sides of a triangle. The triangular ridges are specifically named for the cusps to which they belong. Also present on many posterior teeth is a **transverse ridge**, a collective term given to the joining of two triangular ridges crossing the occlusal table transversely or from the labial to the lingual outline.

Each shallow and wide depression on the occlusal table is a **fossa**. One type of fossa on posterior teeth,

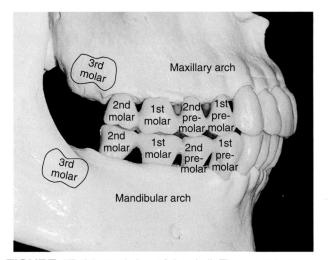

FIGURE 17-1 Lateral view of the skull. The permanent posterior teeth are identified and include the premolars and molars. (Note that the third molars, or "wisdom teeth," have not erupted yet.)

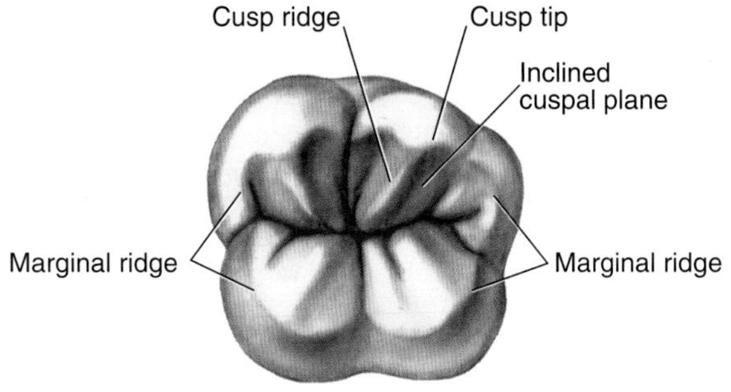

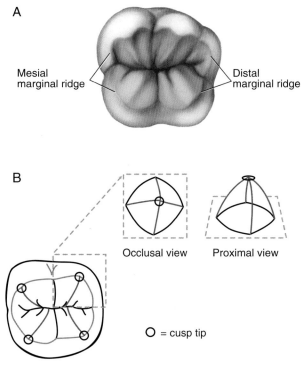

FIGURE 17-3 Occlusal views of a permanent posterior tooth. **A:** Occlusal table highlighted. **B:** Triangular ridges highlighted, with a close-up of the gothic pyramid of the cusp.

FIGURE 17-2 An example of the occlusal surface on a permanent posterior tooth and its features.

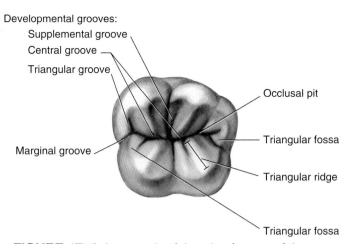

Developmental grooves:
- Supplemental groove
- Central groove
- Triangular groove
- Marginal groove
- Occlusal pit
- Triangular fossa
- Triangular ridge
- Triangular fossa

FIGURE 17-4 An example of the other features of the occlusal table on a permanent posterior tooth, including the central groove.

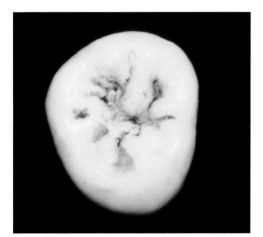

FIGURE 17-5 An example of supplemental grooves on the occlusal surface of a permanent posterior tooth.

the **central fossa,** is located at the convergence of the cusp ridges in a central point, where the grooves meet. Another type of fossa is the **triangular fossa,** which appears to have a triangle shape at the convergence of the cusp ridges and is associated with the termination of the triangular grooves (discussed next). Sometimes located in the deepest portions of the fossae are **occlusal developmental pits.** Each pit is a sharp pinpoint depression where two or more grooves meet.

Developmental grooves, or primary grooves, are also found on the occlusal table. The developmental grooves on each different posterior tooth type are located in the same place and mark the junction among the **developmental lobes.** The grooves are sharp, deep, V-shaped linear depressions. The most prominent developmental groove on posterior teeth is the **central groove,** which generally travels mesiodistally and separates the occlusal table buccolingually.

Other developmental grooves are **marginal grooves,** which cross the marginal ridges and serve as a spillway, allowing food to escape during mastication. Finally, there are **triangular grooves** that separate a marginal ridge from the triangular ridge of a cusp and at their terminations form the triangular fossae.

In contrast, **supplemental grooves,** or secondary grooves, appear as shallower, more irregular linear depressions (Figure 17-5). Supplemental grooves branch from the developmental grooves, but these grooves are not always present in the same pattern on the occlusal table of each different tooth type. In general, the more posterior the tooth, the more supplemental grooves are present, such that the occlusal table appears more wrinkled.

When examined from the buccal and lingual views, the crown outline of the posterior teeth is trapezoidal, or four-sided with only two parallel sides (not including the occlusal surface cusp form of posteriors). Thus

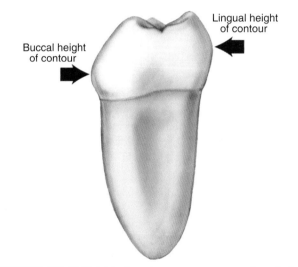

Lingual height of contour

Buccal height of contour

FIGURE 17-6 Height of contour on a permanent posterior tooth.

the longer of the two parallel sides is toward the occlusal aspect. This arrangement is quite important in the functioning of the teeth.

For posterior teeth, the **height of contour** for the crown's buccal surface is in the cervical third, and the lingual surface is in the middle or occlusal third (Figure 17-6). When compared with anterior teeth, the posterior teeth are wider labiolingually than mesiodistally, except for the mandibular molars.

In another comparison with anterior teeth, the **contact area** of each of the posterior teeth is wider, usually located to the buccal of center, and is nearer the same level on each proximal surface. In addition, on each proximal surface is a **cementoenamel junction (CEJ)** curvature that is less pronounced on the posterior teeth than on the anteriors. In fact, the CEJ is often quite straight for posterior teeth.

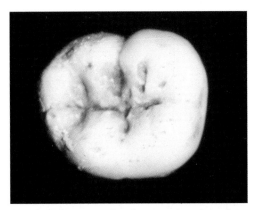

FIGURE 17-7 An example of a complex pit and groove pattern on the occlusal surface of a permanent posterior tooth.

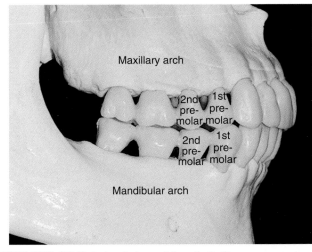

FIGURE 17-8 Lateral view of the skull. The permanent premolars are identified.

 Clinical Considerations for Posterior Teeth

The complex pit and groove patterns on the occlusal surface of permanent posterior teeth can make them susceptible to caries (Figure 17-7). This susceptibility is due to increased bacterial plaque biofilm retention and the weakness of enamel forming the walls of the pits and grooves (see Chapter 12 for more information). All pits and grooves must be checked for decay with an explorer and mirror. Newer devices are being used chairside by clinicians, along with the results of the clinical examination, to detect occlusal and smooth surface caries using a laser-induced fluorescent probe. Posterior teeth with deep pit and groove patterns but without incipient decay should have enamel sealants placed on the occlusal surface shortly after eruption.

PERMANENT PREMOLARS

General Features

The permanent premolars are the most anteriorly placed posterior teeth in the permanent dentition (Figure 17-8 and Table 17-1). Each dental arch has four premolars, two to each quadrant.

There are two types of premolars: the **first premolar** and the **second premolar**. One of each type of premolar is present in each quadrant of each dental arch. The first premolar is closer to the midline at the fourth position from it. The second premolar is next to the first premolar and is in the fifth position from the midline. Both types of premolars are distal to the permanent canine and mesial to the permanent first molar when full eruption of the permanent dentition has occurred. The permanent premolars are succedaneous and replace the primary first and second molars.

As posterior teeth, premolars have a shorter crown than anterior teeth. The buccal surface of the premolars is rounded and has a prominent vertical **buccal ridge** in the center of the crown (Figure 17-9). Two buccal developmental depressions are noted on each side of the buccal ridge. The buccal ridge of premolars is similar to the labial ridge of the canines and may be related to the increased development of the middle buccal lobe. The height of contour, or crest of curvature, of the crown buccally is in the cervical third, as in anterior teeth. Lingually, the height of contour for premolars is in the middle third.

An older dental term for a premolar was **bicuspid** because of the usual presence of two cusps on the occlusal surface, one more cusp than in the canines. However, the permanent mandibular second premolar frequently has three cusps. Thus the name *premolar* is more widely used today because these teeth are always anterior to the molars.

Finally, in addition to the cusps, the occlusal surface of a premolar, similar to all permanent posterior teeth, has marginal ridges, triangular ridges, developmental grooves, and occlusal developmental pits. The boundaries of the occlusal surface, the marginal ridges and cusp ridges, form an inner occlusal table.

In addition, most premolars usually have one **root**, except for the permanent maxillary first premolar, which has two roots. Whether one or two roots are present, premolars have proximal **root concavities.**

Permanent Maxillary Premolars

GENERAL FEATURES

Both types of maxillary premolars resemble each other more than do the mandibular premolars. A maxillary

TABLE 17-1

Anatomical Information on Permanent Premolars

	Maxillary First Premolar	Maxillary Second Premolar	Mandibular First Premolar	Mandibular Second Premolar
Universal number	#5 and #12	#4 and #13	#21 and #28	#20 and #29
General crown features	Occlusal table with marginal ridges and cusps, with tips, ridges, inclined planes, grooves, fossae, pits; buccal ridge.			
Specific crown features	Larger than second, with buccal cusp longer of two, long central groove	Smaller than first, two cusps same length, short central groove, no mesial surface features like first, increased supplemental grooves	Smaller than second, smaller lingual cusp of two, mesial surface features	Larger than first, usually three cusps: Y groove pattern or two cusps: H or U groove pattern, increased supplemental grooves *M/L cusp is larger*
Mesial and distal contact	Just cervical to the junction of occlusal and middle thirds			
Distinguishing right from left	Longer mesial cusp slope, mesial features: marginal groove, developmental depression, deeper CEJ curvature	Lingual cusp offset to the mesial	Shorter mesial cusp slope, mesiolingual groove, deeper mesial CEJ curvature	Distal marginal ridge more cervically located, thus more occlusal surface visible from distal view *mesial CEJ is more cervical*
General root features	Proximal root concavities			
Specific root features	Bifurcated with root trunk; elliptical on cross section	Single-rooted; elliptical on cross section *Can be bifurcated*	Single-rooted; ovoid or elliptical on cross section	

CEJ = cementoenamel junction.

Clinical Considerations for Premolars

The permanent premolars function to assist the molars in grinding food during mastication because of their broad occlusal surface and their prominent cusps. The premolars also assist the canines in piercing and tearing food with those cusps. These teeth, along with the canines, also help maintain the height of the lower third of the vertical dimension of the face and support the facial muscles, especially those muscles in the corners of the mouth. Thus the premolars are involved in aesthetics and speech, less so than the anterior teeth but more so than the molars.

Single, permanent premolars can be extracted in each quadrant for orthodontic purposes to improve dental arch spacing. If a premolar has been extracted, the distinctive pit and groove patterns on the occlusal surface will help in identifying the remaining premolars when the arch space from the extraction is lost if the remaining molars are not restored. First premolars are extracted more often than second premolars during orthodontic treatment. However, orthodontists today tend to expand the jaw instead of removing premolars to retain a more natural shape to the arches. Also, permanent premolars present difficulty in instrumentation of the root because they have proximal root concavities, especially on the mesial of the maxillary first premolar.

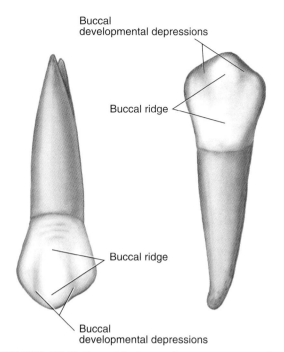

Buccal developmental depressions

Buccal ridge

Buccal ridge

Buccal developmental depressions

FIGURE 17-9 Buccal features of permanent premolars.

first premolar is larger than a maxillary second premolar, but in contrast, a mandibular first premolar is smaller than a mandibular second premolar. Both maxillary premolars erupt earlier than the mandibular premolars.

The crown of a maxillary premolar is shorter occlusocervically than that of a maxillary canine but is slightly longer than that of a molar. The crown outline from the proximal aspect is trapezoidal, or four-sided with only two parallel sides, similar to all maxillary posterior teeth.

The crown is also centered over the root and shows no lingual inclination, unlike the mandibular premolars or other mandibular posterior teeth. The maxillary premolars also have a greater buccolingual width than mesiodistal width compared with the mandibular premolars or other mandibular posterior teeth when viewed from the occlusal. The outline for both maxillary premolars is somewhat hexagonal, or six-sided, and almost oval compared with the round mandibular premolars.

Both maxillary premolars have two cusps of almost equal size. In contrast, the mandibular premolars can have more than two cusps, but any lingual cusps are always smaller. The cusps of all premolars are centered over the long axis of the tooth from either proximal view. The maxillary premolars are composed of four developmental lobes: three buccal and one lingual.

Additionally, the roots of the maxillary premolars are shorter than those of the maxillary canines. The

root length is the same as that of the molars. A maxillary premolar's roots show slight lingual and distal inclination. The roots on cervical cross section are elliptical, or an elongated oval, which may be slightly altered by proximal root concavities.

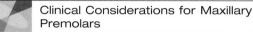

Clinical Considerations for Maxillary Premolars

The roots of maxillary premolars may penetrate the anterior portion of the maxillary sinus as a result of accidental trauma or during tooth extraction because of the close relation of these roots to the sinus walls (see Chapter 11). In addition, the discomfort of sinusitis can be mistakenly interpreted as tooth related (stemming from the maxillary premolar), and vice versa. Thus radiographic study of the tooth or maxillary sinus and other diagnostic tests are necessary to determine the cause of the discomfort.

PERMANENT MAXILLARY FIRST PREMOLARS #5 AND #12

Specific Overall Features (Figure 17-10)

The permanent maxillary first premolars erupt between 10 and 11 years of age (root completion occurs between the ages of 12 and 13). These teeth erupt distal to the primary maxillary canines or their arch space and thus are the succedaneous replacements for the primary maxillary first molars.

The crown of a maxillary first premolar has an angular shape with sharp outlines compared with a maxillary second premolar's more rounded shape. The tooth's two cusps are also sharply defined, with the buccal cusp usually about 1 mm higher than the lingual cusp. The tooth appears bent mesially when viewed from the occlusal compared with the second premolar of the same arch. The central groove on the occlusal surface is also longer on the maxillary first premolar than on the second.

Most maxillary first premolars have two root branches or are **bifurcated** in the apical third, with one buccal root and one lingual or palatal root, unlike the other single-rooted premolars. Maxillary first premolars originate as a single root on the base of the crown, as do other premolars and anterior teeth; this portion is called the **root trunk.**

A cervical cross section of the root trunk follows the form of the crown. The root trunk usually makes up half the length of the entire root, and the root branches make up the other half. The roots are rounded overall and taper to sharp apices. The buccal root of this tooth is larger but not longer than the lingual root. A distinct mesial concavity is present on the root trunk of maxillary first premolar, extending from the contact area to the bifurcation. The mesial surface groove on

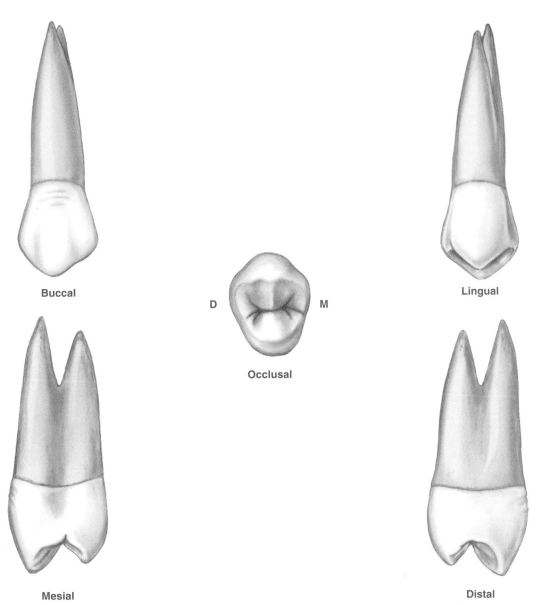

Buccal

D   M

Lingual

Occlusal

Mesial

Distal

FIGURE 17-10 Various views of the permanent maxillary right first premolar.

root makes this tooth periodontally fragile because it allows an increased deposit level. The distal surface has a groove that is reduced in depth, creating a convex or flat surface.

This trunk can also have a fused or laminated root, with very little of the root bifurcated. If a single root is present, which occurs in 20 percent of the population, it is wider buccolingually than mesiodistally, the buccal and lingual surfaces are rounded, and the root is tapered to a blunt apex. In cross-section, the root becomes kidney shaped. A single root also has a deep and wide mesial surface root concavity, which ranges from relatively shallow to deep enough to almost bifurcate the root. Three-rooted, or trifurcated, maxillary first premolars have been noted, with two buccal roots and a single lingual root.

The pulp cavity for a two-rooted tooth usually shows two pulp horns (one for each cusp) and two pulp canals (one for each root) (Figure 17-11). Even if there is only one undivided root, as for the maxillary second premolar, two pulp canals are usually found, although they often combine to form one apical foramen.

Buccal View Features

The crown of a maxillary first premolar is the widest mesiodistally of all the premolars (Figure 17-12). This tooth's crown is wide at the level of the contact areas and more narrow at the CEJ, similar to the maxillary canine. The mesial contact with the maxillary canine

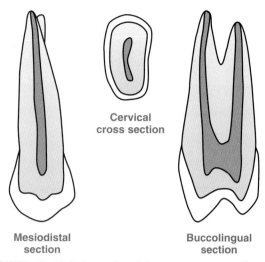

Cervical cross section

Mesiodistal section

Buccolingual section

FIGURE 17-11 Pulp cavity of the permanent maxillary right first premolar.

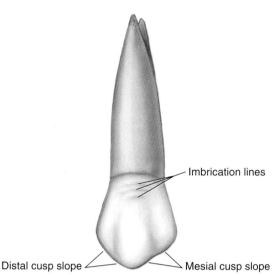

Imbrication lines

Distal cusp slope

Mesial cusp slope

FIGURE 17-12 Buccal features of the permanent maxillary right first premolar.

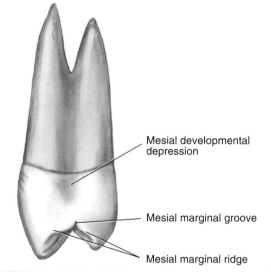

Mesial developmental depression

Mesial marginal groove

Mesial marginal ridge

FIGURE 17-13 Mesial features of the permanent maxillary right first premolar.

is just cervical to the junction of the occlusal and middle thirds. The distal contact with the maxillary second premolar is the same, just cervical to the junction of the occlusal and middle thirds.

The mesial and distal outlines of the crown of the maxillary first premolar are almost straight from the contact areas to the CEJ, but the mesial outline is more rounded. Both these outlines converge more toward the cervical than they do on the maxillary second premolars. Imbrication lines and perikymata are found on the buccal surface, and these extend mesiodistally in the cervical third. The CEJ curvature of the tooth is evenly rounded toward the apex of the tooth and has less depth than on anterior teeth.

The buccal cusp of a maxillary first premolar is high, sharp, and also slightly distal to the long axis of the tooth because the two cusp slopes of the buccal cusp are *not* equal in height. This tooth is the only tooth in the permanent dentition that has a buccal cusp with the mesial cusp slope longer than the distal cusp slope, which *helps to distinguish the right maxillary first premolar from the left*. This relationship of the cusp slopes normally exists upon eruption; attrition may change it. A bulge may be found occasionally on the buccal cusp of this tooth.

Lingual View Features

The lingual surface of the maxillary first premolar is rounded in all directions but is smaller than the buccal surface. The shorter lingual cusp is sharp but not as sharp as the buccal cusp and is offset toward the mesial. Thus the cusp slopes of the lingual cusp are again not equal in length. From the lingual aspect, however, the mesial cusp slope is shorter than the distal cusp slope.

Proximal View Features

On the mesial surface of the crown of a maxillary first premolar, the mesial marginal ridge is present on the concave occlusal margin. A mesial marginal groove is also sometimes present (Figure 17-13). This developmental groove crosses the mesial marginal ridge and extends from the occlusal to the middle third of the crown, lingual to the contact area.

The mesial surface usually also has a mesial developmental depression located cervical to the contact area, across the CEJ, normally extending onto the root. On the root, the depression joins a deep developmental depression between the roots. The CEJ curvature is more occlusally located on the mesial than on the distal surface. All these prominent mesial features from the

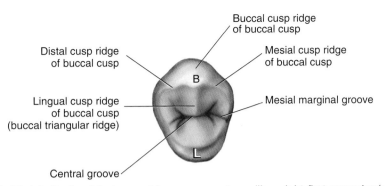

FIGURE 17-14 Occlusal features of the permanent maxillary right first premolar (occlusal table highlighted).

proximal view *help to distinguish the right maxillary first premolar from the left.*

The distal surface is similar to the mesial, except that it does not have a depression and more of the occlusal surface shows because the distal marginal ridge is more cervically located than is the mesial marginal ridge. A distal marginal groove is sometimes located across the distal marginal ridge, but this distal groove is shallower than the groove on the mesial surface. Additionally, the CEJ curvature on the distal surface is not as deep cervically as the mesial.

Occlusal View Features

The outline of the occlusal surface of a maxillary first premolar is somewhat hexagonal or six-sided but is wider buccolingually than mesiodistally (Figure 17-14). The buccal ridge (or buccal cusp ridge of the buccal cusp, as discussed later) is prominent on the buccal margin, and the lingual margin of the occlusal outline is almost a semicircle. The mesial and distal margins are straight as they converge toward the lingual. Thus the lingual portion of the tooth is narrower mesiodistally than the buccal portion. When the mesial marginal groove is prominent, it may create a dip in the mesial outline.

Occlusal Table Components

The buccal cusp of a maxillary first premolar is sharper and higher. The occlusal function of the buccal cusp involves only its lingual surface. Four buccal cusp ridges descend from the buccal cusp tip, each named for its location: buccal, lingual, mesial, and distal. Because this is the first occlusal table of a posterior tooth under discussion, this text provides details on each of the occlusal table features. This information can then be related to the occlusal tables of other posterior teeth.

The buccal cusp ridge of the buccal cusp extends cervically from the cusp tip on the buccal surface and corresponds to the buccal ridge. The lingual cusp ridge extends lingually from the buccal cusp tip to the central groove (also called the *buccal triangular ridge* or *buccal portion of the transverse ridge,* as discussed later). The mesial cusp ridge of the buccal cusp extends mesially from the cusp tip to the mesiobucco-occlusal point angle area. The distal cusp ridge extends distally from the buccal cusp tip to the distobucco-occlusal point angle area.

Between the cusp ridges are four buccal inclined cuspal planes, named for the two cusp ridges between which they lie: mesiobuccal, mesiolingual, distobuccal, and distolingual. However, only the mesiolingual and distolingual inclined cuspal planes function during occlusion.

The lingual cusp of the maxillary first premolar is rounder, less sharp, and shorter. This cusp is also located well to the lingual and offset to the mesial. Again, there are four lingual cusp ridges and four lingual inclined cuspal planes similar to those associated with the buccal cusp, but all the lingual inclined cuspal planes are functional. This is because the entire lingual cusp functions during occlusion, unlike the buccal cusp.

Extending mesiodistally across the occlusal table of the maxillary first premolar is a long central groove, evenly dividing the tooth buccolingually. The central groove is a developmental groove and is also sharply defined, deep, and V-shaped. A few supplemental grooves appear irregular in shape and shallower, and they branch from the central groove. Thus the occlusal surface is relatively smooth compared with the adjacent maxillary second premolar.

The lingual cusp ridge, which runs from the buccal cusp tip to the central groove, is also termed the buccal triangular ridge (Figure 17-15). The buccal cusp ridge of the lingual cusp is also termed the lingual triangular ridge because it runs from the lingual cusp tip to the central groove. Perpendicular to the central groove is a transverse ridge, the collective term given to the joining of the buccal triangular ridge and the lingual triangular ridge.

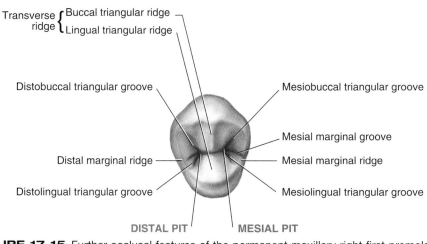

Transverse ⎰ Buccal triangular ridge
ridge ⎱ Lingual triangular ridge

Distobuccal triangular groove

Mesiobuccal triangular groove

Mesial marginal groove

Distal marginal ridge

Mesial marginal ridge

Distolingual triangular groove

Mesiolingual triangular groove

DISTAL PIT   MESIAL PIT

FIGURE 17-15 Further occlusal features of the permanent maxillary right first premolar (fossae highlighted).

The central groove of the maxillary first premolar also crosses to the mesial marginal ridge, which is shorter than the distal marginal ridge. Extending from the central groove, another developmental groove, the mesial marginal groove, crosses the mesial marginal ridge and travels onto the mesial surface of the tooth.

Just inside the distal and mesial marginal ridges, descending down the slope of the buccal cusp are two developmental grooves, the mesiobuccal triangular groove and the distobuccal triangular groove. Across the occlusal table, the lingual cusp also has two developmental grooves, the mesiolingual triangular groove and the distolingual triangular groove.

Each of these triangular grooves ends in a triangular depression called a *triangular fossa*. These fossae are the deeper mesial triangular fossa, which surrounds the mesiobuccal triangular groove, and the shallower distal triangular fossa, which surrounds the distobuccal triangular groove.

The boundaries of the mesial triangular fossa are the mesial marginal ridge, the transverse ridge, and the mesial cusp ridges of the two cusps. The distal triangular fossa has boundaries similar to those of the mesial fossa in a mirror-image fashion. The deepest portions of these fossae are the occlusal developmental pits. These are termed the mesial pit and distal pit, respectively, and they are connected by the central groove.

PERMANENT MAXILLARY SECOND PREMOLARS #4 AND #13

Specific Overall Features (Figure 17-16)

The permanent maxillary second premolars erupt between 10 and 12 years of age (root completion occurs between the ages of 12 and 14). These teeth erupt distal to the permanent maxillary first premolars and thus are the succedaneous replacements for the primary maxillary second molars.

A maxillary second premolar resembles a first premolar, except that its crown is less angular and more rounded. Also, more crown variations, especially in its occlusal surface anatomy, are noted in this tooth compared with maxillary first premolars.

Unlike a maxillary first premolar, a maxillary second premolar usually has only a single root, but it may occasionally have two roots. The dimensions between the maxillary second and the first premolars are usually about the same overall, except for greater root length of the second. The mesial concavity is not as pronounced as in a first premolar. The pulp cavity of this tooth has two pulp horns and one single pulp canal (Figure 17-17).

Buccal View Features

The buccal cusp of a maxillary second premolar is neither as long nor as sharp as that of a maxillary first premolar (see Figure 17-16). All other features of the buccal surface of a maxillary second are similar to those of the first. Again, the mesial contact with a maxillary first premolar is just cervical to the junction of the occlusal and middle thirds on the buccal surface. The distal contact with a maxillary first molar is the same, just cervical to the junction of the occlusal and middle thirds.

LINGUAL VIEW FEATURES

All lingual surface features of a maxillary second premolar are similar to those of a maxillary first premolar. One noteworthy exception is that the lingual cusp is larger, almost the same height as the buccal cusp on a maxillary second premolar. In addition, the lingual cusp is slightly displaced to the mesial, which *helps to distinguish the right maxillary second premolar from the left.* In addition, less of the occlusal surface is seen

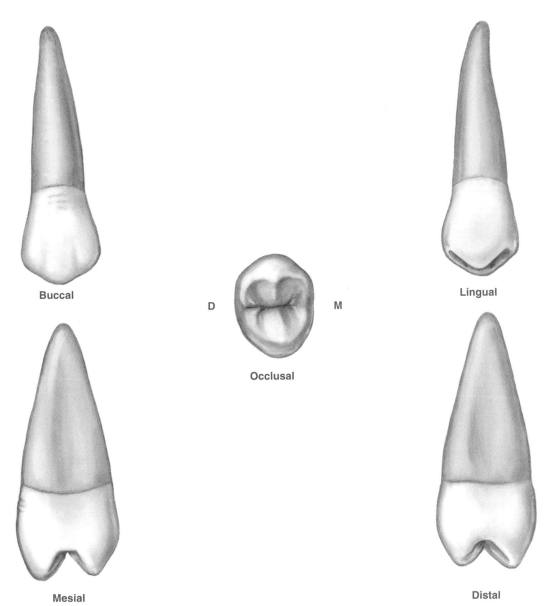

Buccal

D   M

Occlusal

Lingual

Mesial

Distal

FIGURE 17-16 Various views of the permanent maxillary right second premolar.

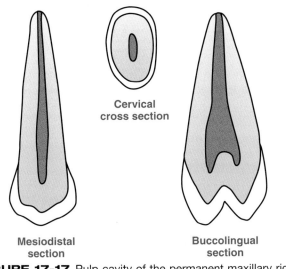

**Cervical
cross section**

**Mesiodistal
section**

**Buccolingual
section**

FIGURE 17-17 Pulp cavity of the permanent maxillary right second premolar.

from this view because the crown is longer on the lingual.

Proximal View Features

The mesial surface of a maxillary second premolar is similar to that of a maxillary first premolar, except that the cusps are closer to being the same size and no mesial developmental depression is present on the crown and root. Instead, this area cervical to the contact area is rounder.

In addition, this tooth has no mesial marginal groove. Both the contact areas and mesial marginal ridge are more cervically located than those on a maxillary first premolar. The distal surface is the same as the mesial surface without any distal marginal groove, but the contact area is larger.

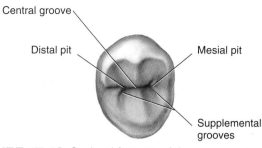
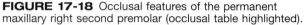

FIGURE 17-18 Occlusal features of the permanent maxillary right second premolar (occlusal table highlighted).

Occlusal View Features

The outline of the occlusal surface of a maxillary second premolar is more rounded and larger overall than that of a maxillary first premolar from the occlusal view. Thus the hexagonal outline of the crown from the occlusal is more difficult to see.

Occlusal Table Components

The central groove is shorter on a maxillary second premolar than on a maxillary first premolar (Figure 17-18). This groove ends in a mesial pit and distal pit, which are closer together and thus more to the middle of the occlusal table.

A maxillary second premolar has numerous supplemental grooves radiating from the central groove. This gives the tooth a more wrinkled appearance compared with a maxillary first premolar. Other features and the overall anatomy of this tooth's occlusal surface are similar to those of a maxillary first premolar.

Permanent Mandibular Premolars

GENERAL FEATURES

Mandibular premolars do not resemble each other as much as do the maxillary premolars. In addition, a mandibular first premolar is smaller than a mandibular second premolar; in contrast, a maxillary first premolar is larger overall than the second. Generally, both mandibular premolars erupt into the oral cavity later than do the maxillary premolars.

Quite distinct from maxillary premolars, the buccal outline of the crown of all mandibular premolars shows a strong lingual inclination when viewed from the proximal, similar to all mandibular posterior teeth. The permanent mandibular premolars also have an equal buccolingual and mesiodistal width when viewed from the occlusal, making the outline almost round. In addition, both types of premolars have a similar buccal outline of both the crown and root.

The mesial and distal contact areas of mandibular premolars are on nearly the same level. Similar CEJ curvatures are also found on both premolars. From each proximal view, both the crown outlines of mandibular premolars are rhomboidal, or four-sided with opposite sides parallel, like all mandibular posterior teeth. The crowns thus incline lingually on their root bases, bringing the cusps into proper occlusion with their maxillary antagonists and the distribution of forces along their long axes.

Unlike the maxillary premolars, both of which have two cusps of almost equal size, the mandibular premolars can have more than two cusps; however, any lingual cusps are always smaller than the buccal cusp.

These teeth usually have a single root. The angulation of the roots of mandibular premolars may show slight distal inclination. The root on cervical cross section is either ovoid (egg-shaped) or elliptical (an elongated oval), shapes that may be slightly altered by the presence of proximal root concavities. These proximal root concavities are most frequently found on the mesial surface of the root.

Clinical Considerations for Mandibular Premolars

Both types of mandibular premolars can present difficulty during instrumentation because they have narrow lingual surfaces combined with the lingual inclination of the crown, which poses special difficulties with subgingival instrument placement. In addition, patients may have problems performing adequate oral hygiene because of the lingual inclination of the crown, which causes some patients to miss the associated lingual gingiva and clean only the occlusal surface with a toothbrush. The nearby tongue also makes oral hygiene and instrumentation more difficult on the lingual surface.

PERMANENT MANDIBULAR FIRST PREMOLARS #21 AND #28

Specific Overall Features (Figure 17-19)

The permanent mandibular first premolars erupt between 10 and 12 years of age (root completion occurs between the ages of 12 and 13). These teeth erupt distal to the permanent mandibular canines and thus are the succedaneous replacements for the primary mandibular first molars.

A mandibular first premolar resembles a mandibular canine in many more ways than it does a mandibular second premolar. This is true despite the fact that a premolar is smaller overall than a canine. However, the buccolingual width of this tooth is similar to that of a mandibular canine. Thus a mandibular first premolar shows a transition in the dental arch from the canine to the molarlike second premolar.

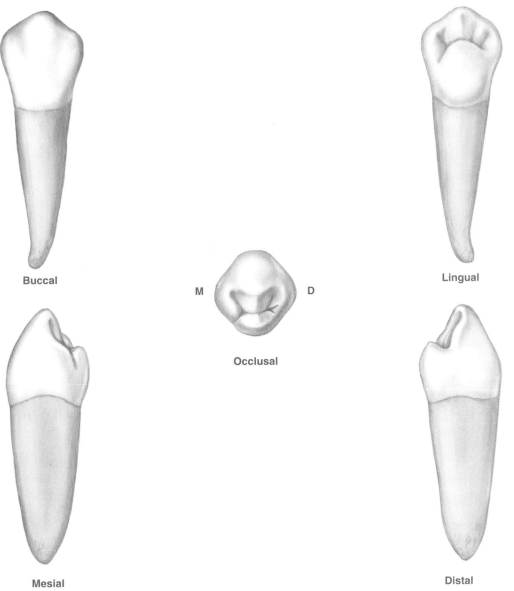

Buccal

Lingual

M   D

Occlusal

Mesial

Distal

FIGURE 17-19 Various views of the permanent mandibular right first premolar.

A mandibular first premolar has a buccal cusp that is long and sharp and is the only functional cusp during occlusion, similar to a mandibular canine. The lingual cusp of a mandibular first premolar is usually small and nonfunctioning. The lingual cusp, then, is similar in appearance to the cingulum found on some maxillary canines, but it can vary considerably. Finally, the occlusal surface of the mandibular first premolar has a similar outline and slopes sharply to the lingual, and the mesiobuccal cusp ridge is shorter than the distobuccal cusp ridge, all similar to the mandibular canine.

A mandibular first premolar has a smaller and shorter root than does a mandibular second premolar, although it is closer to the length of a second premolar than to that of a mandibular canine. The buccal aspect of the root is more conical, but the lingual aspect is tapered. A deep groove may be found on the distal root surface. The tooth occasionally has a bifurcated root, with the root divided into buccal and lingual portions.

The pulp cavity of this tooth consists of two pulp horns and a single pulp canal (Figure 17-20). Each pulp horn is located within a cusp. The buccal pulp horn is more pronounced, and the lingual pulp horn is smaller and less significant.

Buccal View Features

The outline of the crown of a mandibular first premolar from the buccal is nearly symmetrical (see Figure 17-19). The middle developmental lobe is well-developed, resulting in a prominent buccal ridge and

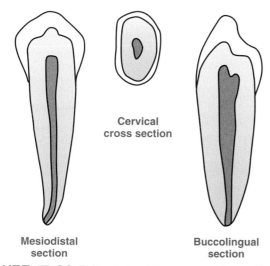

FIGURE 17-20 Pulp cavity of the permanent mandibular right first premolar.

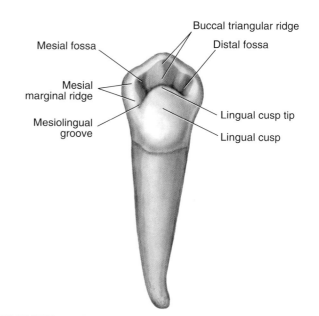

FIGURE 17-21 Lingual features of the permanent mandibular right first premolar (occlusal table highlighted).

a large, pointed buccal cusp, but the buccal ridge is not as prominent as on a maxillary first premolar. Two buccal developmental depressions are often seen among the three buccal lobes. Imbrication lines are not usually found on the buccal surface.

The buccal cusp is also located slightly to the mesial of the center of the crown, again similar to a mandibular canine. Thus the two cusp slopes of a premolar are not equal in length. The mesial cusp slope of the buccal cusp is shorter than the distal cusp slope, which *helps to distinguish the right mandibular first premolar from the left.*

The mesial outline of the mandibular first premolar is slightly concave from the mesial contact to the CEJ. The distal outline is rounder and shorter. Again, the mesial contact with the maxillary first premolar is just cervical to the junction of the occlusal and middle thirds. The distal contact with the maxillary first molar is the same, just cervical to the junction of the occlusal and middle thirds.

Lingual View Features

The lingual surface is much narrower than the buccal on a mandibular first premolar, with the crown tapering to the lingual (Figure 17-21). Most of the mesial and distal surfaces therefore can be seen from the lingual. The lingual cusp is small and nonfunctional during occlusion, and the lingual cusp tip is often pointed.

Because the lingual cusp is small, most of the occlusal surface can be seen from this view. The lingual cusp tip lines up with the buccal triangular ridge. The mesial fossa and distal fossa are on each side of this ridge. A developmental groove, the mesiolingual groove, usually separates the mesial marginal ridge from the mesial cusp slope of the small lingual cusp.

Proximal View Features

From the mesial, the crown of a mandibular first premolar tilts noticeably toward the lingual at the cervix, as do all mandibular posterior teeth (see Figure 17-19). Thus the buccal outline is longer than the lingual outline. This lingual inclination of the crown also places the buccal cusp tip almost over the root axis line. Thus the lingual cusp tip is usually in line vertically with the lingual surface of the cervical portion of the root. The transverse ridge slopes 45 degrees from the buccal cusp tip to the occlusal surface and then nearly flattens out to the lingual cusp tip.

The mesial marginal ridge is nearly parallel to the angulation of the transverse ridge at a more cervical level. The slope of the mesial marginal ridge is similar to that of anterior teeth. The mesiolingual groove again can be seen near the lingual margin. The CEJ curvature is also more occlusal on the mesial surface. Both these mesial surface features *help to distinguish the right mandibular first premolar from the left.*

The distal view of the mandibular first premolar is similar to the mesial, except for the absence of a groove near the lingual margin. The distal marginal ridge is much more developed than that of the mesial, and its continuity is unbroken by any deep developmental grooves. Also, the distal marginal ridge does not show quite as steep a slope toward the lingual, as is present on the mesial.

Occlusal View Features

The crown outline of the mandibular first premolar is diamond-shaped from the occlusal, with a notch in the mesial outline at the mesiolingual groove (Figure

17-22). The prominent buccal ridge is located on the buccal margin. The lingual margin is much shorter than the buccal outline. The mesial margin is slightly rounded to nearly straight, except in the area near the mesiolingual groove. The distal margin is even more rounded than the mesial margin.

Occlusal Table Components

Both the cusps and transverse ridge of the mandibular first premolar are offset to the mesial, leaving the distal portion of the tooth larger than the mesial portion. The larger and functioning buccal cusp of a mandibular first premolar has four buccal cusp ridges and four functioning buccal inclined cuspal planes, all of which are named for their location. The lingual cusp ridge of the buccal cusp is also the buccal triangular ridge.

The lingual cusp of the mandibular first premolar is quite small, usually no more than half the height of the buccal cusp. It also has four lingual cusp ridges and four lingual inclined cuspal planes. The buccal cusp ridge of the buccal cusp is also the lingual triangular ridge.

The transverse ridge is composed of the joining of the buccal triangular ridge of the lingual cusp and the lingual triangular ridge of the buccal cusp. The buccal triangular ridge is longer than the lingual, thus making up a greater part of the transverse ridge. The transverse ridge is perpendicular to the central groove. This groove, which slightly separates the two triangular

ridges, is sometimes rather indistinct, and thus the two triangular ridges appear to be continuous.

The mesial marginal ridge of a mandibular first premolar closely resembles the angulation of the marginal ridges of anterior teeth, especially the canine. This is because it slopes from the buccal to the lingual at a 45-degree angle (Figure 17-23). The mesial marginal ridge is less prominent and shorter than the distal marginal ridge. The distal marginal ridge also does not have quite as steep a slope toward the lingual.

The mesial fossa and distal fossa and associated mesial pit and distal pit are also found on the occlusal table. The mesial fossa is shallower than the distal. Although both are circular, the mesial fossa is slightly more linear. The mesial pit is the junction of the central groove, mesiolingual groove (previously described on the lingual and mesial aspects), and mesiobuccal triangular groove (similar in location to that of the maxillary premolars). The distal pit is the junction of the central groove, distal marginal groove, distolingual triangular groove, and distobuccal triangular groove.

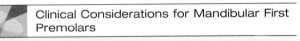

Clinical Considerations for Mandibular First Premolars

When mandibular first premolars have Class I metallic restorations in their mesial and distal fossae, these restorations are sometimes nicknamed "snake eyes" because of the roundness of the two fossae (Figure 17-24). This type of restoration can also be seen on the occlusal surface of mandibular second premolars. Tooth-colored restorative materials are now more commonly placed on the occlusal surface of these smaller posterior teeth to achieve a more attractive appearance.

PERMANENT MANDIBULAR SECOND PREMOLARS #20 AND #29
Specific Overall Features (Figure 17-25)

The permanent mandibular second premolars erupt between 11 and 12 years of age (root completion occurs between the ages of 13 and 14). These teeth erupt distal to the mandibular first premolars and thus are the suc-

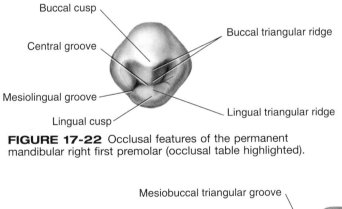

FIGURE 17-22 Occlusal features of the permanent mandibular right first premolar (occlusal table highlighted).

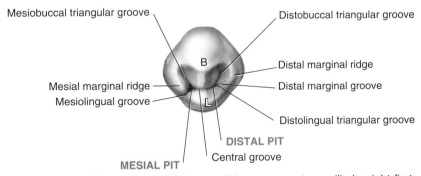

FIGURE 17-23 Additional occlusal features of the permanent mandibular right first premolar (fossae highlighted).

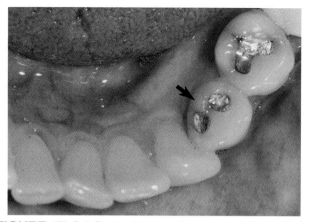

FIGURE 17-24 Restorations on the permanent mandibular first premolar called "snake eyes" *(arrow)*.

cedaneous replacements for the primary mandibular second molars.

There are two forms of the mandibular second premolars: the three-cusp type (tricuspidate form) and two-cusp type (bicuspidate form; Figure 17-26). Unlike mandibular first premolars, the more common (55 percent frequency) three-cusp type has three cusps: one large buccal cusp composed of the three buccal lobes and two smaller lingual cusps composed of the two lingual lobes. Thus the three-cusp type is composed of five developmental lobes: three buccal and two lingual.

Similar to mandibular first premolars, the less common (45 percent frequency) two-cusp type has a larger buccal cusp and a single smaller lingual cusp.

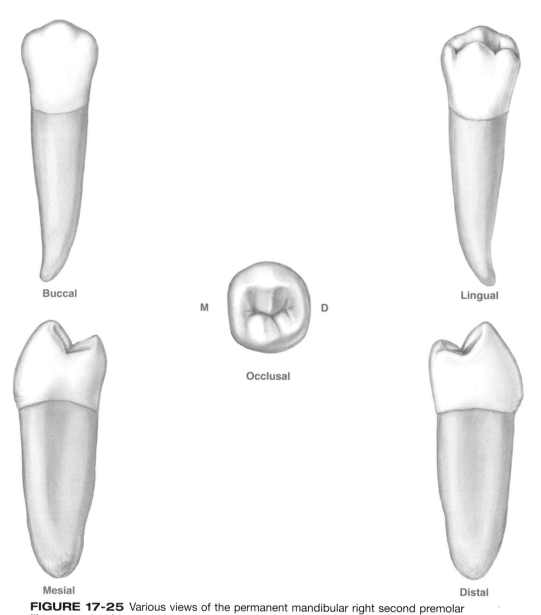

Buccal

Lingual

M   D

Occlusal

Mesial

Distal

FIGURE 17-25 Various views of the permanent mandibular right second premolar (three-cusp type).

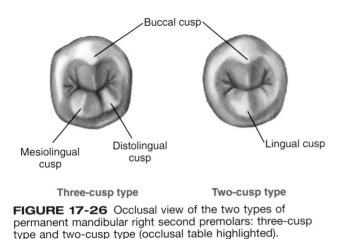

FIGURE 17-26 Occlusal view of the two types of permanent mandibular right second premolars: three-cusp type and two-cusp type (occlusal table highlighted).

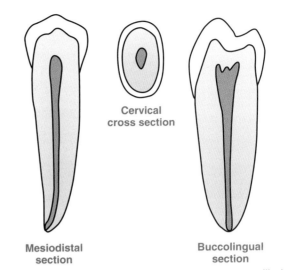

FIGURE 17-27 Pulp cavity of the permanent mandibular right second premolar (three-cusp type).

The two-cusp type is thus composed of four developmental lobes: three buccal and one lingual.

Both types of mandibular second premolars have more supplemental grooves than the first premolar of the same arch. The two types of this tooth differ mainly in their occlusal features, but other surface features are similar. The three-cusp type also appears more angular from the occlusal view, and the two-cusp type appears more rounded.

Although a mandibular first premolar resembles a mandibular canine, the more common three-cusp type of mandibular second premolar resembles a small molar because its lingual cusps are well developed, which places both marginal ridges horizontal and superior on the occlusal table. A more efficient occlusion thus results, with the premolars in the opposite arch, similar to the molars. A mandibular second premolar thus represents a transition from a caninelike first premolar to the molars.

The single root of a mandibular second premolar is larger and longer than that of a first premolar but shorter than those of the maxillary premolars. Proximal root concavities are pronounced. In addition, the apex of this tooth is blunter than that of a first molar or of the maxillary premolars. The pulp cavity of the three-cusp type shows three pointed pulp horns (Figure 17-27). Two pulp horns are present with the two-cusp type. No matter the number of pulp horns, all pulp horns are more pointed in the mandibular second premolar than the first.

Buccal View Features

A mandibular second premolar has a shorter buccal cusp than does a mandibular first premolar (see Figure 17-25). The cusp slopes of the buccal cusp of the mandibular second premolar are also more rounded. The mesial contact and distal contact are wide and at the same location, just cervical to the junction of the occlusal and middle thirds.

Lingual View Features

From the lingual, a mandibular second premolar shows considerable differences from a first premolar (Figure 17-28). The lingual cusp or cusps, depending on the type, are longer. Thus less of the occlusal surface can be seen from this view. Because the lingual cusp is still smaller than the buccal cusp, however, part of the buccal portion of the occlusal surface may be seen.

Differences between the two types can be seen in other features. In the three-cusp type, the mesiolingual cusp is wider and longer than the distolingual cusp. A developmental groove, the lingual groove, is located between the cusps, extending a short distance on the lingual surface and usually distal to the center of the crown because the mesiolingual cusp is wider.

With the two-cusp type of the mandibular second premolar, the single lingual cusp development is at an equal height with the mesiolingual cusp of the three-cusp type but is higher than that of a first premolar. The two-cusp type has no groove lingually but does show a distolingual developmental depression where the lingual cusp ridge joins the distal marginal ridge.

Proximal View Features

From the mesial, a mandibular second premolar has a shorter buccal cusp and is located more to the buccal than a first premolar (see Figure 17-25). Therefore the distance between the cusp tips of this tooth is shorter than for the first. In addition, the crown is wider buccolingually, and the lingual cusp or cusps are larger. The mesial marginal ridge is at almost a right angle, or almost 90 degrees, to the long axis of the tooth. There is no mesiolingual groove.

The distal view is similar, although more of the occlusal surface can be seen from this view because the

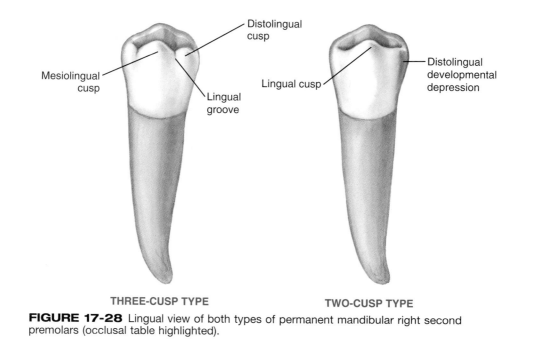

THREE-CUSP TYPE   **TWO-CUSP TYPE**

FIGURE 17-28 Lingual view of both types of permanent mandibular right second premolars (occlusal table highlighted).

distal marginal ridge is more cervically located than the mesial marginal ridge, which *helps to distinguish the right mandibular second premolar from the left.*

Occlusal View Features

The general shape of the crown outline of a mandibular second premolar is more nearly square, especially in the three-cusp type, than a mandibular first premolar (see Figure 17-25). The convergence of the mesial and distal margins toward the lingual is equally severe.

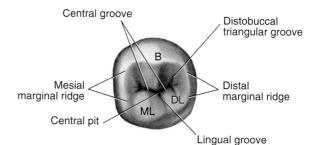

FIGURE 17-29 Occlusal view of the three-cusp type of permanent mandibular right second premolar showing the Y-shaped groove pattern (occlusal table highlighted).

Occlusal Table Components

In both the three-cusp and two-cusp types of mandibular second premolar, the buccal cusp is similar. Thus the two types are the same in that portion of the occlusal table, which is buccal to the mesiobuccal and distobuccal cusp ridges. Each of the cusps has buccal ridges, triangular ridges, and cuspal inclined planes, named for their location and orientation.

On the three-cusp type, the cusps are separated by two developmental grooves, a V-shaped central groove and a linear lingual groove (Figure 17-29). The lingual groove extends lingually between the two lingual cusps and ends on the lingual surface of the crown just below the meeting of the lingual cusp ridges. These two grooves together form a distinctive Y-shaped groove pattern on the occlusal table.

On the three-cusp type, a deep central pit is located at the junction of the central groove and the lingual groove, toward the lingual. The central pit is also more to the distal between the mesial marginal ridge and the

distal marginal ridge because the mesiolingual cusp is wider than the distolingual cusp. Some anatomists prefer to separate the central groove on this tooth into two grooves, a mesial groove and a distal groove.

On the three-cusp type of a second mandibular premolar, the mesial portion of the central groove travels in a mesiobuccal direction and ends in a mesial pit surrounded by a mesial triangular fossa just distal to the mesial marginal ridge, which is often crossed by a mesial marginal groove (Figure 17-30). The distal portion of the central groove travels in a distobuccal direction, is slightly shorter than the mesial groove, and ends in a distal pit surrounded by a distal triangular fossa mesial to the distal marginal ridge.

These triangular fossae are shallow, irregularly shaped, and more linear in form than the triangular fossae of the maxillary premolars. In addition, on the occlusal table is a mesiobuccal triangular groove,

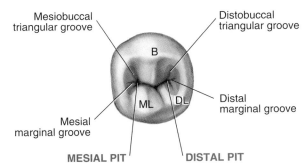

FIGURE 17-30 Additional occlusal features of the three-cusp type of permanent mandibular right second premolar (fossae highlighted).

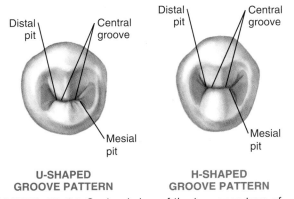

FIGURE 17-31 Occlusal view of the two-cusp type of permanent mandibular right second premolar, showing the U- and H-shaped groove patterns (fossae highlighted).

which extends into the mesial pit. The distobuccal triangular groove, distolingual triangular groove, and possibly a distal marginal groove extend into the distal pit.

In contrast, the two-cusp type is rounder lingual to the buccal cusp ridges (Figure 17-31). The mesial and distal margins converge slightly, making the lingual portion narrower than the buccal but never to the degree of a mandibular first premolar. The larger and longer buccal cusp is seen directly opposite the smaller and shorter lingual cusp. On the two-cusp type, a central groove on the occlusal table travels in a mesiodistal direction.

The central groove is most often crescent-shaped, forming a U-shaped groove pattern on the occlusal table. Less often, the central groove may be straight, forming an H-shaped groove pattern on the occlusal table. The lingual cusp of the type with the H groove pattern is larger and sharper than the one with the U groove pattern and is often offset to the mesial. The buccal cusp for both occlusal groove patterns of the two-cusp type has four functional inclined planes, and the lingual cusp has two.

The central groove of the two-cusp type has its terminal ends centered in the mesial fossa and distal fossa, which are circular depressions having supplemental grooves radiating from them. Some of these teeth have a mesial pit and distal pit centered in mesial and distal fossae instead of an unbroken central groove. Most have a distolingual developmental depression crossing the distolingual cusp ridge. None of the mandibular second premolar has a lingual groove or central pit.

Clinical Considerations for Mandibular Second Premolars

With premature loss of a primary mandibular second molar, the developing permanent mandibular first molar inclines and drifts mesially. The developing permanent mandibular second premolar is prevented from normal eruption because its arch space is nearly closed. This situation can allow the maxillary second premolar to become **impacted** against the first molar. An impacted tooth is an unerupted or partially erupted tooth that is positioned against another tooth, bone, or even soft tissue, making complete eruption unlikely. This problem may be prevented by careful evaluation of patients with mixed dentition and use of preventive orthodontic care such as space maintainers.

Developmental Disturbances with Mandibular Second Premolars

The permanent mandibular second premolars are commonly involved in partial **anodontia** and thus are congenitally missing (see Chapter 6 for more discussion). With this disturbance, the appropriate individual tooth germ (or germs) in the area are absent because of failure of the initiation process during tooth development. This condition can be bilateral or unilateral. This extremely important information must be obtained by careful patient evaluation when primary mandibular second molars are retained in a mixed or mature dentition. Missing permanent teeth may require prosthetic replacement or implant and can result in problems in spacing and occlusion.

Dental professionals should note that these retained primary molars, without the presence of their succedaneous permanent teeth, may not be shed, or exfoliated, for many years. Thus these primary teeth can serve as functioning replacements for the permanent premolar teeth and should not be extracted unless they are involved in root pathology or are uncomfortably mobile.

PERMANENT MOLARS
General Features

The permanent molars are the most posteriorly placed posterior teeth of the permanent dentition, distal to the premolars (Figure 17-32). Molars are also the largest teeth in the dentition. Each dental arch usually has six

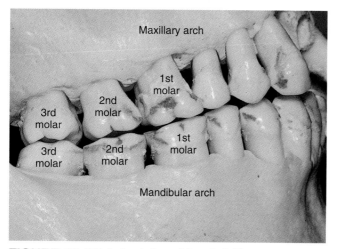

FIGURE 17-32 Lateral view of the skull. The permanent molars are identified.

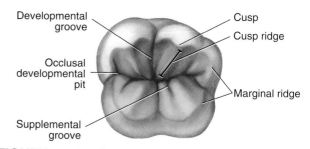

FIGURE 17-33 Occlusal view of a permanent molar (occlusal table highlighted).

molars, three in each quadrant, if all have erupted. The name *molar* comes from the Latin word for grinder, one of the functions of the molar teeth.

There are three types of molars: the **first molars,** the **second molars,** and the **third molars** (see Figure 17-32). The first molars and second molars are called the 6-year molars and 12-year molars, respectively, because of their eruption times.

The third molars, also known as the "wisdom teeth," are extremely variable in their eruption time as well as in their anatomical size and form. They were given this unusual nickname in ancient times when it was thought that only educated men had this important type of molar. Many dental professionals jokingly argue against the wisdom shown, given that these teeth erupt between 17 and 21 years of age.

Eruption of the third molars usually marks the end of the growth of the jawbones. The first molar usually is overall the largest, and the second and third are each progressively smaller. Only the permanent dentition has three types of molars. One of each type of molar is present in each quadrant of each dental arch. The first molars are closer to the midline, at the sixth position from it, and are also distal to the permanent second premolars when full eruption of the permanent dentition has occurred. The second molars are distal to the first molars and are in the seventh position from the midline. Finally, the third molars are distal to the second molars and are in the eighth position from the midline.

All three types of molars erupt in order distal to the primary second molars, long after all the primary teeth have erupted and are functioning. Thus all the permanent molars are nonsuccedaneous, and they do not replace any primary teeth. Because of the continued elongation of the facial bones during development, these teeth usually have enough space as they pro-

gressively erupt (except for third molars in some cases, discussed later).

Each molar has an extremely large crown compared with the rest of the permanent dentition, but the crown is shorter occlusocervically in contrast to the teeth anterior to it. Each buccal surface of a molar has a prominent cervical ridge running mesiodistally in the cervical one third.

Like all posterior teeth, molars have an occlusal surface with usually three or more cusps, of which at least two are buccal cusps (Figure 17-33). Unlike anterior teeth and premolars, molars do not exhibit buccal developmental depressions. Evidence of developmental lobe separation is in the developmental grooves on the occlusal table. In addition to cusps, the occlusal table of the molar is bordered by cusp ridges and marginal ridges. The occlusal table of molars is even more complicated than that of premolars because it has more developmental grooves, supplemental grooves, and occlusal developmental pits. These grooves and pits are located on the occlusal and lingual surfaces of maxillary molars and on the occlusal and buccal surfaces of mandibular molars.

In addition, molars usually are **multirooted.** Maxillary molars usually have three root branches, and mandibular molars have two (Figure 17-34). Molars originate as a single root on the base of the crown, as do anterior teeth. This portion is called the root trunk. The cervical cross section of root trunk follows the form of the crown, but the root then divides from the root trunk into the number of root branches for its type.

Between two or more of these root branches, before they divide from the root trunk, is an area called the **furcation.** The spaces between the roots at the furcation are called **furcation crotches.** Teeth with two roots, such as mandibular molars, have two furcation crotches; teeth with three roots can have three furcation crotches. Such crotches can be either facial and lingual or mesial and distal, depending on tooth type, each with a slightly different individual configuration. The furcation crotches may be close to the CEJ or far from it. **Root concavities** are also found on many of the root branches of molar teeth as well as on the furcal surfaces. In a molar, the root canals join the pulp chamber apical to the CEJ.

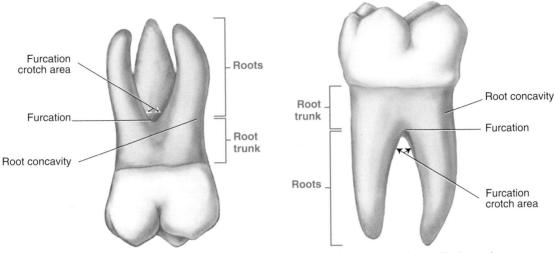

FIGURE 17-34 Buccal root features of a permanent maxillary and mandibular molar.

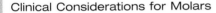

Clinical Considerations for Molars

As the largest and strongest crowns of the permanent dentition, the permanent molars, assisted by the premolars, function in grinding food during mastication. This grinding function is possible because molars have wide occlusal surfaces with prominent cusps. These teeth also support the tissues of the cheek, especially the facial muscles. They maintain the height of the lower third of the vertical dimension of the face and arch continuity. Thus they are involved in aesthetics and speech—but less so than the premolars.

Multiple roots give molars increased periodontal tissue support. However, with the loss of periodontal tissue support caused by advanced periodontal disease, the furcations, furcation crotches, and root concavities of the molars can lose their bony coverage in varying degrees. These areas can be located by probing with a Nabor's probe within a periodontal pocket; if recession has occurred, they can become clinically exposed. Bacterial plaque biofilm and other deposits can be retained in the exposed furcation crotches and root concavities, leading to further periodontal tissue disease (Figure 17-35).

Thus furcation crotches and root concavities on these molars present a challenge during both instrumentation and performance of oral hygiene in the area. Approximately half of molar furcations are too narrow for access by scaler. The furcations of a tooth may be reduced by a dental bur during a minor odontoplasty, possibly after surgically reflecting a gingival flap near the furcation. In addition, when roots are close together, access to interproximals may be even more difficult. The cervical ridge on molars also presents challenges during instrumentation around the cervical area.

In addition, awareness of root trunk dimensions and their relationship to the furcations is critical to the periodontal prognosis of a molar. According to one recent study, short root trunks are most commonly found buccally on both maxillary and mandibular molars. Additionally, short root length was associated with long root trunks, and long root trunks were more commonly found on the second molar than on the first molars. The evidence also suggested a strong correlation between length of root trunk and furcation invasion by periodontal disease.

According to recent statistics, approximately 25 percent of patients will need to have their third molars removed before age 25, a procedure that is still controversial. Often, patients are not even aware of the troubled nature of their third molars. Studies show that more than 40 percent of adult patients who never had their third molars removed during adolescence developed infection, caries, cyst formation, or periodontal disease (discussed later) by age 45, thus requiring extraction. The risk of surgical complications in these adult patients increases by approximately 30 percent compared with the equivalent risk for adolescents. However, surgeons are also now being taught to refrain from removing functioning third molars that are not causing any problems. Thus an evaluation of the third molars by age 25 is generally recommended.

Developmental Disturbances with Molars

Permanent molar teeth, similar to incisors, may be affected in children with congenital syphilis. The spirochete *Treponema pallidum,* a sexually transmitted organism, is passed from an infected pregnant woman to her fetus via the placenta. This organism may cause localized enamel hypoplasia and result in **mulberry molars,** a disturbance that occurs during tooth development. (All disturbances are discussed further in Chapter 6.)

A mulberry molar has a crown with an abnormally shaped occlusal surface characterized by berrylike nodules or tubercles of enamel instead of cusps. Children with this condition may also have other developmental anomalies, such as blindness, deafness, and paralysis caused by congenital syphilis. Treatment using full-coverage crowns may be performed to improve the appearance of these teeth.

Another disturbance associated with molars is the **enamel pearl.** Mainly found on the buccal surfaces of second molars, these deposits of enamel apical to the level on the CEJ have a tapered form and extend into root furcation areas. One study showed that teeth exhibiting these features were found to have deeper root concavities compared with teeth that lacked cervical enamel projections, suggesting a significant impact on furcation involvement. Unlike calculus, which it resembles radiographically, the enamel pearl cannot be removed by scaling. It must be ground away to restore the normal contour of the tooth.

In a more common and separate disturbance, the permanent molars may have one or more **tubercles,** or accessory cusps, on the occlusal surface. Finally, **dilaceration** of the root (or roots) can also occur with the molars, making extraction and endodontic treatment difficult.

Another disturbance is **root fusion,** which creates deep developmental grooves when the roots fuse. These can function as pathways to accumulate deposits that are not easily accessible to professional periodontal therapy or oral hygiene. A recent study shows that the highest prevalence of permanent molars with root fusion occurred in maxillary second molars, followed by mandibular second molars, maxillary first molars, and finally, mandibular first molars. Studies show that females present a higher incidence overall of root fusion than males.

Permanent Maxillary Molars

GENERAL FEATURES

Permanent maxillary molars erupt 6 months to 1 year after the corresponding permanent mandibular molars (Table 17-2). They are usually the first permanent teeth to erupt into the maxillary arch. In addition, maxillary molars are overall the largest and strongest teeth of the maxillary arch. They are usually shorter occlusocervically than are the crowns of teeth anterior to them, but they are larger in all other measurements than other maxillary teeth.

All maxillary molars are wider buccolingually than mesiodistally; in comparison, the mandibular molars are wider mesiodistally. From the occlusal, the outline of the crown of maxillary molars is rhomboidal, or four-sided with opposite sides parallel. Like all maxillary posterior teeth, the crown outline is also trapezoidal from each proximal view—again four-sided but with only two parallel sides. In addition, the crown is also centered over the root and shows no lingual inclination, like all maxillary molars and unlike mandibular molars.

Each maxillary molar usually has four major cusps, with two cusps on the buccal portion of the occlusal table and two on the lingual (Figure 17-36). A unique feature is present on the occlusal table of most maxillary molars except the third molar, an **oblique ridge.** A type of transverse ridge, an oblique ridge crosses the occlusal table obliquely and is formed by the union of the triangular ridge of the distobuccal cusp and distal cusp ridge of the mesiolingual cusp. In contrast, an oblique ridge is never present on mandibular molars.

Maxillary molars usually have three root branches, or are **trifurcated,** unlike mandibular molars, which usually have only two root branches (see Figure 17-34). These roots are the mesiobuccal, distobuccal, and lingual (or palatal). The lingual root is usually the largest and longest. The farther distal a molar is in the maxillary arch, the shorter and more varied in size, shape, and curvature are the roots. The roots also become less divided or divergent as the tooth is located farther distally. Thus a first molar has longer, more divergent roots than a third molar and has more consistency in the root's size, shape, and curvature. Roots of maxillary molars show great lingual and moderate distal inclination within the alveolar bone.

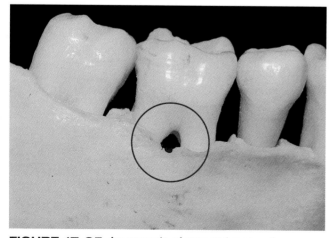

FIGURE 17-35 An example of exposed root surface on permanent molars, with furcation area and its crotch exposed on mandibular first molar (see *circle*).

TABLE 17-2

Anatomical Information on Permanent Maxillary Molars

	Maxillary First Molar	Maxillary Second Molar	Maxillary Third Molar
Universal number	#3 and #14	#2 and #15	#1 and #16
General crown features	Occlusal table with marginal ridges, cusps with tips, inclined planes, ridges, grooves, fossae, and pits; buccal cervical ridge		
Specific crown features	Largest tooth in arch, largest crown in dentition; four major cusps, with buccal cusps almost equal in height; fifth minor cusp of Carabelli associated with mesiolingual cusp and prominent oblique ridge	Smaller crown than first, heart-shaped or rhomboidal crown outline, thus three or four cusps; oblique ridge less prominent, with mesiobuccal cusp longer than distobuccal cusp and no fifth cusp; distolingual cusp smaller than on first or absent	Smaller crown than second, variable in form, heart-shaped or rhomboidal crown outline, thus three or four cusps
Mesial contact	Junction of occlusal and middle thirds	Middle third	Middle third
Distal contact	Middle third	Middle third	None
Distinguishing right from left	Mesiolingual cusp outline longer and larger but not as sharp as distolingual cusp	Mesiolingual cusp outline longer and larger but not as sharp as distolingual cusp	Distobuccal cusp shorter than mesiobuccal cusp and roots curved distally
Root features	Trifurcated roots, with furcations, root trunks, and root concavities		Usually fused roots, curving distally
	Divergent roots; furcations well removed from the CEJ	Less divergent roots	

CEJ = cementoenamel junction.

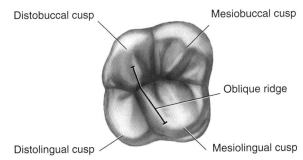

Distobuccal cusp
Mesiobuccal cusp
Oblique ridge
Distolingual cusp
Mesiolingual cusp

FIGURE 17-36 Occlusal view of a permanent maxillary molar.

Because maxillary molars are trifurcated, the three furcations are usually located on the mesial, buccal, and distal surfaces. All furcations on maxillary teeth usually begin near the junction of the cervical and middle thirds of the root. The buccal furcation is located midway between the mesial and distal sur-

faces. The mesial and distal furcations are located more to the lingual than the buccal surface. Root concavities are found on the mesial surface of the mesiobuccal root, the lingual surface of the lingual root, and all three furcal surfaces.

Clinical Considerations for Maxillary Molars

The roots of maxillary molars may penetrate the middle and posterior portions of the maxillary sinus as a result of accidental trauma or during tooth extraction because of the close relation of these roots to the sinus walls (see Chapter 11). In addition, the discomfort of sinusitis can be mistakenly interpreted as tooth related (stemming from the maxillary molars), and vice versa. Thus radiographic study of the tooth or maxillary sinus and other diagnostic tests become necessary to determine the cause of the discomfort in this area.

Because of the arch position of permanent maxillary molars, with the natural overhang of the cheek, instrumentation and oral hygiene of the buccal surface may be difficult. Instrumentation and oral hygiene of the proximal furcation crotch areas of the maxillary molars

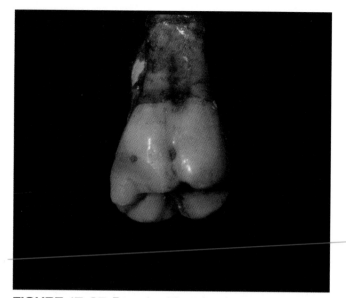

FIGURE 17-37 Example of lingual surface anatomy of a lingual pit on the crown of the permanent maxillary molar; note the view of palatal root.

have the easiest access from the lingual because the furcations are located closer to the lingual surface.

A possible lingual pit on the lingual surface of permanent maxillary molars is susceptible to caries (Figure 17-37). This susceptibility to caries results from both increased bacterial plaque biofilm retention and the thinness of enamel forming the walls of the pit (see Chapter 12 for more information on enamel features). Enamel sealants should be placed on the lingual surface of any teeth with deep pits shortly after eruption. However, because of the histology of enamel in the area, pit sealants are not as successful on the lingual surface as they are on the occlusal surface.

Developmental Disturbances with Maxillary Molars

The maxillary molars are some of the most common teeth of the permanent dentition to be involved in **concrescence.** (See Chapter 6 for more information.) Concrescence is the union of the root structure of two or more teeth through the cementum only. The teeth involved were originally separate but join because of excessive cementum deposition in one or more teeth following eruption. Concrescence occurs as a result of traumatic injury or crowding of the teeth in the area during the apposition and maturation stage of tooth development. This disturbance may present problems during extraction and endodontic treatment; thus preoperative radiographs are important.

PERMANENT MAXILLARY FIRST MOLARS #3 AND #14

Specific Overall Features (Figure 17-38)

The permanent maxillary first molars erupt between 6 and 7 years of age (root completion occurs between

ages 9 and 10). Thus these teeth are the first permanent teeth to erupt into the maxillary arch. They erupt distal to the primary maxillary second molars and thus are nonsuccedaneous.

The maxillary first molar is the largest tooth in the maxillary arch and also has the largest crown in the permanent dentition. It has a much more complex crown form than do the nearby maxillary premolars. Of all the maxillary permanent molars, the first is the least variable in form.

This tooth is composed of five developmental lobes: two buccal and three lingual. These are named in the same manner as their associated cusps: mesiobuccal, distobuccal, mesiolingual, distolingual, and an additional minor cusp on the lingual (discussed later). Evidence of lobe separation can be found in the developmental grooves on the occlusal surface.

The roots of maxillary first molars are larger and more divergent than those of the second molars and are more complex in form than those of the maxillary premolars. The roots are twice as long as the crown. Thus the furcations are well removed from the cervical area of the tooth. The distal furcation crotch is wider than the mesial crotch.

The lingual, or palatal, root is the largest and longest, inclines lingually, and extends beyond the crown outline. The lingual root has a bananalike curvature toward the buccal. A vertical depression may be present on the palatal surface of the root that is more pronounced at the cervical third.

Both the mesiobuccal and distobuccal roots have an extreme curvature that makes them together look like the handles of a set of pliers. The mesiobuccal root is the second largest and longest, is inclined mesially and buccally, and has its apical third curving distally. The distobuccal root is the smallest, shortest, and thus the weakest of the three. This root inclines distally and buccally, and its apical one third curves mesially. The buccal furcation is about 4 mm apical to the CEJ.

The mesial furcation is 3 mm from the CEJ and not centered. Its entrance is dictated by the size of mesiobuccal root and located two thirds of the buccolingual width of the root trunk from the buccal and one third of the buccolingual width of the root trunk from the lingual. The mesial furcation is wider buccolingually than mesiodistally. The distal furcation is 5 mm from the CEJ and is predisposed to develop periodontal disease owing to the proximity of the divergent distobuccal root to the adjacent second molar.

The pulp cavity of a maxillary first molar usually has one pulp horn for each major cusp (Figure 17-39). Thus the four pulp horns are mesiobuccal, distobuccal, mesiolingual, and distolingual. Three main pulp canals are usually present, one for each of the three roots. The lingual pulp canal is the largest, the distobuccal the smallest, and the mesiobuccal between these two in size. A maxillary first molar sometimes

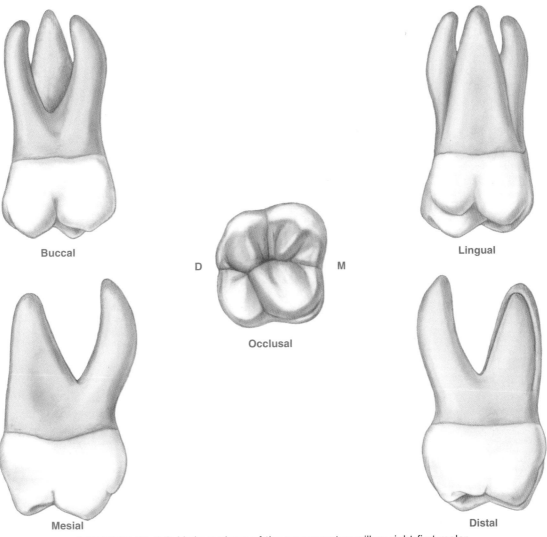

FIGURE 17-38 Various views of the permanent maxillary right first molar.

has four pulp canals, with two pulp canals in the mesiobuccal root.

Buccal View Features

The general shape of a maxillary first molar from this view is trapezoidal, with the longer parallel side toward the occlusal (see Figure 17-38). The entire buccal surface is larger than that of the adjacent premolar. Despite this fact, the occlusocervical measurement is slightly smaller.

Parts of all four major and functioning cusps are seen from this view: the mesiobuccal cusp, distobuccal cusp, mesiolingual cusp, and distolingual cusp (because the two lingual cusps are slightly offset to the distal relative to the buccal cusps). The occlusal outline of the mesiobuccal cusp is wider, but the distobuccal cusp tip is sharper. However, the two buccal cusps are nearly the same height, and the mesiolingual cusp tip is seen between them.

The occlusal outline of a maxillary first molar is divided symmetrically by the buccal groove. This developmental groove extends between the two buccal cusps, runs apically about halfway to the CEJ, and is parallel with the long axis of the tooth. There it can fade out, but it may end in a buccal pit. In addition, the buccal groove may end in two short, slanting grooves with or without a buccal pit.

The mesial outline is flat from the CEJ occlusally to the mesial contact. The mesial contact is at the junction of the occlusal and middle thirds. The mesial contact is initially with a primary maxillary second molar, until that tooth is exfoliated, or shed. The mesial contact is then with a permanent second premolar when it erupts. Occlusally from the mesial contact, the mesial outline is rounded.

Instead of being flat like the mesial, the distal outline of the maxillary first molar is rounded or convex from the CEJ to the occlusal surface. The distal contact is in the middle third. However, no distal

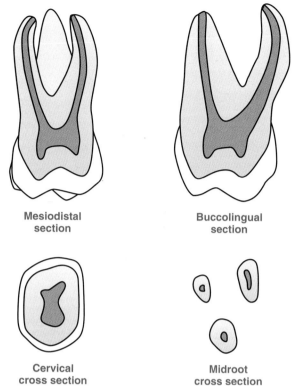

Mesiodistal section

Buccolingual section

Cervical cross section

Midroot cross section

FIGURE 17-39 Pulp cavity of the permanent maxillary right first premolar.

contact occurs until the permanent maxillary second molars erupt. The CEJ is slightly and irregularly curved apically but with less curvature than that on teeth anterior to it. A sharp dip or point may be observed just occlusal to the furcation area.

Lingual View Features

The lingual surface of the maxillary first molar is almost as wide mesiodistally as the buccal surface and is also trapezoidal. However, the lingual surface is more rounded or convex than the buccal. Both the mesial and distal outline and CEJ curvature are about the same, except that the distal outline is shorter because the distolingual cusp is smaller than the distobuccal cusp.

Similar to the buccal surface, the lingual surface has a distolingual groove that divides the occlusal outline into two asymmetrical portions. Dissimilar to the buccal surface, only the two lingual cusps can be seen from this view. Being the largest cusp on the occlusal surface, the mesiolingual cusp outline is much longer and larger, but the cusp is not as sharp as the distolingual cusp, which *helps to distinguish the right maxillary first molar from the left.* The distolingual groove usually ends in a lingual pit in the middle of the lingual surface, but it may fade out.

Commonly arising from the lingual surface of the mesiolingual cusp of the maxillary first molar is a fifth

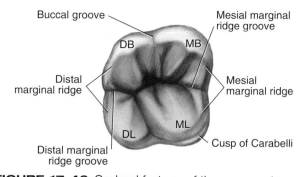

FIGURE 17-40 Occlusal features of the permanent maxillary right first molar (occlusal table highlighted).

nonfunctioning cusp called the **cusp of Carabelli.** This minor cusp is set apart from the rest of the mesiolingual cusp by its associated **cusp of Carabelli groove.** This small cusp, named after the dentist who described it, and its equally small groove varies in prominence from tooth to tooth. Its presence can be variable; it is not present in all dentitions.

Proximal View Features

The only two cusps of the maxillary first molar that are seen from the mesial are the mesiobuccal cusp and mesiolingual cusp. A mesial marginal groove usually notches the mesial marginal ridge about midway along its length. The contact area on the mesial is situated slightly to the buccal.

The distal view is the same as the mesial, except that the mesial cusp tips are seen projecting beyond the outline of the distobuccal cusp and distolingual cusp from proximal. The distal marginal ridge is less prominent and dips farther cervically than on the mesial, with a distal marginal groove halfway along its length. On both views, the CEJ usually curves slightly toward the occlusal and on the distal may even be a straight line on some teeth.

Occlusal View Features

The overall rhomboidal outline of the occlusal surface of a maxillary first molar is seen from this occlusal view (Figure 17-40) because it is four-sided with opposite sides parallel. The buccal outline is divided unequally into two parts by the buccal groove, and the mesial portion is longer than the distal portion. The lingual outline is also divided unequally into two parts by the distolingual groove, with the mesial portion longer and less rounded than the distal portion. The mesial marginal ridge is longer and more prominent than the distal marginal ridge. Both marginal ridges are crossed by a mesial marginal ridge groove and distal marginal ridge groove, respectively. Because this is the first molar a student will study, a detailed discussion of the occlusal table follows.

Occlusal Table Components

The two marginal ridges and the mesial and distal cusp ridges of the four major cusps on the buccal and lingual border the occlusal table of the maxillary first molar (Figure 17-41). Each major cusp has a triangular ridge and three other cusp ridges. Also present are four inclined cuspal planes with each major cusp.

The mesiobuccal cusp has a sharp cusp tip and is the second largest cusp. It has a mesial cusp ridge that extends from the cusp tip to the mesiobuccal occlusal point angle. The distal cusp ridge runs from the cusp tip to the buccal groove. The buccal cusp ridge passes from the cusp tip to the CEJ on the buccal surface. Finally, the lingual cusp ridge runs from the cusp tip to the central groove and is the triangular ridge of the mesiobuccal cusp. The mesiobuccal cusp has four inclined planes, with all the lingual portions functional.

The distobuccal cusp has the sharpest cusp tip and is the third largest cusp. Its triangular ridge, cusp ridges, and inclined planes are named similarly to those of the mesiobuccal cusp.

The mesiolingual cusp is the largest cusp of the maxillary first molar, with a rounded cusp tip. Its cusp ridges are similar to those of the other cusps, except that the distal triangular ridge extends from the mesiolingual cusp tip in an oblique distobuccal direction. There the distal triangular ridge meets the lingual triangular ridge of the distobuccal cusp to form a prominent oblique ridge. The mesiolingual cusp also has four inclined planes, all of which are functional. A typical transverse ridge is also present on the occlusal table of the maxillary first molar. It is formed by the buccal triangular ridge of the mesiolingual cusp and the lingual triangular ridge of the mesiobuccal cusp.

The smallest cusp, when present on the maxillary first molar, is the minor and nonfunctional cusp, the cusp of Carabelli, with its cusp of Carabelli groove.

The distolingual cusp is the smallest of the major cusps and is the most variable of this group. The triangular ridge, cusp ridges, and inclined planes are similar to those of other cusps, except that all the inclined planes are functional.

Four fossae are also present on a maxillary first molar, along with associated developmental grooves and occlusal pits: central, mesial triangular, distal triangular, and distal. The central fossa is mesial to the oblique ridge. The central fossa has the central pit in its most central, deepest portion. The central pit divides the central groove into two portions, the mesial groove and distal groove. Thus the central pit is at the junction of three developmental grooves: buccal, mesial, and distal. Along with the central groove and other developmental grooves, supplemental grooves can be present.

Three triangular grooves are present: the mesiobuccal triangular groove, mesiolingual triangular groove, and distobuccal triangular groove. The buccal groove extends onto the buccal surface. The mesial groove, as part of the central groove, extends from the central pit to the mesial pit. The mesial pit is in the mesial triangular fossa, distal to the mesial marginal ridge. Thus the mesial pit is at the junction of four developmental grooves: the mesial, mesiobuccal triangular, mesiolingual triangular, and mesial marginal.

As part of the central groove, the distal groove usually extends from the central pit across the oblique ridge to the distal pit and is sometimes referred to as the transverse groove of the oblique ridge. The distal pit is in the distal triangular fossa, mesial to the distal marginal ridge. Thus the distal pit is at the junction of five developmental grooves: the distal, distolingual, distobuccal triangular, distal marginal, and distal lingual triangular. The last fossa is the distal fossa, a linear rather than circular depression that is distal and parallel to the oblique ridge and thus is in the distolingual groove.

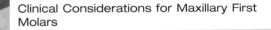

Clinical Considerations for Maxillary First Molars

Because of their arch position and because the permanent maxillary first molars are the first permanent teeth to erupt in the maxillary arch, they are considered important in the development of occlusion (see Chapter 20 for more discussion). The importance of this role in occlusion is shown if this tooth is lost (Figure 17-42). Today, loss of this tooth commonly results from periodontal disease, whereas in the past it resulted from caries.

Loss of the tooth is followed by mesial inclination and drift of the maxillary second molar into the open arch space. The mandibular first molar, if present, also supererupts. Occlusion and then mastication are disabled, and predisposition to further periodontal disease around the irregularly spaced teeth is greatly increased. Prosthetic replacement is an important way to prevent these situations.

The distobuccal surfaces of the permanent first molars may have increased supragingival tooth deposits such as bacterial plaque biofilm, calculus, and stain. This buildup of deposits is mainly due to the maxillary first molars' position in the oral cavity, opposite the duct openings of the parotid salivary glands on the inner cheek. Saliva, with its mineral content, is released from these glands and causes the bacterial plaque biofilm to mineralize faster into calculus.

PERMANENT MAXILLARY SECOND MOLARS #2 AND #15

Specific Overall Features (Figure 17-43)

The permanent maxillary second molars erupt between 12 and 13 years of age (root completion occurs between ages 14 and 16). These teeth erupt distal to the

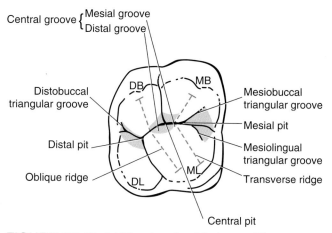

Central groove { Mesial groove
                 Distal groove

Distobuccal triangular groove

Distal pit

Oblique ridge

DB   MB

DL   ML

Mesiobuccal triangular groove

Mesial pit

Mesiolingual triangular groove

Transverse ridge

Central pit

FIGURE 17-41 Additional occlusal features of the permanent maxillary right first molar (fossae highlighted).

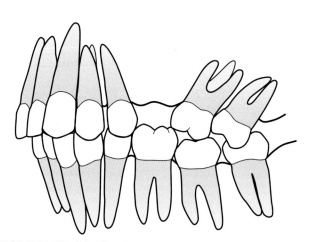

FIGURE 17-42 The changes that can occur in the permanent dentition when the maxillary first molar is lost: mesial inclination and drift of the maxillary second molar into the open oral space and supereruption of the mandibular first molar.

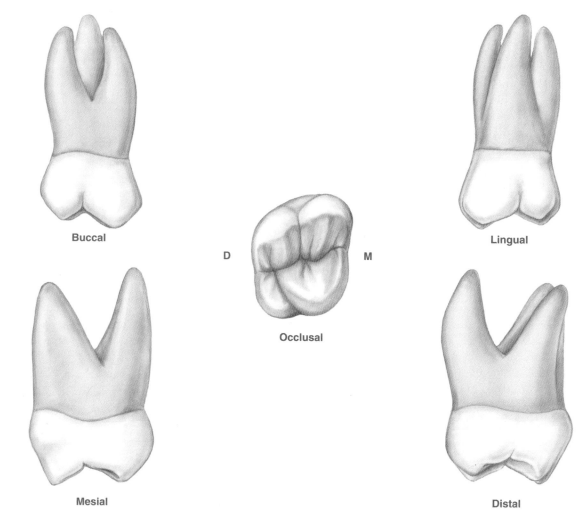

Buccal

Lingual

D   M

Occlusal

Mesial

Distal

FIGURE 17-43 Various views of the permanent maxillary right second molar (rhomboidal crown outline).

permanent maxillary first molars and thus are non-succedaneous.

Much variation in the form of the maxillary second molars is observed, especially in the size of the distolingual cusp. The crown usually has four cusps similar to the four major cusps of the first molar, but it can have three cusps. This tooth is composed of four developmental lobes, all named in the same manner as their associated cusps. Evidence of lobe separation can be found in the developmental grooves on the occlusal surface.

The three roots on maxillary second molars are smaller than those on the first molars. They are also less divergent and more parallel than on the first molars. The lingual root is still the largest and longest and extends beyond the crown outline, but it is usually straighter and not as curved toward the buccal as the lingual root of the maxillary first molars. The furcation notches are narrower than those in the first molars, and all depressions are shallower. The chance of fusion, especially of the buccal roots or even of all three roots, is greater for the second than for the maxillary first molars.

The pulp cavity of a maxillary second molar consists of a pulp chamber and three main pulp canals, one for each of the three roots (Figure 17-44). Each major cusp usually has one pulp horn, for a total of four pulp horns: mesiobuccal, distobuccal, mesiolingual, and distolingual.

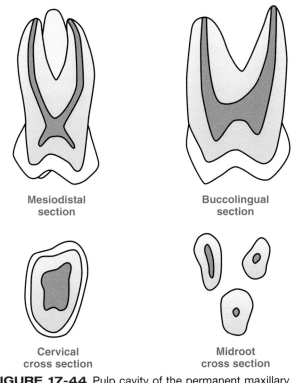

Mesiodistal section

Buccolingual section

Cervical cross section

Midroot cross section

FIGURE 17-44 Pulp cavity of the permanent maxillary right second molar (rhomboidal crown outline).

Buccal View Features

A maxillary second molar is shorter occlusocervically and narrower mesiodistally than a first molar (see Figure 17-43). The buccal groove is located farther distally on the buccal surface of the second than the first. The mesiobuccal cusp is longer and has a less sharp cusp tip than the distobuccal cusp. Both the mesial contact and distal contact are in the middle third.

Lingual View Features

The distolingual cusp of the maxillary second molar is smaller and shorter than on the first molar and is sometimes not present. Thus the outline of the largest cusp of the occlusal surface, the mesiolingual cusp, is much longer and larger, but the cusp is not as sharp as the distolingual cusp, which *helps to distinguish the right maxillary second molar from the left*. In addition, a fifth cusp (or cusp of Carabelli) usually does not exist. From this view, the cusp tips of the distobuccal cusp and the mesiobuccal cusp can be seen.

A lingual pit is usually present at the end of the distolingual groove, which does not extend as far mesially or cervically as the groove on the first molar. Thus the distolingual groove ends at a point that is occlusal and distal to the center of the lingual surface.

Proximal View Features

From the mesial, the mesial contact area of a maxillary second molar is larger and the cervical flattening or concavity is never as pronounced as in a maxillary first molar. From the distal, the distobuccal cusp and distolingual cusp are smaller on a second than a first molar, thus showing more of the occlusal surface. Note that no distal contact area is present until possibly the third molar erupts and moves into occlusion.

Occlusal View Features

The outline of the crown of a maxillary second molar is narrower mesiodistally than that of a maxillary first molar but is about the same width buccolingually. Two crown outline types are possible on this tooth when viewed from the occlusal: rhomboidal and heart-shaped (Figure 17-45). The rhomboidal type of crown outline on the second molar has four sides with opposite sides parallel and is the most common. The rhomboidal type is similar to that of the first molar but even more accentuated. The heart-shaped type is the less common occlusal outline and is similar to the typical maxillary third molar.

Occlusal Table Components

With the rhomboidal type of occlusal outline on a maxillary second molar, the cusps present are similar to the major cusps of a maxillary first molar. With the heart-shaped type, the distolingual cusp is quite small, with the other three cusps completely overshadowing it. The distolingual cusp is sometimes absent in the heart-shaped type, and the distolingual groove is confined to the occlusal table.

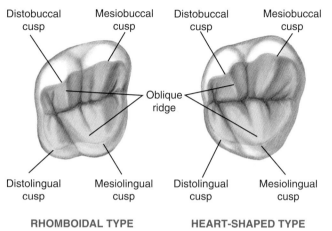

Distobuccal cusp   Mesiobuccal cusp   Distobuccal cusp   Mesiobuccal cusp

Oblique ridge

Distolingual cusp   Mesiolingual cusp   Distolingual cusp   Mesiolingual cusp

RHOMBOIDAL TYPE   **HEART-SHAPED TYPE**

FIGURE 17-45 Occlusal view of the two types of crown outlines of the permanent maxillary right second molars: rhomboidal and heart-shaped types (occlusal table highlighted).

The cusp ridges, triangular ridges, transverse ridge, oblique ridge, developmental grooves, fossae, and occlusal pits for both types of a second molar are similar to those of the first molar of the same arch. However, the oblique ridge is less prominent on the second than on the first molar. Instead, more supplemental grooves are usually present on the occlusal table of the second.

PERMANENT MAXILLARY THIRD MOLARS #1 AND #16
Specific Overall Features (Figure 17-46)

The permanent maxillary third molars may erupt between 17 and 21 years of age (root completion occurs between the ages of 18 and 25). If they erupt (see the later section on clinical considerations), they erupt distal to the permanent maxillary second molars and thus are nonsuccedaneous. The tooth's mesial contact is in the middle third, but it does not have a distal tooth contact.

No standard form is observed for this tooth, and describing a typical maxillary third molar is therefore difficult. This tooth is the smallest molar and the tooth

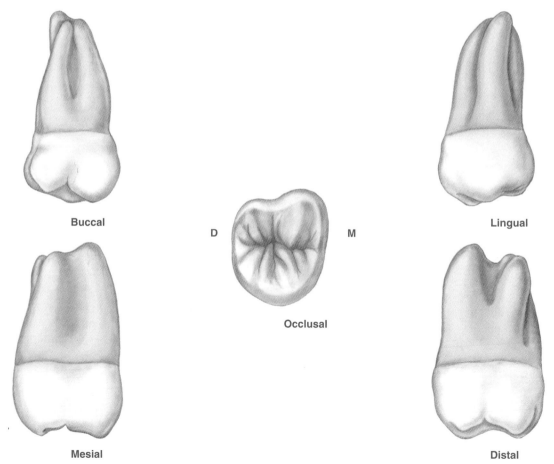

Buccal

D   M

Lingual

Occlusal

Mesial

Distal

FIGURE 17-46 Various views of the permanent maxillary right third molars (heart-shaped occlusal outline).

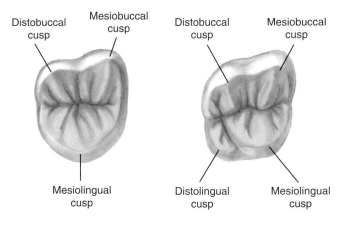

FIGURE 17-47 Occlusal views of the two types of crown outlines of the permanent maxillary right third molars: heart-shaped and rhomboidal types (occlusal table highlighted).

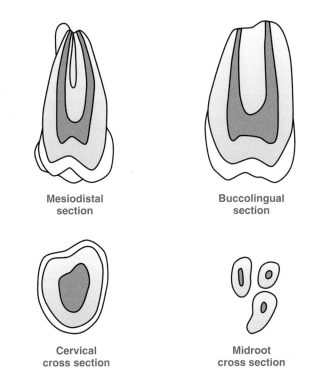
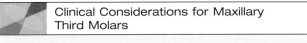

FIGURE 17-48 Pulp cavity of the permanent maxillary right third molar.

most variable in shape in the permanent dentition. Thus it is smaller in all dimensions than a second maxillary molar. The crown of a maxillary third molar is poorly developed compared with the other maxillary molars. The tooth is composed of four developmental lobes.

There are two types of occlusal outlines for a maxillary third molar (Figure 17-47). The most common occlusal outline for the tooth is heart-shaped, similar to a maxillary second molar but with more supplemental grooves on the occlusal table. Generally, with the heart-shaped occlusal outline, the tooth has only three cusps: mesiobuccal, distobuccal, and mesiolingual, with an absent distolingual cusp.

If a fourth cusp is present, the occlusal outline is a rhomboidal type, with a small and nonfunctioning distolingual cusp. No oblique ridge is present. For both types of occlusal forms, the distobuccal cusp is much shorter than the mesiobuccal cusp, which *helps to distinguish the right maxillary third molar from the left.*

Like other maxillary molars, the maxillary third molars are trifurcated. However, the roots are sometimes so close together that they are fused, either partially or fully, and thus may give the appearance of a single root. All roots of a third molar are also poorly developed, like the crown, and shorter than that of a second molar. The distobuccal root usually is the smallest and often is found tucked under the crown. The roots are curved distally, which *helps to distinguish the right maxillary third molar from the left.*

The pulp cavity of a maxillary third molar may have a pulp chamber and three pulp canals (Figure 17-48). The tooth may sometimes have one large pulp canal, if the root is fused, to as many as four pulp canals, if there are four roots. The number of pulp horns varies and depends on the number of cusps; if there are three cusps, there are three pulp horns.

Clinical Considerations for Maxillary Third Molars

The permanent maxillary third molars may also fail to erupt and remain impacted within the alveolar bone. An impacted tooth is an unerupted or partially erupted tooth that is positioned against another tooth, bone, or even soft tissue in such a way that complete eruption is unlikely. This impaction usually occurs because the maxilla is underdeveloped and space or arch length is insufficient to accommodate these teeth because they are the last to erupt in the maxillary arch. Surgical removal may be necessary. Any oral hygiene procedures or instrumentation may also be difficult when these teeth are erupted because of their posterior arch position.

Developmental Disturbances with Maxillary Third Molars

The permanent maxillary third molars, along with the mandibular third molars, commonly exhibit partial anodontia and thus are congenitally missing (all disturbances are discussed further in Chapter 6). With this disturbance, the appropriate individual tooth germ in the area is missing owing to failure of the initiation process during tooth development. This situation usually has no harmful consequences, however.

This tooth also commonly exhibits partial microdontia. This disturbance leads to a smaller molar crown with one cusp, or **peg third molar,** either unilaterally or bilaterally, owing to failure in the proliferation process during tooth development (Figure 17-49). This tooth may also have accessory roots that complicate extraction procedures. Finally, developmental cyst formation may occur within the dental tissues of an impacted crown of a maxillary third molar, resulting in a **dentigerous cyst.**

= micro-dont [handwritten annotation]

Permanent Mandibular Molars

GENERAL FEATURES

Permanent mandibular molars erupt 6 months to 1 year before the corresponding permanent maxillary molars (Table 17-3). The crown of a mandibular molar has four or five major cusps, of which there are always

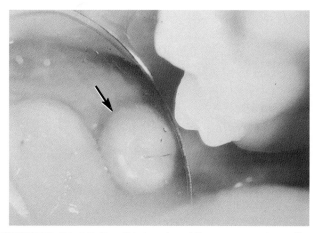

FIGURE 17-49 Peg third molar of the permanent maxillary arch *(arrow).*

two lingual cusps of about the same width. All mandibular molars are wider mesiodistally than buccolingually, similar to anterior teeth. In comparison, maxillary molars are wider buccolingually, as are all posterior teeth. Thus from an occlusal view, the outline of the crown of a mandibular molar is also rectangular, with four sides, or pentagonal, with five sides.

Quite distinct from maxillary molars, the buccal crown outline of all mandibular molars also shows a strong lingual inclination when viewed from the proximal, like the nearby premolars. Thus from each proximal view, the crown outline is rhomboidal, or four-sided with opposite sides parallel, like all mandibular posterior teeth. The crown is thus inclined lingually on the root base, bringing the cusps into proper occlusion with their maxillary antagonists and distributing the forces along the long axis.

Mandibular molars usually have two roots, or are bifurcated, with a mesial root and distal root (see Figure 17-34). Both these roots on mandibular molars show great to moderate distal root inclination. Because these teeth are bifurcated, the two furcations are located on the buccal and lingual surfaces midway between the proximal surfaces. These furcations are at a level of one fourth the root length from the CEJ. Root

TABLE 17-3

Anatomical Information on Mandibular Molars

	Mandibular First Molar	Mandibular Second Molar	Mandibular Third Molar
Universal number	#19 and #30	#18 and #31	#17 and #32
General crown features	Occlusal table with marginal ridges, cusps with tips, inclined planes, ridges, grooves, fossae, and pits		
Specific crown features	First permanent tooth to erupt, with widest crown mesiodistally of dentition; five cusps, with Y groove pattern and with buccal groove possibly ending in buccal pit	Smaller crown than first; four cusps with cross-shaped groove pattern	Smaller crown than second
Mesial and distal contact	Junction of occlusal and middle thirds	Middle third	Mesial: middle third Distal: none
Distinguishing right from left	Distal cusp smallest, with a sharp cusp	Difference in height of contour for buccal and lingual from each proximal surface; wider on the mesial than distal	Wider buccolingually on mesial than on distal
General root features	Bifurcated roots, with root trunks, furcation, and root concavities		Fused root, irregularly curved, with sharp apices
Specific root features	Divergent roots, with furcations well removed from the CEJ	Less divergent roots, with furcations closer to CEJ	

CEJ = cementoenamel junction.

concavities are also found on the mesial surface of the mesial root and on furcal surfaces of both the mesial and distal roots. The root concavities on the mesial root are especially prominent if this root also has two root canals.

Clinical Considerations for Mandibular Molars

All three types of mandibular molars can present difficulty in instrumentation because of their narrow lingual surfaces combined with the lingual inclination of the crown; therefore placement of instruments subgingivally can be difficult.

In addition, patients may have difficulty in performing oral hygiene because of the lingual inclination of the crown. They may miss the associated lingual gingiva and clean only the occlusal surface with a toothbrush. The proximity of the tongue also makes oral hygiene and instrumentation more difficult on the lingual surface.

PERMANENT MANDIBULAR FIRST MOLARS #19 AND #30

Specific Overall Features (Figure 17-50)

The permanent mandibular first molars erupt between 6 and 7 years of age (root completion occurs between the ages of 9 and 10). These teeth are usually the first permanent teeth to erupt in the oral cavity. They erupt distal to the primary mandibular second molars and thus are nonsuccedaneous.

The crown of a mandibular first molar usually has five cusps: three buccal and two lingual. Thus these teeth are usually composed of five developmental lobes, like the maxillary first molars but unlike the other mandibular molars, which have four. The lobes are named for their associated cusps. Separational evidence of the lobes is also found in the developmental grooves on the occlusal surface. Occasionally, the distal

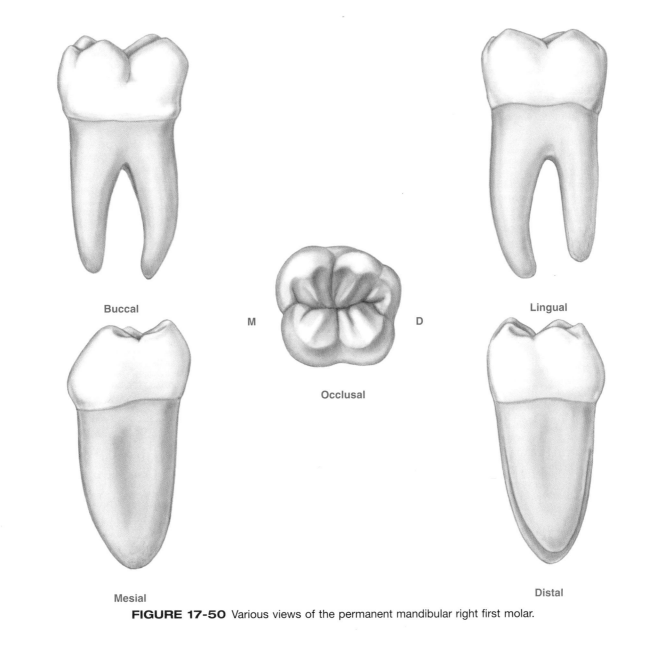

Buccal

Mesial

M   Occlusal   D

Lingual

Distal

FIGURE 17-50 Various views of the permanent mandibular right first molar.

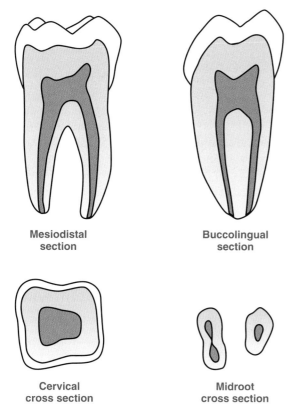

Mesiodistal
section

Buccolingual
section

Cervical
cross section

Midroot
cross section

FIGURE 17-51 Pulp cavity of the permanent mandibular right first molar.

cusp is missing. More rarely, in large molars the distal cusp is joined by a sixth cusp.

The two roots, mesial and distal, of a mandibular first molar are larger and more divergent than those of a second molar, leaving the roots widely separated buccally. The root trunk of the first is also shorter than that of the second. Both roots are usually the same length, but if one is longer, it is the mesial root. The mesial root is also the wider and stronger of the two. If this molar has three roots, it is because the mesial root has both buccal and lingual branches.

Fluting, an elongated developmental depression, is noted on many surfaces of the root branches, especially on the mesial surface of the mesial root, but none is observed on the distal surface of the distal root. Furcations are well removed from the CEJ. The buccal furcation entrance diameter is smaller than that of the lingual furcation and is 3 mm from the CEJ. The lingual furcation is 4 mm from the CEJ.

The pulp cavity of a mandibular first molar is more likely to have three root canals: distal, mesiobuccal, and mesiolingual, and five pulp horns (Figure 17-51). The distal pulp canal is much larger than the other two canals and is usually the only canal in the distal root. The mesial root usually has two pulp canals, the mesiobuccal and mesiolingual. Rarely, these two mesial canals join into one single apical foramen or only one pulp canal is found in the mesial root. Again

rarely, two canals are present in the distal root, just as with the mesial root.

Buccal View Features

The crown of a mandibular first molar is larger mesiodistally than occlusocervically (see Figure 17-50). It is the widest tooth mesiodistally of any permanent tooth because it has a fifth major cusp. From this view, at least some portion of all five cusps is visible.

The mesiobuccal cusp is the largest, widest, and highest cusp on the buccal portion. The distobuccal cusp is slightly smaller, shorter, and sharper than the mesiobuccal cusp. The distal cusp, despite its name, is considered a buccal cusp; it is the lowest cusp and slightly sharper than the other two. The occlusal outline is divided into three sections by the two grooves, as they pass into the buccal surface: the mesiobuccal groove and distobuccal groove. These sections of the crown surface decrease in size distally. These buccal grooves on a first mandibular molar are important in classifying the dentition in relation to the maxillary arch (see Chapter 20 for more information).

The mesiobuccal groove on a mandibular first molar extends straight cervically to a point about midway occlusocervically but slightly mesial to the center mesiodistally. The mesiobuccal groove almost always ends in the buccal pit. Also, the mesiobuccal groove may end in two short, slanting grooves or may fade out after a short distance. The distobuccal groove extends cervically, similarly to the mesiobuccal groove, but is slightly distal to the center mesiodistally. The distobuccal groove usually ends in a distobuccal pit but sometimes just fades out.

A buccal cervical ridge, which is a mesiodistally oriented roundness in the cervical third of the buccal surface, is apparent. It is usually more prominent in its mesial portion. In addition, a shallow concavity may extend mesiodistally in the middle third.

The mesial outline is slightly concave from the contact area cervically and is rounded occlusal to the contact. The distal outline is more rounded than the mesial. Both the mesial contact and distal contact are at the junction of the occlusal and middle thirds.

Lingual View Features

The lingual surface of a mandibular first molar is smaller than the buccal surface. The mesial and distal outlines of the lingual are similar to the buccal. The occlusal outline is divided by the lingual groove between the mesiolingual cusp and the distolingual cusp.

Proximal View Features

The crown of a mandibular first molar is smaller buccolingually than mesiodistally and cervico-occlusally.

The crown is also inclined toward the lingual, as are the other mandibular posterior teeth. Additionally, the crown outline is an imperfect rhomboid, having four sides with opposite sides parallel, because the surface is wider at the cervical than the occlusal.

The buccal margin on the mesial surface is usually rounded, especially at the buccal cervical ridge. The buccal cervical ridge is in the cervical third, where the height of contour is also located. The lingual margin on the mesial is either straight or slightly rounded from the CEJ to the height of contour in the middle third. It is then rounded from the height of contour to the occlusal. The CEJ is either straight or slightly curved occlusally but always is located at a more occlusal level on the lingual portion of the mesial surface.

The mesial marginal groove notches the mesial marginal ridge. The tooth has a flattened or slightly concave area centrally located in the gingival third, comparable to the mesial concavity of a maxillary first premolar.

The distal surface of a mandibular first molar is similar to the mesial but smaller, especially in the buccolingual dimension. The distal marginal ridge is notched by the distal marginal groove. The distal marginal ridge is located more cervically than the mesial marginal ridge.

Occlusal View Features

The crown outline of the mandibular first molar is roughly pentagonal, with the fifth side created by the distal cusp. The distal portion of the buccal outline converges toward the distal to create the fifth side of the outline. The buccal outline has rounded line angles and is divided into three portions by the two buccal grooves, the mesiobuccal groove and the distobuccal groove. The length of the buccal cusps decreases distally as noted from the buccal view.

The lingual outline is divided into two portions by the lingual groove. The mesial outline is divided into two portions by the mesial marginal groove. The distal outline, the shortest of the five sides, is divided by the distal marginal groove.

Occlusal Table Components

The mandibular first molar usually has five functional cusps, which if listed from largest to smallest are mesiobuccal, mesiolingual, distolingual, distobuccal, and distal (Figure 17-52). The order of the cusps from highest to lowest is mesiolingual, distolingual, mesiobuccal, distobuccal, and distal cusp. Each cusp has four cusp ridges, a triangular ridge, and four inclined cuspal planes.

The mesiobuccal cusp is the bulkiest cusp, although it has a blunt tip. Except for the distal cusp, the disto-

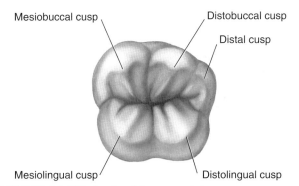

FIGURE 17-52 Occlusal features of the permanent mandibular right first molar.

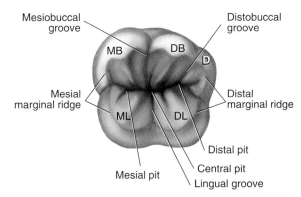

FIGURE 17-53 Additional occlusal features of the permanent mandibular right first molar (occlusal table highlighted).

buccal cusp is the smallest of the cusps and has a rounded tip. The mesiolingual cusp is second in size to the mesiobuccal cusp and has the sharpest tip. The distolingual cusp is also quite sharp but is slightly smaller than the mesiolingual cusp. The distal cusp is the smallest and has a sharp cusp, which *helps to distinguish the right mandibular first molar from the left.*

This tooth has the most complex developmental groove pattern of all the permanent mandibular molars (Figure 17-53). A Y-shaped groove pattern is formed on the occlusal table of a mandibular first molar around the cusps by the mesiobuccal groove, distobuccal groove, and lingual groove. Two marginal ridges border the occlusal table, the mesial marginal ridge and the distal marginal ridge. No transverse ridges are found on the occlusal, unlike a maxillary first molar and a mandibular second molar.

The occlusal table also has three fossae: the large central fossa and the smaller mesial triangular fossa and distal triangular fossa. Three pits are associated with the fossae: the mesial pit, central pit, and distal pit. The central pit is the also the deepest pit and divides the central groove into two grooves, the mesial groove and distal groove.

The central pit is the junction of three grooves: mesiobuccal, distobuccal, and lingual. The mesial pit is the junction of four grooves: mesial, mesiobuccal tri-

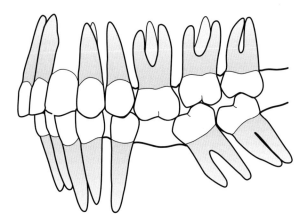

FIGURE 17-54 The changes that can occur in the permanent dentition with the loss of the mandibular first molar: inclination and mesial drift of the mandibular second molar and possibly third molar and supereruption of the maxillary first molar into the space.

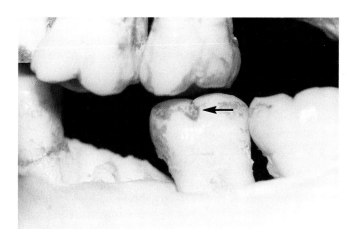

FIGURE 17-55 An example of a buccal pit *(arrow)* on the permanent mandibular first molar on a skull.

angular, mesiolingual triangular, and mesial marginal. The distal pit is the junction of three grooves: the distal, the distolingual, and distal marginal.

Clinical Considerations with Mandibular First Molars

Because of their arch position and because the permanent mandibular first molars are the first permanent teeth to erupt in the mandibular arch, they are considered important in regard to the development of occlusion (see Chapter 20 for more information).

The importance of the role of this tooth in occlusion is shown when the tooth is lost (Figure 17-54). This loss may easily occur because this tooth is the first permanent tooth to erupt into the oral cavity. It has a greater chance of being affected by caries because child patients are just beginning to master oral hygiene and diet restrictions. In addition, early dental restorative intervention of the caries may be neglected.

With the loss of the tooth, the mandibular second molar and possibly the third molar incline and drift mesially into the newly opened arch space. The maxillary first molar also supererupts into the space. Occlusion and then mastication are disabled, and predisposition to further caries and possibly periodontal disease around the irregularly spaced teeth is greatly increased. Orthodontic care is important to prevent these situations after tooth loss.

Buccal pits that may occur on the buccal surface of permanent mandibular first molars are susceptible to caries because of both increased bacterial plaque biofilm retention and the thinness of enamel forming the walls of the pit (Figure 17-55; see also Chapter 12 for more information). Enamel sealants should be placed on the buccal surface of mandibular first molars shortly after they erupt. Sealants on the buccal pit do not bond as well as they do on the occlusal surface, however, because of the histology of the area. If caries does occur, tooth-colored restorative materials can be used to achieve a more aesthetic appearance, and thus the buccal pit may not be easy to discern.

PERMANENT MANDIBULAR SECOND MOLARS #18 AND #31

Specific Overall Features (Figure 17-56)

The permanent mandibular second molars erupt between 11 and 12 years of age (root completion occurs between the ages of 14 and 15). These teeth erupt distal to the permanent mandibular first molars and thus are nonsuccedaneous.

The crown measurements of a mandibular second molar are generally smaller than those of a first molar. The four cusps of a second are nearly equal in size compared with the five cusps of differing sizes of a first molar.

Like the mandibular third molars, the mandibular second molars are usually composed of four developmental lobes, unlike the mandibular first molars, which have five lobes. The lobes are named for the associated cusps, and the developmental grooves on the occlusal surface show lobe division.

The two roots of a second molar are smaller, shorter, less divergent, and closer together than those of a first molar. The root trunk of a second molar is also longer than that of a first molar. The mesial root of the second is not as broad as that of a first molar, but the furcation is farther to the CEJ. All root depressions are shallower. Overall, root variability is greater than in the first molar.

Although the pulp cavity of a mandibular second molar can have two pulp canals (one for each root), it is more likely to have three pulp canals, similar to a mandibular first molar (Figure 17-57). These are the distal, mesiobuccal, and mesiolingual canals (the latter two being together in the mesial root). The tooth usually has only four pulp horns, which correspond to the four cusps.

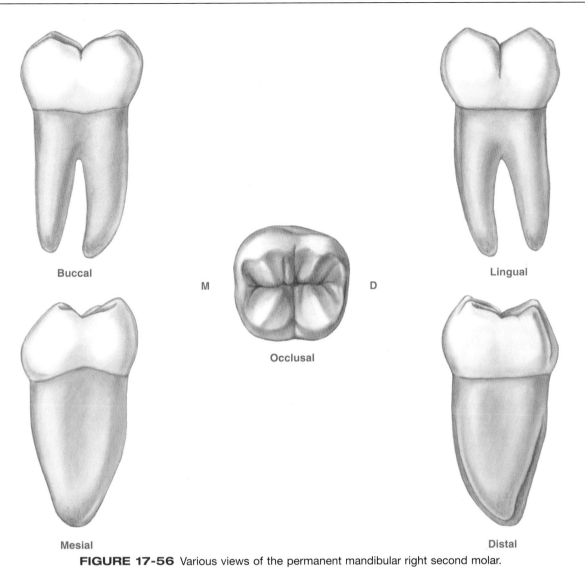

Buccal

M

D

Occlusal

Lingual

Mesial

Distal

FIGURE 17-56 Various views of the permanent mandibular right second molar.

Buccal View Features

The buccal groove divides the same-size mesiobuccal cusp and distobuccal cusp of a mandibular second molar (see Figure 17-56). The mesial contact is at the junction of the occlusal and middle third. The distal contact is slightly more cervical but still is at the junction of the occlusal and middle third.

Lingual View Features

The mesiolingual cusp and distolingual cusp have the same size and shape as the buccal cusps, although they have sharper cusp tips. Because the crown converges lingually, a portion of the mesial and distal surfaces can be seen from this view.

Proximal View Features

The buccal height of contour is in the cervical third, and the lingual height of contour is in the middle third

for the second molar. The crown also tapers distally when viewed from the mesial aspect. That is because the molar is also wider buccolingually on the mesial surface than on the distal. Both these mesial surface features *help to distinguish the right mandibular second molar from the left.* The buccal cervical ridge is less pronounced on the second molar than on the first or the proximal.

The CEJ curvature on both proximal surfaces of a mandibular second molar is less pronounced than that of a first molar. Neither the mesial nor distal marginal ridge is divided by a marginal groove.

Occlusal View

The outline of the crown of a mandibular second molar is rectangular (Figure 17-58). The tooth has four cusps, two buccal and two lingual: the mesiobuccal, distobuccal, mesiolingual, and distolingual. With this view, the occlusal surface of a second molar is considerably

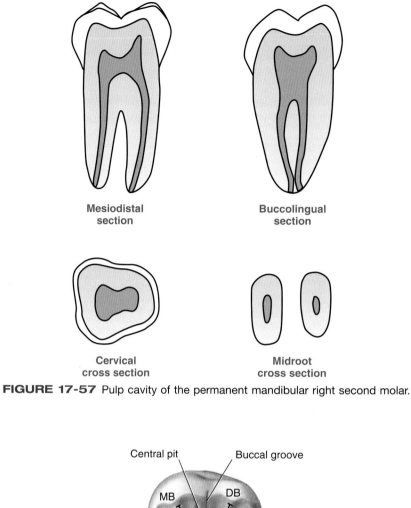

Mesiodistal section

Buccolingual section

Cervical cross section

Midroot cross section

FIGURE 17-57 Pulp cavity of the permanent mandibular right second molar.

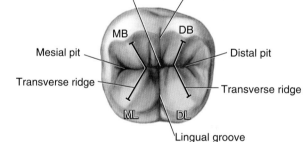

Central pit

Buccal groove

MB

DB

Mesial pit

Distal pit

Transverse ridge

Transverse ridge

ML

DL

Lingual groove

FIGURE 17-58 Occlusal features of the permanent mandibular right second molar (occlusal table highlighted).

different from that of a first because there is no distal cusp and all cusps are of equal size.

Components of the Occlusal Table

A cross-shaped groove pattern is formed where the well-defined central groove is crossed by the buccal groove and lingual groove, dividing the occlusal table into four parts that are nearly equal. The three occlusal pits are the central pit, the mesial pit, and the distal pit. Cusp slopes on a second molar are less smooth than on a first because second molars have more supplemental grooves.

Unlike a mandibular first molar, this tooth has two transverse ridges. The triangular ridges of the mesiobuccal and mesiolingual cusps meet to form a transverse ridge, as do the distobuccal and distolingual cusps.

PERMANENT MANDIBULAR THIRD MOLARS #17 AND #32

Specific Overall Features (Figure 17-59)

The mandibular third molars may erupt between 17 and 21 years of age (root completion occurs between

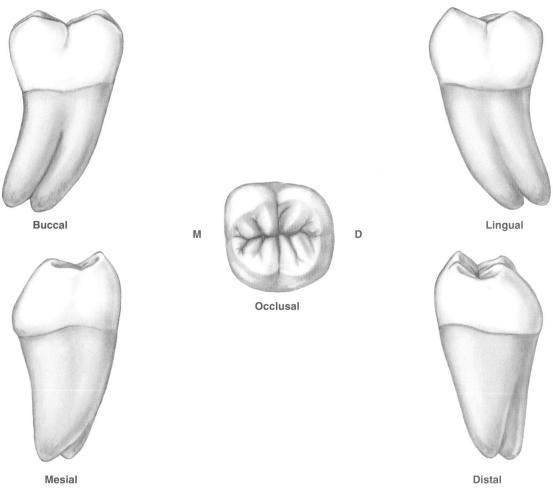

Buccal

M   D

Occlusal

Lingual

Mesial   Distal

FIGURE 17-59 Various views of the permanent mandibular right third molar.

the ages of 18 and 25). If they erupt (see the later section on clinical considerations), they erupt distal to the permanent mandibular second molars.

Similar to maxillary third molars, the mandibular third molars are variable in shape, having no standard form. Thus a typical mandibular third molar is difficult to describe. This molar usually is smaller in all dimensions than the second molar. It sometimes is the same size as the first molar.

Like the mandibular second molars, the mandibular third molars are usually composed of four developmental lobes, unlike the mandibular first molars, which have five lobes. The lobes are named for the associated cusps, and the developmental grooves on the occlusal surface show lobe division.

The crown of a mandibular third molar tapers distally when viewed from the mesial aspect. That is because the molar is also wider buccolingually on the mesial surface than on the distal surface, which *helps*

to distinguish the right mandibular third molar from the left, like all mandibular molars. The crown is usually smaller in all dimensions than that of a second molar.

The occlusal outline of the crown is more oval than rectangular, although the crown usually resembles that of a second molar. The two mesial cusps are larger than the two distal cusps. The occlusal surface appears quite wrinkled, with an irregular groove pattern, numerous supplemental grooves, and occlusal pits; if an excess of these features exists, the occlusal surface is described as *crenulated*.

A mandibular third molar usually has two roots that are fused, irregularly curved, and shorter than those of a mandibular second molar. Additionally, the roots are usually smaller in proportion to the crown and have sharp apices. The pulp cavity of the tooth is usually similar to that of the second molars, with four pulp horns and two or three pulp canals (Figure 17-60).

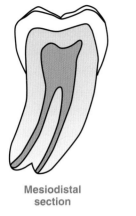
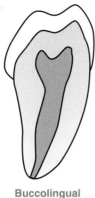

Mesiodistal
section

Buccolingual
section

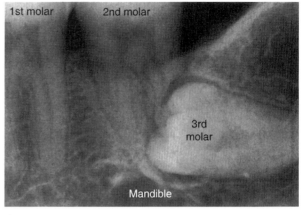

FIGURE 17-61 Radiograph of an impacted permanent mandibular third molar.

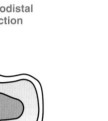

Cervical
cross section

Midroot
cross section

FIGURE 17-60 Pulp cavity of the permanent mandibular right third molar.

 ### Clinical Considerations for Mandibular Third Molars

The permanent mandibular third molars may also fail to erupt and remain impacted within the surrounding alveolar bone (Figure 17-61), which occurs more frequently than with the maxillary counterparts. An impacted tooth is an unerupted or partially erupted tooth that is positioned against another tooth, bone, or even soft tissue, making complete eruption unlikely. This impaction usually occurs because the mandible is underdeveloped and space or arch length is insufficient to accommodate these teeth, which are the last to erupt in the mandibular arch. Surgical removal may be necessary. The third molars may also be partially erupted, making the gingiva surrounding and possibly overlying the crown susceptible to periodontal infections caused by poor oral hygiene of the area.

 ### Developmental Disturbances with Mandibular Third Molars

The permanent mandibular third molars, along with the maxillary third molars, are permanent teeth commonly involved in partial anodontia, being congenitally missing either unilaterally or bilaterally. (All disturbances are discussed further in Chapter 6.) With this disturbance, the appropriate individual tooth germ in the area is missing because of a failure in the initiation process during tooth development. However, anodontia usually has no harmful consequences.

These teeth may also have accessory roots, which complicate extraction procedures. Finally, developmental cyst formation may occur within the dental tissues of an impacted crown of a mandibular third molar, resulting in a dentigerous cyst.

CHAPTER 18

Primary Dentition

This chapter discusses the following topics:

- Primary teeth
  - Primary incisors
  - Primary canines
  - Primary molars

After studying, this chapter, the reader should be able to:

1. Use the correct name and universal designation letter for each primary tooth when examining a diagram and a patient.
2. Demonstrate the correct location of each primary tooth on a diagram and a patient.
3. Define and pronounce the key terms when discussing the primary teeth.
4. Describe the general features of primary teeth and of each primary tooth type.
5. Describe the specific features of each primary tooth.
6. Discuss the important clinical considerations and developmental disturbances based on the anatomy of the primary teeth.
7. Integrate the knowledge of dental anatomy of the primary teeth into the dental treatment of patients.

Key Terms

Cervical ridge	Primary dentition	Primate spaces

PRIMARY TEETH

The first set of teeth is the **primary dentition** (Figure 18-1). The primary dentition is exfoliated, or shed, and replaced by the permanent dentition. There are 20 primary teeth, 10 per dental arch. These include incisors, canines, and molars (Figure 18-2). These are designated in the Universal Tooth Designation System by the capital letters *A* through *T*.

Calcification of the primary teeth begins in utero at 13 to 16 weeks. By 18 to 20 weeks prenatally, all the primary teeth have started to calcify. There are usually no primary teeth visible in the oral cavity at birth. The first eruption of a primary tooth, a primary mandibular central incisor, occurs at an average age of 6 to 10 months, and the rest follow (Table 18-1).

The primary dentition takes between 2 and 3 years to be completed, beginning with the initial calcification

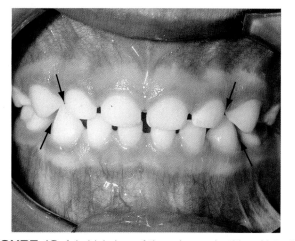

FIGURE 18-1 Labial view of the primary dentition. Note the attrition of the masticatory surgaces of the dentition, which may normally be present with the primary dentition. Primate spaces of the primary dentition are indicated by the arrows. (From Bird DL, Robinson DS. Modern Dental Assisting, ed 8. WB Saunders, Philadelphia, 2005.)

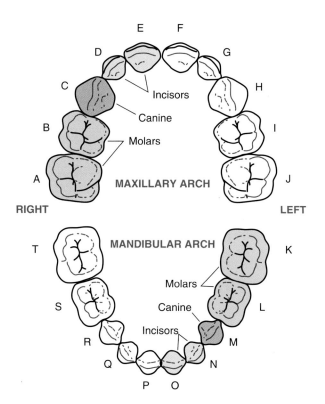

FIGURE 18-2 Occlusal views of the primary teeth showing the maxillary and mandibular arches.

of the primary mandibular central incisors and being completed in the roots of the primary maxillary second molar (see Figure 6-26, *A* for the chronological order of primary tooth eruption and shedding). A 6-month delay or acceleration is considered normal. If you see a child who is unusually early or late in getting their teeth, inquire about family dental history. However, tooth types tend to erupt in pairs so that if there is any asymmetry, a radiograph of the area may be required.

TABLE 18-1

Approximate Eruption and Shedding Ages for Primary Teeth

Maxillary Teeth	Eruption	Shedding
Central incisor	8-12 months	6-7 years
Lateral incisor	9-13 months	7-8 years
Canine	16-22 months	10-12 years
First molar	13-19 months	9-11 years
Second molar	25-33 months	10-12 years
Mandibular Teeth	**Eruption**	**Shedding**
Central incisor	6-10 months	6-7 years
Lateral incisor	10-16 months	7-8 years
Canine	14-18 months	9-12 years
First molar	17-23 months	9-11 years
Second molar	23-31 months	10-12 years

Adapted from Ash MM. *Wheeler's Dental Anatomy, Physiology and Occlusion*, ed 8. WB Saunders, Philadelphia, 2002

Females shed their primary teeth and receive their permanent teeth slightly earlier than males, possibly reflecting the earlier overall physical maturation achieved. The actual dates are not as important as the eruption sequence because a great deal of variation exists in the actual dates of eruption, although the sequence is uniform.

Also considered normal are certain interproximal spaces between the primary teeth because space is necessary for the proper alignment of the future permanent dentition. These spaces are called the primate spaces and mainly involve spaces between the primary maxillary lateral incisor and canine and between the primary mandibular canine and first molar (see Figure 18-1; see also Chapter 20 for more discussion). They are called *primate spaces* because they are most marked in the dentitions of primates. Primate spaces occur in about 50 percent of children.

The primary teeth are not just little permanent teeth because important differences occur in the structure of primary teeth compared with that of permanent teeth. The primary teeth are smaller overall and have whiter enamel than the permanent teeth because of the increased opacity of the enamel, which covers the underlying yellow dentin (see Figure 18-1). Other differences between these two dentitions are also evident (Figures 18-3 to 18-5). The crown of any primary tooth is short in relation to its total length.

The crowns are also more constricted, or narrower, at the cementoenamel junction (CEJ), making them appear bulbous. The masticatory surface may show significant attrition as a result of grinding (bruxism), but this finding may not be a predictor of this habit as an adult (see Figure 18-1). A **cervical ridge** is present on both the labial and lingual surfaces of anterior teeth and on buccal surfaces of the molars (see Figure 18-5). These ridges are much more prominent than any similar structure on permanent molars.

The roots of primary teeth are also narrower and longer than the crown length (see Figures 18-3 to 18-5). Roots may also show partial resorption radiographically as the teeth begin to exfoliate. The crown : root ratios are smaller than their permanent counterparts.

The pulp cavity on primary teeth shows that pulp chambers and pulp horns are relatively large in proportion to those of the permanent teeth, especially the mesial pulp horns of the molars (Figure 18-6). Overall, the dentin of the primary dentition is thinner than that of the permanent counterparts. However, the dentin thickness between the pulp chambers and the enamel is increased, especially in the primary mandibular second molar. The enamel is also relatively thin but has consistent thickness overlying the dentin of the crown.

Primary Incisors

GENERAL FEATURES

Each dental arch has four primary incisors. As in the permanent dentition, each quadrant has two incisor types, the central and the lateral. Both primary incisors resemble their permanent successor, with some exceptions. Both have the same arch position, function, and general shape as the permanent counterpart and function as such for about 5 years.

Dental professionals sometimes note extensive wear of the incisal edges of the primary incisors and the formation of an edge-to-edge relationship between the arches resulting from bruxism (grinding of the teeth). The significance of this finding and its possible relevance to later adult habits are unknown (see Figure 18-1 and Chapter 20).

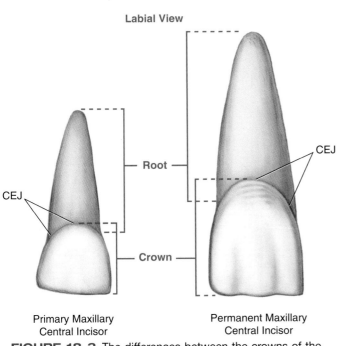

Labial View

Primary Maxillary
Central Incisor

Permanent Maxillary
Central Incisor

FIGURE 18-3 The differences between the crowns of the primary and permanent teeth (note especially the different crown/root ratios). CEJ = cementoenamel junction.

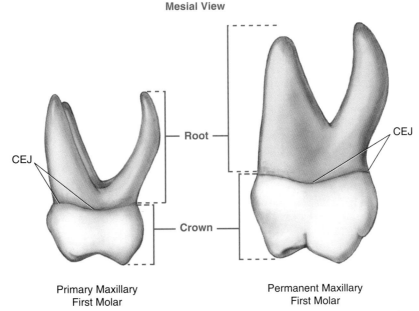

Mesial View

Primary Maxillary
First Molar

Permanent Maxillary
First Molar

FIGURE 18-4 The differences between the crowns and roots of the primary and permanent teeth (note especially the differences at the cementoenamel junction [CEJ]).

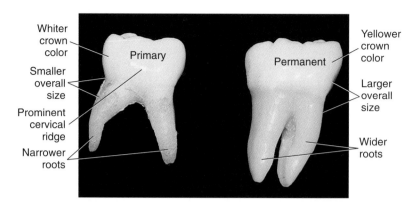

FIGURE 18-5 Extracted teeth showing the differences between the primary and permanent teeth.

Clinical Considerations for the Primary Dentition

Child patients and their caregivers sometimes discount the importance of the teeth of the primary dentition, believing that they are temporary and will soon be replaced. It is true that a 70-year-old person will have spent 91 percent of his or her life chewing on permanent teeth but only 6 percent of his or her chewing career with the deciduous dentition. The primary dentition generally functions in aesthetics, mastication, and speech for a child for only 5 to 12 years. However, these teeth also serve to hold the eruption space for the succedaneous permanent teeth, which will replace the primary teeth. Individually, each primary tooth functions in the same way as its permanent counterpart.

In the past, many carious primary teeth were extracted instead of repaired, resulting in crowding and potential occlusal problems in the permanent dentition (see Chapter 20 for more discussion). Worse still, many carious primary teeth were ignored, resulting in serious oral infections and discomfort for the child patient.

Today the value of primary teeth is more realistically appreciated, and more are saved from caries because of early dental care. Still, the value of these teeth must be imparted to the caregivers and child patient. Supervised oral hygiene must begin early, as the first primary teeth erupt into the oral cavity, to prevent premature loss of the primary teeth. Because the enamel and dentin are thinner, the risk of endodontic complications is greater for the primary dentition. The pulp chamber and horns are also larger, increasing the possibility of pulpal exposure during cavity preparation. These factors can be coupled with the increased possibility of poor oral hygiene in the child patient, especially without any supervision. Nighttime use of a baby bottle or sugar on a pacifier must also be considered in a child with extensive acute caries of the primary teeth, which is generally called "baby bottle mouth" (Figure 18-7) or early childhood caries.

Bulging of the cervical ridge of primary teeth must also be taken into account when these teeth are involved in any restorative procedure. Extensive extrinsic staining of the primary teeth may be attributed to Nasmyth's membrane (see Chapter 6 for more information).

A child's first dental appointment should occur within 6 months of the eruption of the first primary tooth and no later than 12 months of age. The intent of this recommendation is to provide information to caregivers, which will help to establish positive preventive behaviors, prevent serious dental problems, and allay concerns. This early initial visit affords the dental professional the opportunity to provide basic, timely information and to do this in 6-month increments.

Early dental care is important not only for keeping the primary dentition healthy but also for assessing appropriate preventive orthodontic intervention when needed. Preventive measures such as space maintainers, retainers, removal of any extraneous bulbous proximal crown width, and removal of retained primary teeth as needed may allow for the correct eruption sequence and alignment of the permanent teeth later (see Chapter 20). Extraction procedures of primary teeth should always be performed with caution and with radiographic confirmation of a permanent replacement, especially with primary molars. If primary teeth are retained too long, possibly ankylosed, missing (anodontia), or impacted permanent teeth may be present.

In addition, if severe periodontal inflammation and destruction in the primary dentition are found, either locally or generally, early aggressive periodontitis (formerly known as *prepubertal periodontitis*) must be suspected. Early intervention with this severe yet uncommon periodontal disease can prevent further periodontal destruction.

Mesiodistal Section

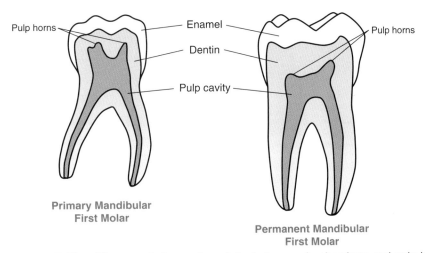

Primary Mandibular
First Molar

Permanent Mandibular
First Molar

FIGURE 18-6 The differences between the relatively large pulp chambers and pulp horns of the primary teeth and those of permanent teeth, which are relatively smaller.

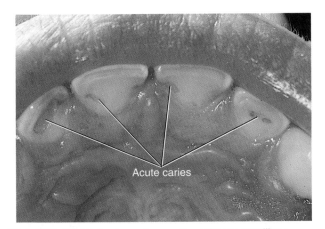

FIGURE 18-7 Acute caries on the primary maxillary anterior teeth caused by "baby bottle mouth" or extreme childhood caries. This condition is associated with putting the baby to bed with a bottle.

PRIMARY MAXILLARY CENTRAL INCISOR *E* AND *F*

Specific Features (Figure 18-8)

From the labial aspect, the crown of the primary maxillary central incisor appears wider mesiodistally than incisocervically, the opposite of its permanent successor. In fact, it is the only anterior tooth of either dentition with this crown dimension. Additionally, its mesial and distal outlines are more rounded than the permanent central incisor as a result of the cervical constriction. The incisal outline is relatively straight from this view, but it slopes toward the distal with attrition.

Unlike their permanent successors, the primary maxillary central incisors have no mamelons, leaving the labial surface smooth. Rarely, these teeth have developmental depressions or imbrication lines. No pits are evident on the lingual surface. The cingulum and marginal ridges on the lingual surface all are more prominent than on the permanent successor, and the lingual fossa is deeper.

Both proximal surfaces of the maxillary central incisor appear similar. Because of the short crown and its wide labiolingual measurement, the crown appears thick, even at the incisal third. The CEJ curves distinctly toward the incisal but not as much as on its permanent successor. This curvature is less distal than mesial, as in the permanent successor. From the incisal surface, the crown appears wider mesiodistally than labiolingually, and the incisal edge appears nearly straight. The single root is generally round and tapers evenly to the apex. It is longer, relative to crown length, than the permanent central incisor.

PRIMARY MAXILLARY LATERAL INCISOR *D* AND *G*

Specific Features (Figure 18-9)

The crown of the primary maxillary lateral incisor is similar to the central incisor but is much smaller than the central in all dimensions. The lateral is also longer incisocervically than mesiodistally, exactly the opposite of the central. The incisal angles are also more rounded than the central. The root is also similar to that of the central, but the lateral's root is longer in proportion to its crown compared with the same proportions of the central, and its apex is sharper.

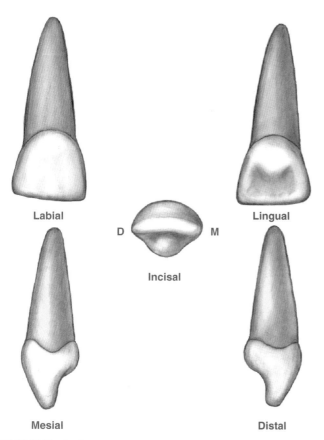

Labial

Lingual

D — M

Incisal

Mesial

Distal

FIGURE 18-8 Various views of the primary maxillary right central incisor.

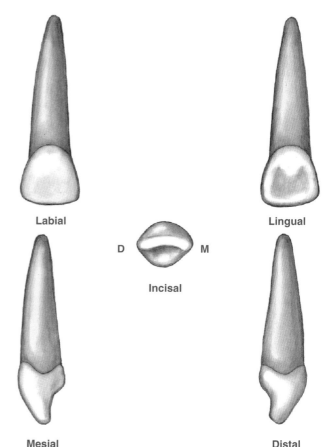

Labial

Lingual

D — M

Incisal

Mesial

Distal

FIGURE 18-9 Various views of the primary maxillary right lateral incisor.

PRIMARY MANDIBULAR CENTRAL INCISOR *O* AND *P*

Specific Features (Figure 18-10)

The crown of the primary mandibular central incisor looks more like the primary mandibular lateral incisor than its permanent successor or any other primary maxillary incisor . This tooth is also quite symmetrical, however, similar to its permanent successor. It is also not as constricted at the CEJ as the primary maxillary central incisor. From the labial aspect, the crown appears wide compared with its permanent successor. Its mesial and distal outlines from the labial aspect also show that the crown tapers evenly from the contact areas.

The lingual surface of the primary mandibular central incisor appears smooth and tapers toward the prominent cingulum. The marginal ridges are less pronounced than those of the primary maxillary incisor, however, and the lingual fossa is shallow. Again, the CEJ curvature on the mesial side is greater than on the distal. From the mesial aspect, this tooth is much wider labiolingually than its permanent successor.

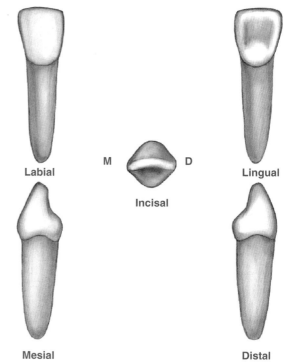

Labial

M — D

Incisal

Lingual

Mesial

Distal

FIGURE 18-10 Various views of the primary mandibular right central incisor.

The incisal edge of the primary mandibular central incisor is centered over the root from the proximal and incisal views and divides the labial and lingual into equal halves. The root is single, long, and slender. The labial and lingual surfaces of the root are rounded, but the proximal surfaces are slightly flattened.

PRIMARY MANDIBULAR LATERAL INCISOR *Q* AND *N*

Specific Features (Figure 18-11)

The crown of the primary mandibular lateral incisor is similar in form to the central incisor of the same arch, but the crown is wider and longer than that of the central. The cingulum is also more developed, and the lingual fossa is slightly deeper than that of the central incisor.

The incisal edge slopes distally, and its distoincisal angle is more rounded, as is the distal margin. From the incisal aspect, the crown is not as symmetrical as is the central, because the cingulum is offset toward the distal. This is the same cingulum position as in its permanent successor. The root may have a distal curvature in its apical third, and it usually has a distal longitudinal groove.

Primary Canines

GENERAL FEATURES

There are four primary canines, two in each dental arch. These primary canines resemble the outline of their permanent successors, with some exceptions.

PRIMARY MAXILLARY CANINE *C* AND *H*

Specific Features (Figure 18-12)

The crown of the primary maxillary canine has a relatively longer and sharper cusp than that of its permanent successor when first erupted. The mesial and distal outlines of the primary maxillary canine are rounder, however, and greatly overhang the cervical line. The mesial cusp slope is longer than the distal cusp slope on this tooth, just the opposite of the

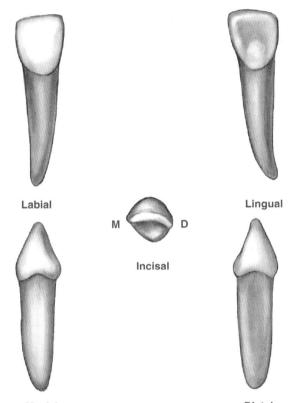

Labial   **Lingual**

M   D

Incisal

Mesial   **Distal**

FIGURE 18-11 Various views of the primary mandibular right lateral incisor.

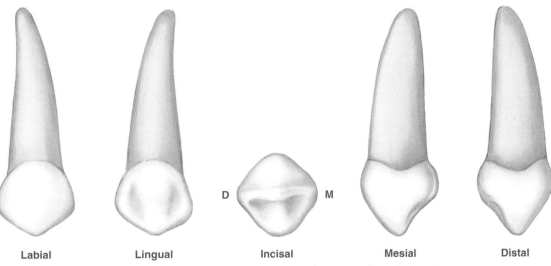

Labial   **Lingual**   **Incisal**   **Mesial**   **Distal**

FIGURE 18-12 Various views of the primary maxillary right canine.

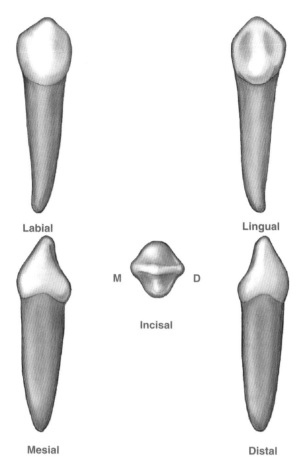

Labial

Lingual

M   D

Incisal

Mesial

Distal

FIGURE 18-13 Various views of the primary mandibular right canine.

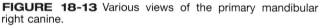

primary mandibular canine and the opposite of the permanent counterpart also.

On the lingual surface of the maxillary canine, the cingulum is well developed, as are the lingual ridge and marginal ridges. The lingual ridge extends from the cingulum to the cusp tip and divides the lingual surface into a shallow mesiolingual fossa and distolingual fossa. A tubercle is often present on the cingulum, extending from the cusp tip to the cingulum.

From the incisal aspect, the crown is diamond-shaped and the cusp tip is slightly offset to the distal. The root is twice as long as the crown and more slender than that of its permanent successor, and it is inclined distally.

PRIMARY MANDIBULAR CANINE
M AND *R*

Specific Features (Figure 18-13)

The crown of the primary mandibular canine resembles that of the primary maxillary canine, although some dimensions are different. This tooth is much smaller labiolingually. The distal cusp slope is much longer than the mesial cusp slope, as is the case on its permanent counterpart.

The lingual surface of the primary mandibular canine is smoother than the primary maxillary canine and is marked by a shallow lingual fossa. The incisal edge of the primary mandibular canine is straight and is centered over the crown labiolingually. The root is long, narrow, and almost twice the length of the crown, although shorter and more tapered than that of a primary maxillary canine.

Primary Molars
GENERAL FEATURES

There are eight primary molars, with two types, a first and second. One of each type is located in each quadrant of both dental arches. Both have the similar arch position, function, and general shape as the permanent counterpart and function as such for approximately 9 years. Primary molars are replaced when exfoliated by the permanent premolars. However, none of the primary first molars resembles any other tooth in either dentition, but the crown of each primary second molar in both arches resembles the permanent first molars that will erupt distal to them. Each molar crown is shorter occlusocervically than mesiodistally.

The occlusal table of a primary molar is more constricted buccolingually than with permanent molars, rather like a rope around a corral (see Figure 18-14 as an example). This constriction is due to the buccal and lingual surfaces of a primary molar being flatter occlusal to the CEJ curvatures, thus narrowing the occlusal table. The occlusal anatomy of the cusps is also not as pronounced as on the permanent successors.

The roots of the molars are flared beyond the crown outlines, widely separating the roots (see Figure 18-14 as an example). Additional space is thus created between the roots for the developing permanent premolar crowns. The primary molars have a short root trunk, as with permanent posterior teeth; the roots branch a short distance from the base of the crown. Again, this arrangement creates more space for the developing permanent premolar crowns.

PRIMARY MAXILLARY FIRST MOLAR
B AND *I*

Specific Features (Figure 18-14)

The crown of the maxillary first molar does not resemble any other crown of either dentition. From the buccal aspect, the mesial and distal outlines are rounded and constricted at the CEJ. The CEJ on the mesial half of the buccal surface curves around an extremely prominent buccal cervical ridge. The height of contour on the buccal is at the cervical one third and for the lingual at the middle one third.

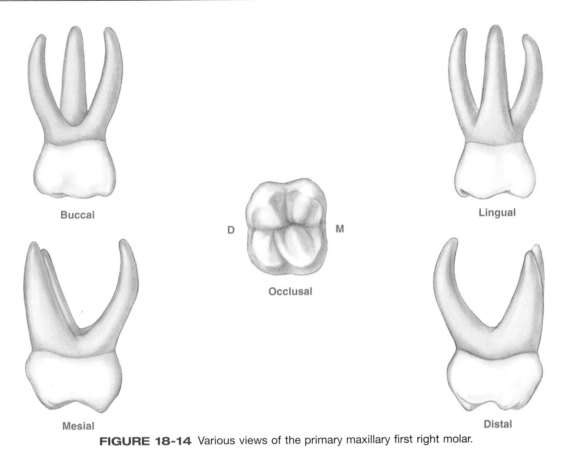

Buccal

Lingual

D   M

Occlusal

Mesial

Distal

FIGURE 18-14 Various views of the primary maxillary first right molar.

The occlusal table of the maxillary first molar can have four cusps: mesiobuccal, mesiolingual, distobuccal, and distolingual, with the two mesial cusps being the largest and the two distal cusps being quite small. It commonly has only three cusps because the distolingual cusp may be absent. The occlusal table also has an extremely prominent transverse ridge. Additionally, an oblique ridge extends between the mesiolingual cusp and the distobuccal cusp; however, it is not as prominent as the one on its permanent counterpart.

The tooth also has an H-shaped groove pattern and three fossae: central fossa, mesial triangular, and distal triangular. The central groove connects the central pit with the mesial pit and distal pit, at each end of the occlusal table.

The buccal groove on the maxillary first molar originates in the central pit and extends buccally, separating the mesiobuccal and distobuccal cusps. The distal triangular fossa contains the disto-occlusal groove, which extends obliquely and is parallel to the oblique ridge just distal to it. Both the buccal and disto-occlusal grooves remain on the occlusal table, unlike its permanent counterpart.

The primary maxillary first molars do have the same number and position of the roots of the primary first molars as the permanent maxillary molars. The three root branches are thinner and have greater flare

than on the permanent molar, and the root trunk is short. The mesiobuccal root is wider buccolingually than the distobuccal root. The lingual root is the longest and most divergent.

PRIMARY MAXILLARY SECOND MOLAR *A* AND *J*
Specific Features (Figure 18-15)
The primary maxillary second molar is larger than the primary maxillary first molar. This tooth most closely resembles the form of the permanent maxillary first molar but is smaller in all dimensions. Thus it usually has a cusp of Carabelli, the minor fifth cusp, as does its permanent counterpart.

PRIMARY MANDIBULAR FIRST MOLAR *L* AND *S*
Specific Features (Figure 18-16)
Unlike any other tooth of either dentition, the primary mandibular first molar has a crown. The tooth does have a prominent buccal cervical ridge, also on the mesial half of the buccal surface, similar to other primary molars. The height of contour on the buccal is at the cervical one third and for the lingual is in the

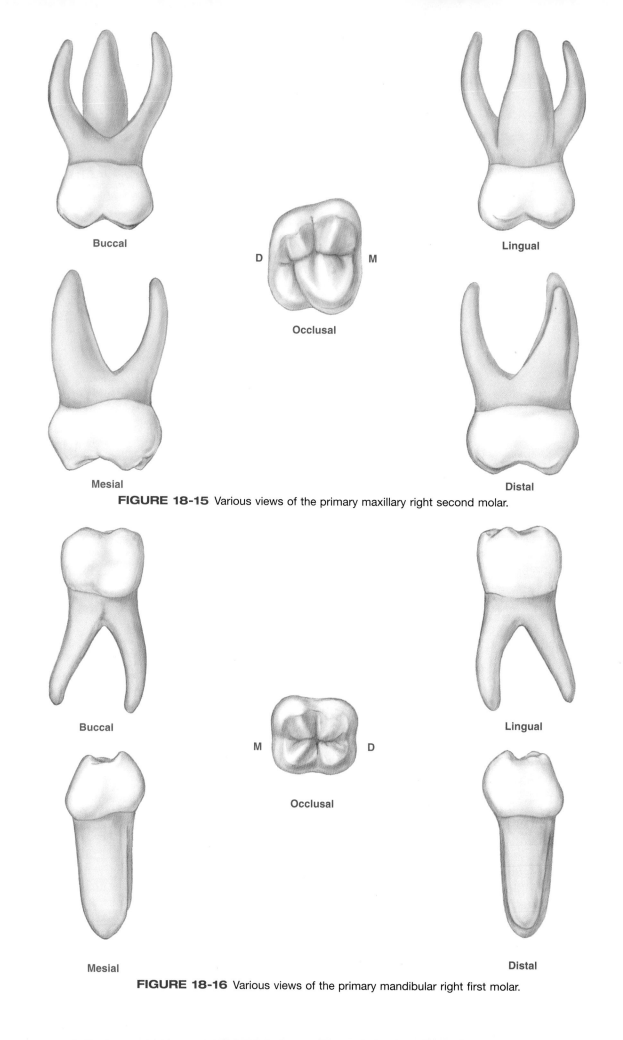

Buccal

D M

Occlusal

Lingual

Mesial

Distal

FIGURE 18-15 Various views of the primary maxillary right second molar.

Buccal

M D

Occlusal

Lingual

Mesial

Distal

FIGURE 18-16 Various views of the primary mandibular right first molar.

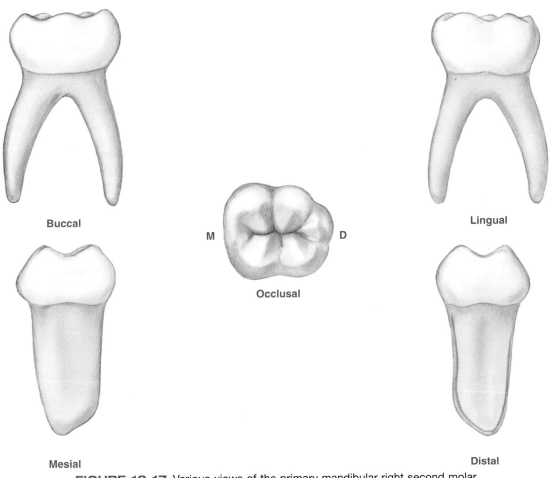

Buccal

Lingual

M   D

Occlusal

Mesial

Distal

FIGURE 18-17 Various views of the primary mandibular right second molar.

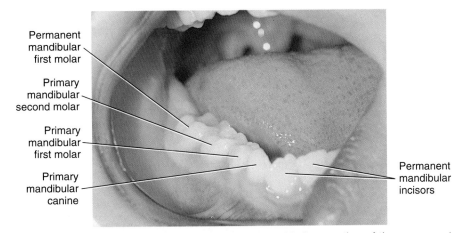

Permanent
mandibular
first molar

Primary
mandibular
second molar

Primary
mandibular
first molar

Primary
mandibular
canine

Permanent
mandibular
incisors

FIGURE 18-18 Clinical view of the mixed dentition with the eruption of the permanent mandibular first molar distal to the primary mandibular second molar. The eruption of the permanent molar is difficult to discern because it looks so much like the primary molar.

middle one third. The mesiolingual line angle of the crown is rounder than any other line angles.

The tooth has four cusps; the mesial cusps are larger. The mesiolingual cusp is long, pointed, and angled in on the occlusal table. A transverse ridge passes between the mesiobuccal and mesiolingual cusps. The tooth does have two roots, which are positioned similarly to those of other primary and permanent mandibular molars.

PRIMARY MANDIBULAR SECOND MOLAR *K* AND *T*
Specific Features (Figure 18-17)

The primary mandibular second molar is larger than the primary mandibular first molar. The tooth most closely resembles the form of the permanent mandibular first molar that erupts distal to it because it has five cusps. The three buccal cusps are nearly equal in size, however, and the primary mandibular second molar has an overall oval occlusal shape.

Clinical Considerations with Primary Molars

Child patients in the mixed dentition period and their caregivers may not notice the presence of the newly erupted permanent first molar of either arch because when it erupts, it appears just like a larger primary second molar that is adjacent to it (Figure 18-18). These children and their caregivers must be reminded that to last a lifetime, these new posterior permanent teeth require careful oral hygiene and possibly enamel sealants on the occlusal surface.

The greater root spread of primary molars, along with their narrow shape and lack of root trunk, make primary molars susceptible to fracture during extraction procedures. Dental professionals should also remember that shedding of primary teeth is an intermittent process, with resorption of the dental tissues being followed by apposition. A loose primary tooth may tighten and thus may not be ready for extraction (see Chapter 6 for more information on tooth exfoliation).

CHAPTER 19

Temporomandibular Joint

This chapter discusses the following topics:

- Temporomandibular joint (TMJ)
- Bones of the joint
  - Temporal Bone
  - Mandible
- Joint capsule
- Disc of the joint
- Jaw moments of the joint
- Disorders of the joint

■ ■ ■

After studying this chapter, the reader should be able to:

1. Define and pronounce the key terms in this chapter.
2. Locate and identify the specific anatomical landmarks of the temporomandibular joint on a diagram, a skull, and a patient.
3. Describe the histology of each component of the temporomandibular joint.
4. Describe the movements of the temporomandibular joint.
5. Discuss the disorders of the temporomandibular joint.
6. Integrate the knowledge of the anatomy and histology of the temporomandibular joint into the dental treatment of the patient.

■ ■ ■

Key Terms

Articular eminence (ar-tik-you-ler), fossa
Articulating surface of the condyle (ar-tik-you-late-ing kon-dyl)
Depression of the mandible (de-presh-in)
Disc of the joint

Elevation of the mandible (el-eh-vay-shun)
Joint capsule
Lateral deviation of the mandible (de-vee-ay-shun)
Protrusion of the mandible (pro-troo-zhin)

Retraction of the mandible (re-trak-shun)
Subluxation (sub-luk-say-shun)
Synovial (sy-no-vee-al) fluid, cavities, membrane
Temporomandibular (tem-poh-ro-man-dib-you-lar) disorder, joint

TEMPOROMANDIBULAR JOINT (TMJ)

The **temporomandibular joint (TMJ)** is a joint on each side of the head that allows for movement of the mandible for mastication, speech, and respiratory movements. The TMJ can be palpated just anterior to each ear. The TMJ develops in the eleventh to twelfth week of prenatal development, during the growth of the associated ligaments, muscles, and bones of the joint.

Patients may have a disorder associated with one or both of their TMJs (discussed later). Thus dental

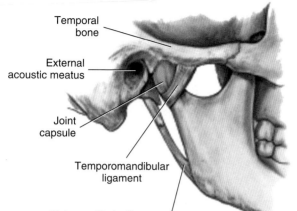

FIGURE 19-1 The temporomandibular joint and its associated bony components. (From Fehrenbach MJ, Herring SW. *Illustrated Anatomy of the Head and Neck,* ed 2. WB Saunders, Philadelphia, 2002.)

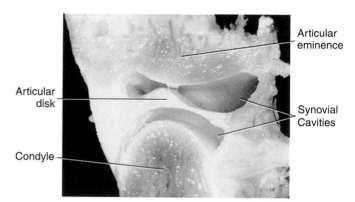

FIGURE 19-2 Block dissection of the temporomandibular joint. (From Nanci A. *Ten Cate's Oral Histology*, ed 6. Mosby, St. Louis, 2003.)

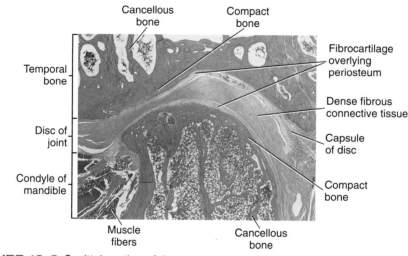

FIGURE 19-3 Sagittal section of the temporomandibular joint, including the articulating area of the temporal bone, the articulating surface of the condyle, and the disc and capsule of the joint. (Courtesy of Dr. Major M. Ash, Jr. BS, DDS, MS, MD hc, University of Michigan, Ann Arbor, MI.)

professionals must understand the anatomy, histology, and normal movements of the TMJ before being able to understand any possible disorders associated with the joint.

BONES OF THE JOINT

The TMJ is the articulation of the temporal bone and the mandible on each side of the head (Figure 19-1). A review of the basic anatomy of the bones may be necessary before the histology and actions of the TMJ can be discussed.

Temporal Bone

The articulating area on the temporal bone of the TMJ is located on the bone's inferior aspect (Figure 19-2).

This articulating area includes the bone's articular eminence and the articular fossa. The **articular eminence** is positioned anterior to the articular fossa and consists of a smooth, rounded protuberance on the inferior aspect of the zygomatic process.

The **articular fossa,** or mandibular fossa, is posterior to the articular eminence and consists of a depression on the inferior aspect of the temporal bone, posterior and medial to the zygomatic arch, the bony portion of the cheek. Posterior to the articular fossa is a sharper ridge, the postglenoid process.

The temporal bone consists of compact bone overlying cancellous bone (Figure 19-3; see Chapter 8). The outermost surface of compact bone is covered by periosteum. Like all bones, the innermost portion of the bone consists of endosteum and the medullary cavity with its bone marrow. The articulating bony

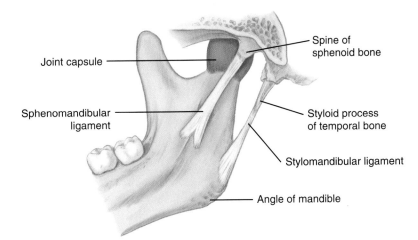

FIGURE 19-4 The joint capsule of the temporomandibular joint. (From Fehrenbach MJ, Herring SW. *Illustrated Anatomy of the Head and Neck,* ed 2. WB Saunders, Philadelphia, 2002.)

surface of the joint is covered by fibrocartilage immediately overlying the periosteum.

Mandible

The mandible articulates with each temporal bone at the heads of the condyle of the mandible with their **articulating surface of the condyle.** In a mature adult, each condyle consists of compact bone overlying cancellous bone (see Figure 19-2). Periosteum overlies the compact bone of the condyle, and the endosteum and bone marrow are located on the innermost portion of the bone. Fibrocartilage overlies the periosteum.

A growth center is located in the head of each condyle before an individual reaches maturity. This growth center consists of hyaline cartilage underneath the periosteum on the articulating surface of the condyle. This is the last growth center of bone in the body.

This area of cartilage within the bone grows in length by appositional growth as the individual grows to maturity. Over time, the cartilage is replaced by bone via endochondral ossification (see Chapter 8). When an individual reaches full maturity, the growth center of bone within the condyle has disappeared. This mandibular growth center in the condyle allows for the increased length of the mandible needed for the larger permanent teeth as well as for the larger brain capacity of the adult. This growth of the mandible also influences the overall shape of the face and thus is charted and used during orthodontic therapy (see Chapter 20).

JOINT CAPSULE

A **joint capsule** completely encloses the TMJ (see Figure 19-3 and Figure 19-4). The capsule wraps around the margin of the temporal bone's articular

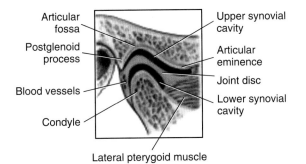

FIGURE 19-5 The disc of the temporomandibular joint and its synovial cavities. (From Fehrenbach MJ, Herring SW. *Illustrated Anatomy of the Head and Neck,* ed 2. WB Saunders, Philadelphia, 2002.)

eminence and articular fossa superiorly. Inferiorly, the capsule wraps around the circumference of the mandibular condyle, at the level of the condyle's neck.

The joint capsule has two layers. The outer layer is a firm, fibrous connective tissue supported by the surrounding ligaments associated with the joint. The inner layer is a **synovial membrane,** which consists of a thin connective tissue that contains nerves and blood vessels. The blood vessels in the synovial membrane produce **synovial fluid.** Synovial fluid is a thick substance that fills the joint, lubricates it, and provides nutrition to the avascular portions of the disc (discussed next).

DISC OF THE JOINT

A **disc of the joint** is located on each side between the temporal bone and condyle of the mandible (Figure 19-5 and see Figures 19-2 and 19-3). On section, each disc appears caplike on the mandibular condyle, with its superior aspect concavoconvex from anterior to posterior and its inferior aspect concave. This shape of the disc conforms to the shape of the adjacent articu-

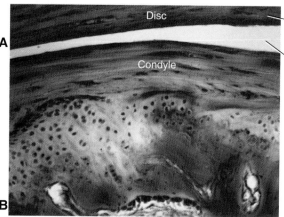

FIGURE 19-6 Microscopic appearance of the temporomandibular joint. **A:** Section of disc of the joint. **B:** Section of condyle of the mandible. (Courtesy of Dr. Major M. Ash, Jr. BS, DDS, MS, MD hc, University of Michigan, Ann Arbor, MI.)

lating bones of the TMJ and is related to normal joint movements.

The disc completely divides the TMJ into two compartments. These two compartments are **synovial cavities,** an upper and a lower synovial cavity. The synovial membrane lining the joint capsule produces the synovial fluid that fills these cavities.

The disc is attached to the lateral and medial poles of the mandibular condyle. The disc is not attached to the temporal bone anteriorly, except indirectly through the capsule. Posteriorly, the disc is divided into two areas. The upper division of the posterior portion of the disc is attached to the temporal bone's postglenoid process, and the lower division attaches to the neck of the condyle. The disc blends with the capsule at these points. This posterior area of attachment of the disc to the capsule is one of the places where nerves and blood vessels enter the joint.

The disc consists of dense fibrous connective tissue (Figure 19-6). Few cells are present, but fibroblasts and white blood cells are among these. The central area of the disc is avascular and lacks innervation, and the peripheral region has blood vessels and nerves. The central area is also thinner but of denser consistency than the peripheral region, which is thicker but has a more cushioned consistency. The synovial fluid in the synovial cavities provides the nutrition for the central area of the disc. With age, the disc thins and may undergo addition of cartilage in the central portion, changes that may lead to impaired movement of the joint (discussed later).

JAW MOVEMENTS OF THE JOINT

Two basic types of movement of the mandible are performed by the joint and its associated muscles of mastication: a gliding movement and a rotational movement (Figures 19-7 and 19-8 and see also Tables 19-1, 19-2, and 19-3).

The gliding movement of the TMJ occurs mainly between the disc and the articular eminence of the temporal bone in the upper synovial cavity, with the disc plus the condyle moving forward or backward, down and up the articular eminence. The gliding movement allows the lower jaw to move forward or backward. Bringing the lower jaw forward involves **protrusion of the mandible.** Bringing the lower jaw backward involves **retraction of the mandible.**

The rotational movement of the TMJ occurs mainly between the disc and the condyle of the mandible in the lower synovial cavity. The axis of rotation of the disc plus the condyle is transverse, and the movements accomplished are depression or elevation of the mandible. The **depression of the mandible** is the lowering of the lower jaw. The **elevation of the mandible** is the raising of the lower jaw.

With these two types of movements, gliding and rotation, and with the right and left TMJs working together, the finer movements of the jaw can be accomplished. These include opening and closing the jaws and shifting the lower jaw to one side.

Opening the jaws, which occurs during mastication, speech, and respiratory movements, involves both depression and protrusion of the mandible. When the jaws close, both elevation and retraction of the mandible occur. Thus the natural opening and closing of the jaws involve a combination of gliding and rotational movements of the TMJs in their respective joint cavities. The disc plus the condyle glides on the articular fossa in the upper synovial cavity, moving forward or backward on the articular eminence. At approximately the same time, the condyle of the mandible rotates on the disc in the lower synovial cavity.

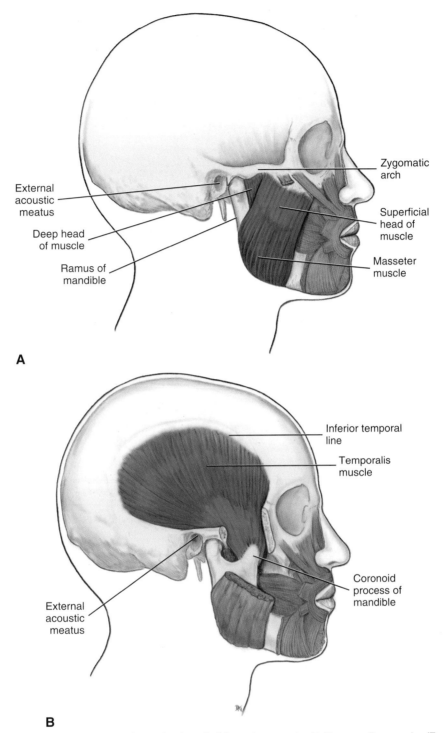

FIGURE 19-7 Muscles of mastication. **A:** Masseter muscle. **B:** Temporalis muscle. (From Fehrenbach MJ, Herring SW. *Illustrated Anatomy of the Head and Neck,* ed 2. WB Saunders, Philadelphia, 2002.)

Continued

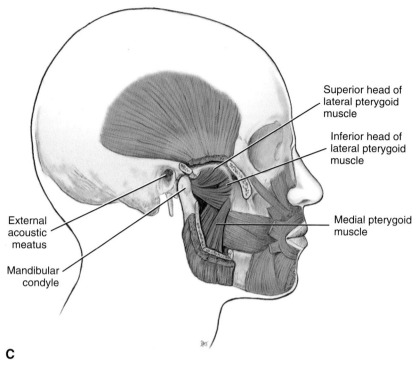

C

FIGURE 19-7, cont'd **C:** Medical and lateral pterygoid muscles.

TABLE 19-1

The Origin and Insertion of the Muscles of Mastication

Muscles	Origin	Insertion
Masseter	**Superficial head:** anterior two-thirds of the lower border of the zygomatic arch **Deep head:** posterior one-third and medial surface of zygomatic arch	**Superficial head:** angle of mandible **Deep head:** ramus of mandible
Temporalis	Temporal fossa	Coronoid process of mandible
Medial pterygoid	Pterygoid fossa of the sphenoid bone	Angle of mandible
Lateral pterygoid	**Superior head:** greater wing of sphenoid bone **Inferior head:** lateral pterygoid plate from the sphenoid bone	**Both heads:** pterygoid fovea of the condyle of the mandible

(From Fehrenbach MJ, Herring SW. *Illustrated Anatomy of the Head and Neck,* ed 2. WB Saunders, Philadelphia, 2002.)

Lateral deviation of the mandible, or lateral excursion, which involves shifting the lower jaw to one side, occurs during mastication. Thus lateral deviation involves both gliding and rotational movements of opposite TMJs in their respective joint cavities. During lateral deviation, one disc plus the condyle glides forward and medially on the articular eminence in the upper synovial cavity, while the other condyle and disc remain relatively stable in position in the articular fossa. These actions produce rotation around the more stable condyle.

During mastication, the power stroke (when the teeth crunch the food) involves a movement from a laterally deviated position back to the midline. If the food is on the right side of the mouth, the mandible is deviated to the right. The power stroke returns the mandible to the center, and thus the movement is to the left and involves retraction of the left side. The reverse situation occurs if the food is on the left.

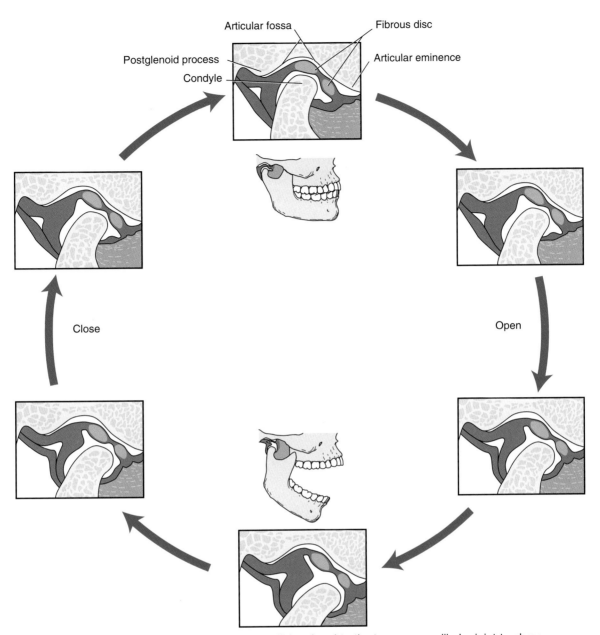

FIGURE 19-8 Movements of the mandible related to the temporomandibular joint to show opening and closing of the mouth.

TABLE 19-2

The Muscles of Mastication with Associated Movements of Mandible

Muscles of Mastication	Movements of Mandible
Masseter	Elevation of mandible (during jaw closing)
Temporalis	Elevation of mandible (during jaw closing) Retraction of mandible (lower jaw backward)
Medial pterygoid	Elevation of mandible (during jaw closing)
Lateral pterygoid	**Inferior heads:** slight depression of mandible (during jaw opening) **One muscle:** lateral deviation of mandible (to shift the lower jaw to the opposite side) **Both muscles:** protrusion of mandible (lower jaw forward)

(From Fehrenbach MJ, Herring SW. *Illustrated Anatomy of the Head and Neck*, ed 2. WB Saunders, Philadelphia, 2002.)

TABLE 19-3

Movements of the Mandible and Temporomandibular Joint

Mandibular Movements	Temporomandibular Joint Movements
Protrusion of mandible, moving lower jaw forward	Gliding in both upper synovial cavities
Retraction of mandible, moving lower jaw backward	Gliding in both upper synovial cavities
Elevation and retraction of mandible, closing the jaws	Gliding in both upper synovial cavities and rotation in both lower synovial cavities
Depression and protrusion of the mandible, opening the jaws	Gliding in both upper synovial cavities and rotation in both lower synovial cavities
Lateral deviation of mandible, to shift lower jaw to the opposite side	Gliding in one upper synovial cavity and rotation in the opposite upper synovial cavity

(From Fehrenbach MJ, Herring SW. *Illustrated Anatomy of the Head and Neck*, ed 2. WB Saunders, Philadelphia, 2002.)

DISORDERS OF THE JOINT

Patients may have a disorder associated with one or both of their TMJs, or a temporomandibular disorder (TMD). Patients may experience chronic joint tenderness, swelling, and painful muscle spasms. They may also have difficulties in moving the joint, such as a limited or deviated mandibular opening.

Recognition of TMD includes palpation of the joint as the patient performs all the movements of the joint. Also palpated are the related muscles of mastication. All signs and symptoms related to the TMD, such as the amount of mandibular opening and facial pain, should be recorded, as should any parafunctional habits and related systemic diseases. To aid in diagnosis, traditional skull radiograph or magnetic resonance imaging (MRI) of the joint may be used (Figure 19-9). This noninvasive procedure for imaging soft tissue uses no ionizing radiation.

Many controversies are associated with the etiology of these disorders. TMD is a heterogeneous, complex disorder involving many factors such as behavioral stressors and parafunctional habits such as clenching and grinding or bruxism (see Chapter 20). Trauma to the jaw may cause TMD with the disc having adhesions to the bony surfaces, but it is not the most common etiological factor. Systemic diseases such as osteoarthritis may involve portions of the TMJ and contribute to TMD. Aging of the disc that causes wear and hardening may also be a factor in TMD; however, TMD does not become worse with age.

Not all patients with TMD have abnormalities in the joint disc or the joint itself. Most symptoms seem to originate from the muscles. Most recent studies do not support the role of TMD in directly causing headaches, neck pain, or back pain or instability. However, cyclic episodes of TMD and other incidents of chronic body pain are commonly encountered in the population with TMD.

Joint sounds can occur because of disc derangement as the posterior portion of the disc becomes caught between the condyle head and the articular eminence. Joint sounds are not a reliable indicator of TMD because they can change over time in a patient. The clicking, grinding, and popping of the joint during movement that are commonly present with TMD are also found in persons without TMD.

Many controversies surround the treatment of TMD, and fewer than half of patients with TMD seek treatment for their disorder. Most recent studies have determined that malocclusion and occlusal discrepancies are not involved in most cases of TMD. Thus occlusal adjustment, repositioning the jaw, and orthodontic treatment are not the treatments of choice for all patients with TMD, nor do these treatments seem to prevent TMD.

Most cases of TMD improve over time with inexpensive and reversible treatments, including patient-based or prescription pain control, relaxation therapy, stress management, habit control, moderate

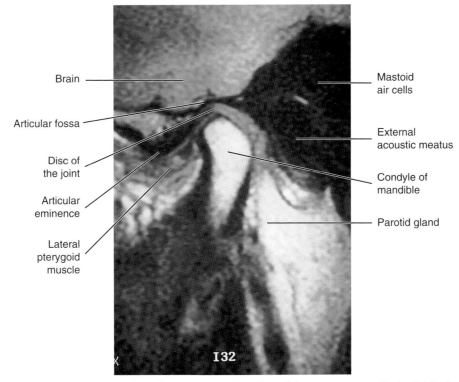

Brain

Articular fossa

Disc of
the joint

Articular
eminence

Lateral
pterygoid
muscle

Mastoid
air cells

External
acoustic meatus

Condyle of
mandible

Parotid gland

I 32

FIGURE 19-9 Coronal magnetic resonance imaging of the temporomandibular joint of an aysmptomatic individual (From Quinn PD. *Color Atlas of Temporomandibular Joint Surgery.* Mosby, St. Louis, 1998.)

home-based muscular exercises, and flat plane nonrepositioning oral splints. These inexpensive and reversible treatments are now showing the same success as more expensive and irreversible treatments. Thus only a few patients with TMD require surgery or other extensive treatment. Surgery of the TMJ can now make use of arthroscopy with an endoscope and lasers.

An acute episode of TMD can occur when a patient opens too wide, causing maximal depression and protrusion of the mandible, as when yawning or receiving prolonged dental care. This causes **subluxation,** or partial dislocation of both joints. Subluxation occurs when the head of each condyle moves too far anteriorly past the articular eminence. Then, when the patient tries to close and elevate the mandible, the condylar heads cannot move posteriorly because both the bony relationships prevent it and the muscles have become spastic.

Treatment of subluxation consists of relaxation of these muscles and careful movement of the mandible downward and back. The condylar heads can then assume the normal posterior position in relation to the articular eminence by the muscular action of the elevating muscles of mastication. These patients must in the future refrain from extreme depression of the mandible.

CHAPTER 20

Occlusion

This chapter discusses the following topics:

- Occlusion
- Normal occlusion
- Centric occlusion
  - Arch form
  - Dental curvatures and angulations
  - Centric stops and relation
  - Lateral and protrusive occlusion
- Mandibular rest position
- Malocclusion
  - Classification of malocclusion
  - Parafunctional habits
  - Skeletal considerations
  - Myofunctional considerations

After studying this chapter, the reader should be able to:

1. Define and pronounce the key terms in this chapter.
2. Describe centric occlusion and its relationship to movement of the mandible.
3. Describe Angle's classification of malocclusion.
4. Discuss parafunctional habits, myofunctional and skeletal considerations, and occlusal trauma and their relationship to occlusion.
5. Integrate the knowledge of occlusion into the dental treatment of a patient.

Key Terms

Abfraction (ab-frak-shen)
Angle's classification of
  malocclusion (mal-ah-kloo-zhun)
Balancing interference
Bruxism (bruk-sizm)
Canine rise
Centric stops, relation
Clenching
Contact areas
Crossbite
Curve of Spee, Wilson
Distal step
End-to-end bite
Flush terminal plane

Gnathic index (nath-ick)
Golden Proportion
Group function
Interocclusal clearance (in-ter-
  ah-kloo-zhal)
Leeway space
Malocclusion (mal-ah-kloo-zhun):
  Class I, Class II, Class III, division
  I, division II
Mesial drift, step
Mesognathic (me-so-nath-ik)
Occlusal trauma
Occlusion (ah-kloo-zhun): centric,
  lateral, primary, protrusive

Open bite
Overbite
Overjet
Parafunctional habits
  (pare-ah-funk-shun-al)
Premature contacts
Primate spaces
Prognathic (prog-nath-ik)
Retrognathic (ret-row-nath-ik)
Root axis line
Side: balancing, working
Supporting cusps
Terminal plane
Vertical dimension of the face

OCCLUSION

Occlusion is the contact relationship between the maxillary and mandibular teeth when the jaws are in a fully closed position, as well as the relationship between the teeth in the same arch. Occlusion develops in a child as the primary teeth erupt. During this time, oral motor behavior develops and masticatory skills are acquired. Occlusion of the erupting permanent teeth is dependent on the occlusion of the primary teeth as they are being shed.

Interrelated factors are involved in the development of the occlusion, such as the associated musculature, neuromuscular patterns, and temporomandibular joint functioning (see Chapter 19 for more information). Thus occlusion is only one aspect of an entire developing masticatory system that includes these other factors. The teeth in proper alignment are self-cleansing by action of check musculature and saliva flow over the smooth tooth surfaces.

When the teeth are not aligned properly, they lose the ability to self cleanse. More importantly, when teeth of either dentition are not occluding properly, the teeth and periodontium may not be able to perform the functions for which they were designed, and unnatural occlusal stress is placed on them, possibly resulting in occlusal disharmony. Occlusal disharmony may then lead to **occlusal trauma.** The teeth and the periodontium are able to withstand many of these daily stresses, but these stresses are often excessive, such as with parafunctional habits (discussed later). Microscopic changes within the periodontium can occur with occlusal trauma (see Chapter 14 for more information).

Dental professionals must remember that occlusal trauma does not directly cause periodontal disease, although it may be an adverse factor in an already weakened and diseased periodontium. Occlusal trauma can usually be stopped if the etiological factors are removed or the involved teeth are protected from these stresses. Unfortunately, the effects of occlusal trauma may not be reversible. These occlusal disharmonies also should be considered during dental treatment.

Occlusal therapy should not be initiated unless signs or symptoms indicate harmful effects from these occlusal disharmonies. The effects on a patient's occlusion must also be kept in mind during all phases of dental treatment, especially during restorative treatment.

NORMAL OCCLUSION

An ideal occlusion rarely exists, but the concept of a normal occlusion provides a basis for treatment. The optimum 138 occlusal contacts for the permanent den-

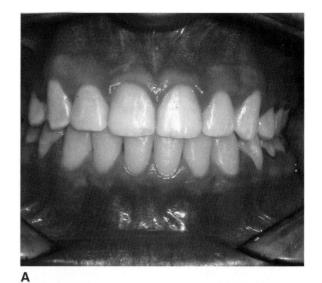

A

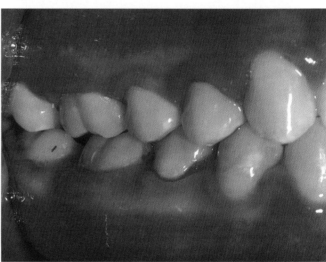

B

FIGURE 20-1 Permanent dentition in centric occlusion. **A:** Facial view. **B:** Buccal view. A normal level of overjet is also present, observed as the horizontal overlap between the two arches. Also shown is a normal amount of overbite, which is the vertical overlap between the two arches. Note the three different segments of each arch, which are used when describing arch form: anterior, middle, and posterior. (Courtesy of Dr. Dona M. Seely, DDS, MSD, Orthodontic Associates, Bellevue, Washington.)

tition in the closure of 32 teeth are seldom, if ever, achieved. When occlusion is considered, the position of the dentition in centric occlusion serves as the basis for reference. Thus centric occlusion serves as the standard for describing a normal occlusion. To prevent occlusal disharmony, all patients should have an occlusal evaluation before and after completion of their dental treatment plan.

CENTRIC OCCLUSION

Centric occlusion (CO), or habitual occlusion, is the voluntary position of the dentition that allows the

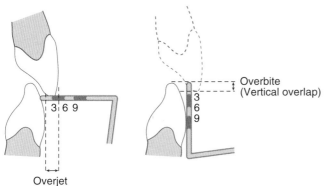

FIGURE 20-2 A comparison of overjet, the horizontal overlap between the two arches, and overbite, the vertical overlap between the two arches.

maximum contact when the teeth occlude (Figure 20-1). Centric occlusion is related to the functioning of the dentition. However, even when the teeth are in full closure, discrepancy between the relationships of the mandible or temporomandibular joints and the maxilla may be significant (skeletal discrepancies are discussed later).

When the teeth of a normal occlusion are in the position of centric occlusion, each tooth of one arch is in occlusion with two others in the opposing arch, except for the mandibular central incisors and maxillary third molars. This structure serves to equalize the forces of impact in occlusion. Another benefit of this arrangement is that if a tooth is lost in one jaw, the alignment of the opposing jaw is not immediately disturbed. One antagonist remains until adequate restorative treatment can be performed.

If a tooth is lost for a longer period, the neighboring teeth usually tip in an effort to fill the edentulous space. The teeth become inclined, and supereruption of the tooth opposing the space then occurs (discussed in Chapter 17 with the loss of the maxillary or mandibular first molars). Thus loss of one tooth disturbs the contact relationships in that area as well as those in the opposing arch, possibly causing changes in the occlusion of the entire dentition. Patients must understand when discussing tooth replacement that teeth are like building blocks: Pull one out of the construction, and they all fall down, possibly resulting in occlusal disharmonies.

When the teeth normally occlude in centric occlusion, the maxillary dental arch naturally overhangs the mandibular arch facially, a position called **overjet** (Figure 20-2). This normal amount of horizontal overlap between the two arches associated with overjet allows for the extensions of movement in the mandible and keeps the soft tissue of the oral cavity out of the way during mastication.

Overjet is measured in millimeters with the tip of a periodontal probe once a patient is in centric occlusion. The probe is placed at a right angle to the labial surface of a mandibular incisor at the base of the incisal edge of a maxillary incisor. The measurement is taken from the labial surface of the mandibular incisor to the lingual surface of the maxillary incisor. Note that the labiolingual width of the maxillary incisor is not included in the measurement.

In centric occlusion, the maxillary incisors also overlap the mandibular incisors, a position called **overbite** (see Figure 20-2). This normal amount of vertical overlap between the two arches allows for contact between the posterior teeth during mastication. Both overjet and overbite tend to decrease with age as a result of attrition, and excessive amounts of either are classified as a malocclusion (discussed later).

Overbite is measured in millimeters with the tip of a periodontal probe after a patient is placed in centric occlusion. The probe is placed on the incisal edge of the maxillary incisor at right angles to the mandibular incisor. As patients open their mouths or depress their jaws, the probe is then placed vertically against the mandibular incisor to measure the distance to the incisal edge of the mandibular incisor. Studies show that overjet measurements were equally distributed among males and females, but overbite was noted more often in females. However, neither measurement was predictably associated with any particular craniofacial pattern. Both overjet and overbite tend to diminish with age, initially because of mandibular growth and later because of wear.

Within each dental arch, the teeth also create **contact areas** as they contact their same-arch neighbors on their proximal surfaces (except the last tooth in each arch of each dentition, which lacks a distal contact). This contact between neighboring teeth serves two purposes: It protects the interdental gingiva or papillae and stabilizes each tooth in the dental arch. These contacts have been discussed with regard to the individual permanent teeth in Chapters 16 and 17.

Open contacts allow for areas of food impaction from opposing cusps, called plunging cusps, resulting in trauma to the interdental gingiva. Open contacts also do not allow for mesiodistal stability between the teeth. Correct restorative treatment should not allow any open contacts unless tooth position and tooth loss make this impossible. Although the practice is controversial, periodontal splints are often placed in the mouth lingually with tooth-colored resins and wires to simulate this stability needed for the teeth within the dental arch. All prosthetic treatment within the mouth, including the placement of bridges, implants, and removable dentures, is an attempt to simulate this stability.

Certain topics must be considered when studying centric occlusion: arch form and its development, dental curvatures and angulations, centric stops, centric relation, lateral and protrusive occlusion, and mandibular rest position.

Arch Form

Each arch of the permanent dentition is divided into three segments when describing arch form: anterior, middle, and posterior (see Figure 20-1). The anterior segment includes the anterior teeth, the middle segment includes the premolars, and the posterior segment includes the molars. The concept of arch segments allows the arches to overlap slightly so that canines and first molars are cooperating in more than one segment. This arrangement serves to indicate that the canines and first molars function as anchor supports for both arches.

The anterior segment of each dental arch is curved and ends at the labial ridges of the canines. The middle segment is straight and extends from the distal portion of the canines to the buccal cervical ridge of the mesiobuccal cusp of the first molar in each arch. The posterior segment creates a straight line, starting from the buccal cusps of the first molars and remaining in contact with the buccal surfaces of the second and third molars.

PHASES OF ARCH DEVELOPMENT

Each dental arch goes through phases of development as the permanent teeth erupt and the primary teeth are being shed (see Figure 6-26 for the chronological timetable for eruption of both dentitions). During this time, the jaw develops and undergoes lengthening to achieve its mature form and accommodate the larger permanent teeth.

Phase one occurs when the permanent first molars erupt. These teeth add dramatically to the chewing efficiency and jaw development during a period of rapid growth of the child. They help support the jaws while the primary anterior teeth are being shed and the other permanent teeth are erupting. The primate spaces in the primary dentition are still present (as noted in Chapter 18) to allow for future space for the permanent teeth.

Phase two occurs with eruption of the permanent anterior teeth near the midline of the oral cavity. First the centrals, then the laterals generally erupt lingually to the primary anterior roots. However, shedding of the primary teeth and jaw growth finally place them labial to the position of the primary teeth they replaced.

In addition, the permanent location of the anterior teeth is not established until the development of the arch form is complete. Thus some degree of transient anterior crowding may occur at approximately 8 or 9 years of age and persist until the emergence of the canines, when the space for the teeth is adequate again. However, incisor crowding that persists into a permanent dentition is considered a type of malocclusion (discussed later).

Phase three in the development of the form of the dental arches begins when the premolars erupt anterior to the permanent molars. Developmentally, this is quite significant because the premolars are so much smaller than the primary molars they replace. This difference in size mesiodistally between the two types of teeth is called the **leeway space** (Figures 20-3 and 20-4). The contour of the bone covering the narrower roots of the premolars, in addition to the state of flux of the bone formation in this area, furnishes adjustment for dental arch measurements, making the middle segment of the arches important architecturally. Thus this space allows for the future forward movement of the molars (discussed later with regard to the occlusion of the primary teeth).

If the second molars erupt before the premolars, the arch perimeter is significantly shortened and occlusal disharmony is likely to occur, as is malocclusion (discussed later). A fixed or removable space maintainer may be used to save this leeway space from the primary molars for the premolars.

Phase four begins when the canines wedge themselves between the lateral incisors and the first premolars. Contact relations between the teeth are established, and the arch is complete from the first molar forward. Simultaneously, the second molars are due to emerge distally to the first molars and support them during the wedging activity of the canines.

Phase five is the final phase of the development of the dental arch form and consists of eruption of the third molars. Often the jaw length is not sufficient for eruption of these last teeth (see Chapter 17).

Thus the sequence for eruption of both the primary and permanent dentition is favorable (Figures 20-5 and 20-6). Keeping this sequence in mind for each dentition is part of the treatment to prevent disruption in patients with primary and mixed dentition. Disruption of this sequence, with overretention or early loss of primary teeth, may allow for problems to occur with the eruption of the permanent dentition. Proper treatment of these cases with disruption in the eruption sequence and early orthodontic referral increase the chances for a normal occlusion. It is important to note that attrition of the proximal surfaces also reduces the mesial-distal dimensions of the teeth and significantly reduces arch length over a lifetime. Some crowding or spacing may also occur after the age of 40 years.

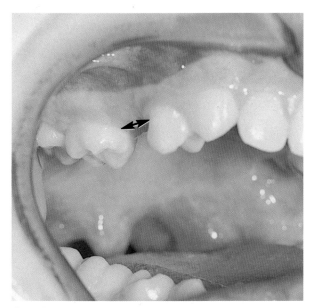

FIGURE 20-3 Leeway space in the maxillary arch is evident (*double-headed arrow*) during the mixed dentition period and in phase three of the development of the dental arches. This space is due to the difference in size mesiodistally between the primary molars and the permanent premolars.

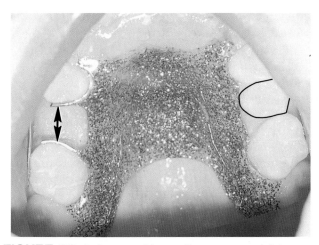

FIGURE 20-4 A removable maxillary space maintainer (sparkle variety) to hold the leeway space from the primary maxillary molar (*double-headed arrow*) for future eruption of the permanent premolars because the permanent maxillary second molar has already erupted. Note that the permanent maxillary second premolar on the opposite side is fully erupted (*outlined*), and no leeway space needs to be maintained.

Dental Curvatures and Angulations

A common mistake is to assume that the forces of occlusion act on squared and flat teeth in straight lines or planes and that the axes of the teeth are at right angles to their masticatory surfaces. Many dental curvatures and angulations are present in normal occlusion and must be considered.

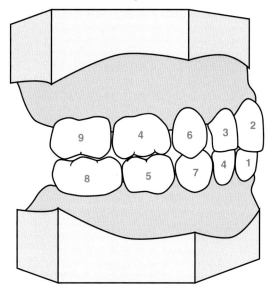

FIGURE 20-5 Favorable sequence of eruption (1-9) for both arches of the primary dentition.

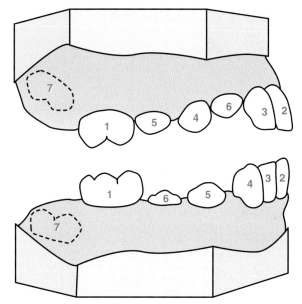

FIGURE 20-6 Favorable sequence of eruption (1-6) per arch of the permanent dentition.

If imaginary planes are placed on the masticatory surfaces of each dental arch, the arches do not conform to these flat planes (Figure 20-7). The maxillary arch is convex occlusally, and the mandibular arch is concave. This anteroposterior curvature is called the **curve of Spee.** The curve of Spee is produced by the curved alignment of all the teeth (especially evident when viewing the posterior teeth from the buccal).

Another curve is the **curve of Wilson** (see Figure 20-7). This concave curve results when a frontal section is taken through each set of both maxillary and

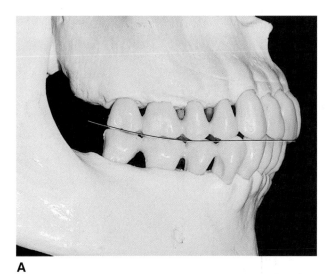

A

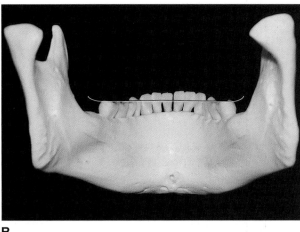

B

FIGURE 20-7 Curves noted in the dental arch. **A:** Curve of Spee noted in the permanent dental arches, with the maxillary arch convex and the mandibular arch concave. **B:** Curve of Wilson noted in the permanent mandibular arch, which is a concave curve that results when a frontal section is taken through each set of molars.

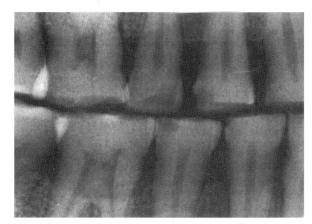

FIGURE 20-8 Attrition, or wear, of the masticatory surfaces of the teeth noted on a radiograph. The result is a loss of the curvatures of the teeth.

mandibular molars, the firsts, seconds, and then thirds. These imaginary dental curvatures are interesting, but it is important to note that modern dentistry does not use these often in practice because they have only a remote association with functional relationships. Both these curves tend to be lost with age as a result of attrition (Figure 20-8).

Individual teeth also exhibit some forms of curvature. Curves are found in the basic form of each tooth. Every third of a tooth represents a curved surface, except where a tooth is worn or fractured. These curvatures of the teeth should be noted when drawing them and especially as one takes the average measurements of the teeth and assigns them to drawing paper, hoping to achieve lifelike drawings. These curves also must be noted when restoring the teeth for proper function and aesthetics.

When a tooth is bisected by its **root axis line (RAL),** angulations of each tooth's root (or roots) within the alveolar bone are noted (discussed per tooth type in Chapters 16 and 17; Figure 20-9). This angled arrangement of the teeth allows for proper spacing between the roots for blood and nerve supply and for securing anchorage of the roots in the jawbones.

Each tooth is placed at the angle that best withstands the lines of forces brought against it during function in normal occlusion. The angle at which it is placed depends on the function that the tooth must perform. If the tooth is placed at a disadvantage because of misalignment in the dental arch, its functional efficiency is limited and the permanence of its position is endangered. The anteriors seem to be placed at a disadvantage because they are more vertically situated in the alveolar bone, but their function is only the momentary biting and cutting of food, not the full force of chewing that occurs in the posterior teeth, which usually have more angulation.

The masticatory surface of teeth does not have any flat planes unless some are created by wear or accident. Therefore during occlusion, the curved surface of one tooth always comes into contact with the curved surfaces of another tooth. Escapement space for food during mastication is provided by the form of the cusps and ridges, sulci and developmental grooves, and the embrasures when the teeth come together in occlusion. These escapement spaces are necessary for efficient occlusion during mastication.

The location and form of the escapement spaces are immediately changed when the occlusal relation is changed, as with attrition or restorative treatment. Whether these changes are related in any form to loss of function of the teeth or masticatory system is controversial. However, knowing the angulation of the roots within the alveolar bone is essential for the

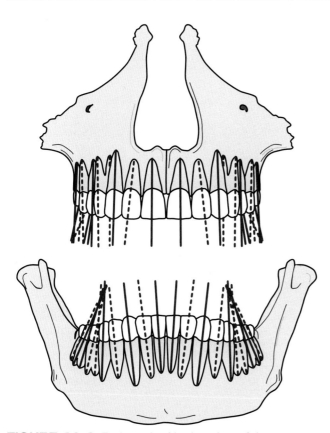

FIGURE 20-9 Each tooth of both arches of the permanent dentition is bisected by its root axis line, showing the angulations of the root within the alveolar bone of the arch.

proper adaptation during radiographs and instrumentation. This measurement is also considered when evaluating a patient's smile.

Centric Stops

When the teeth are in centric occlusion, they should have maximal interdigitation with locking of the two arch positions. The three areas of centric contacts, or **centric stops,** between the two arches are height of cusp contour, marginal ridges, and central fossae (Figure 20-10). Those cusps that function during centric occlusion are called the **supporting cusps** and include the lingual cusps of the maxillary posterior teeth and the buccal cusps of the mandibular posterior teeth. The incisal edges of the mandibular anterior teeth are usually included as supporting cusps.

These centric stops and supporting cusps are checked using articulating paper when restorative or prosthetic treatment is performed (Figure 20-11). An occlusal adjustment involving the removal of restorative, prosthetic, or natural tooth material may be necessary, depending on the results of the occlusal evaluation.

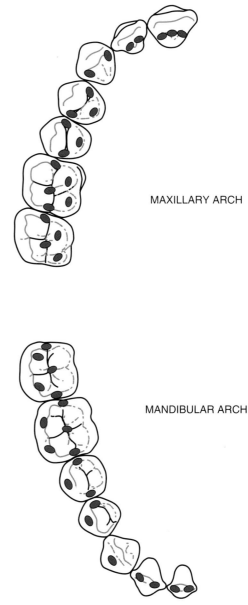

MAXILLARY ARCH

MANDIBULAR ARCH

FIGURE 20-10 The ideal centric stops between the two arches are highlighted. Note that the stops include the height of cusp contour, marginal ridges, and central fossae of the teeth.

A dental manikin with unworn teeth may help show the location of these centric stops and supporting cusps if articulating paper is used and mastication is simulated. The relationship of centric stops to the masticatory surfaces is not rigidly set and may vary considerably among individuals. Centric stops are often in the central fossa and are related to the inner surface of the marginal ridges rather than the embrasure surfaces of the ridges, as indicated in an ideal mapping of centric stops.

These contact relationships change with wear of the dentition. With advancing attrition, the supporting

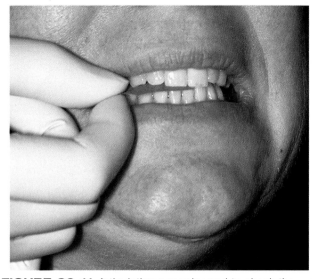

FIGURE 20-11 Articulating paper is used to check the centric stops after restorative treatment.

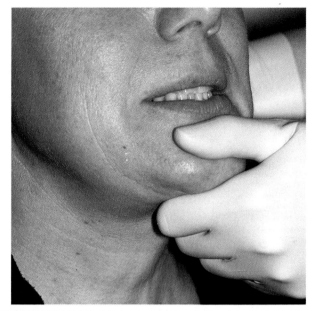

FIGURE 20-12 Attaining centric relation in a patient. The clinician must establish the hinge movement of the mandible by gently arcing the mandible with the fingers in a closing and opening manner several times before attempting placement of the loosened jaw into centric relation, the end point of closure of the mandible in which the mandible is in the most retruded position.

cusps are seated closer and closer to the bottoms of the opposing fossae. This process continues until the development of numerous flat surface contacts, which are termed *occlusal wear facets*. This process can result in the loss of a definite locking of the two jaws in centric occlusion.

The position of the centric stops helps determine the height of the lower one third of the **vertical dimension of the face** when the teeth are in centric occlusion (see Chapter 1). This dimension cannot be exactly measured in patients with teeth, and thus its loss requires clinical judgment. It is based on the **Golden Proportion** as it relates to the face, as discussed in Chapter 1. This dimension is involved in the proper functioning of the teeth and jaws and the aesthetic appearance of a patient. Loss of this portion of the vertical dimension is based on alveolar bone loss and attrition and is discussed in Chapter 14.

Centric Relation

Centric relation (CR) is the end point of closure of the mandible; the mandible is in the most retruded position to which it can be carried by the musculature and ligaments (see Chapter 19 for more information). Even though a patient is rarely in centric relation, except sometimes when swallowing, centric relation is a base measurement from which to evaluate a patient's occlusion because it can be easily repeated.

To attain centric relation, the mandible must undergo complete retraction (Figure 20-12). Centric relation must be determined by the clinician without a patient's muscle participation. To do this, the clinician must gently establish the hinge movement of the mandible on the patient by gently arcing the mandible

with the fingers in a closing and opening manner several times, before attempting placement of the loosened jaw into centric relation. Researchers are currently exploring various ways of clinically relaxing patients' jaws to determine this position of the mandible more precisely.

Ideally, when the mandible is in centric relation, the dentition should be in centric occlusion (thus centric relation equals centric occlusion, or CR=CO). Therefore no major shift of the dentition from centric relation occlusion to centric occlusion should occur. However, the average distance of shift or slide from a patient's occlusion in centric relation to centric occlusion is approximately 1 mm.

Centric occlusion can be attained by having a patient who is in centric relation squeeze his or her teeth together after achieving centric relation. The amount and pathway of shift in the dentition can then be recorded during the occlusal evaluation. This procedure can be simulated by clinicians with their own dentition by putting the head back (centric relation) and then closing their teeth when they bring their head forward (centric occlusion).

The slide or shift in the position of the dentition from centric relation to centric occlusion (centric relation does not equal centric occlusion or CR ≠ CO) should be noted. It is most often caused by **premature contacts** where one or two teeth initially contact before the other teeth. This premature contact may cause occlusal disharmony. Additional slide between the teeth in centric relation to centric occlusion is also associated with tooth malalignment, improper intercuspation of the teeth, improper restorative treatment, and inherited arch lengths and relationships.

Lateral and Protrusive Occlusion

Masticatory movement entails not only the mandible going through elevation and depression but also excursions from side to side and forward, such as lateral deviation and protrusion (see Chapter 19 for a discussion of mandibular movements). Therefore other movements besides centric occlusion and its relationship to the teeth must be evaluated.

Evaluation of **lateral occlusion** is made by moving the mandible either to the right or to the left until the canines on that side are in a cusp-to-cusp relationship (Figure 20-13). Before the canines contact on each side, no other individual teeth should be contacting during lateral occlusion. The side to which the mandible has been moved is called the **working side.** Two working sides are noted in an occlusal evaluation: right lateral and left lateral. The side of the arch opposite to the working side during lateral occlusion is called the **balancing side.**

In normal occlusion, the canine should be the only tooth in function during lateral occlusion; this is called **canine rise,** or *cuspid rise.* Thus the mandible is moved to the working side when checking lateral occlusion until the opposite arch canines are edge to edge. If other teeth are involved in function during lateral occlusion, they must be noted; for example, the first molars may present problems for the dentition.

If the canine rise does not exist on the working side because of cusp wear caused by parafunctional habits or tooth malalignment, it is acceptable that most of the entire posterior quadrant functions during lateral occlusion. This is called **group function** because all opposite arch posterior teeth are sharing the occlusal stress during function.

No teeth should make contact on the opposite balancing side during lateral occlusion. If teeth are in contact on the balancing side, this is called a **balancing interference.** Balancing interference can be involved in occlusal disharmonies. For further confirmation of any balancing interferences during lateral deviation, floss can be placed over the occlusal surfaces on the appropriate side (Figure 20-14).

With the mandible in **protrusive occlusion,** all eight of the most anterior teeth (centrals and laterals) of both arches are normally in contact as the mandible undergoes protrusion (Figure 20-15). If only one or two assume the stress of protrusion, occlusal disharmony may occur.

Mandibular Rest Position

The physiological rest position of the mandible is achieved when the mandible is being held in a relaxed

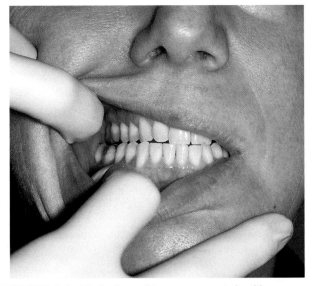

FIGURE 20-13 Patient with a permanent dentition undergoing lateral deviation or excursion to check the lateral occlusion on the working side (side to which the mandible has been moved) and balancing side (other side of the arch from working side). Note that the mandible is being moved until the opposite arch canines are edge to edge so that they are in canine rise.

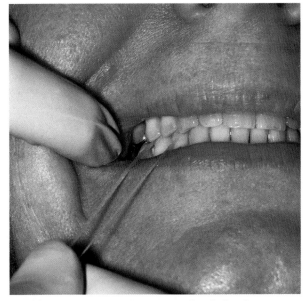

FIGURE 20-14 Using floss to confirm balancing interferences where teeth contact on the balancing side during lateral occlusion.

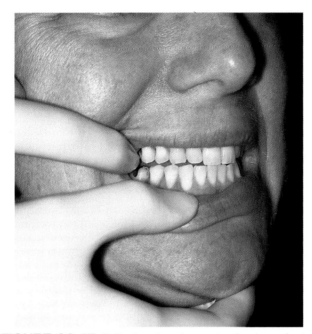

FIGURE 20-15 Patient undergoing protrusion to evaluate protrusive occlusion.

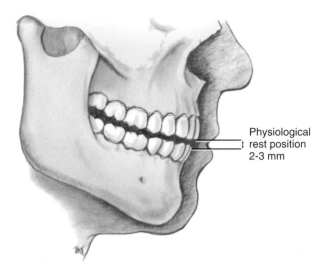

Physiological rest position 2-3 mm

FIGURE 20-16 The physiological rest position of the mandible, or interocclusal clearance of about 2 to 3 mm.

state and is not being used in mastication, speech, or respiratory movements (Figure 20-16). With this rest position, an average space of 2 or 3 mm is noted between the masticatory surfaces of the maxillary and mandibular teeth. This space between the arches when the mandible is at rest is the **interocclusal clearance,** or freeway space.

This position of the mandible at rest is considered fairly stable, although it can be influenced by posture, fatigue, and tension. Thus failure to assume this position when the jaws are not at work may mean that the patient is temporarily tense or has parafunctional habits such as clenching or grinding (bruxism), which may be involved in occlusal problems (discussed later).

MALOCCLUSION

Malocclusion is related to lack of an overall ideal form in the dentition while in centric occlusion. Rarely, malocclusion is directly associated with severe occlusal trauma. Malocclusion may affect patients by having a negative impact on their appearance and increasing their difficulty with oral hygiene procedures. Poor oral hygiene favors bacterial plaque biofilm retention and increases the possibility that periodontal disease will affect the dentition with a malocclusion. Many malocclusions stem from hereditary factors.

An orthodontist working with other specialists, such as speech therapists, can correct most malocclu-

sions related only to the teeth and not to the rest of the masticatory system (see the discussion of orthodontic movement in Chapter 14). However, even during correction of a malocclusion to achieve a more ideal form for the dentition, the occlusal functioning of the dentition also must be considered. Early intervention in the primary and mixed dentitions can prevent many malocclusions.

Approximately 80 percent of children and teenagers show some degree of malocclusion. The most common problems are crowding, a type of malocclusion that affects 40 percent of children and 80 percent of teenagers. The second most common type of malocclusion is excessive overjet of the maxillary incisors, which affects approximately 15 percent of children and teenagers. Other factors are also involved in the consideration of smile design, such as gender, symmetry of color or shape, and position of teeth about the midline. A negative space (dark area) is also a consideration within an ideal smile and highlights the rest of the smile. The back of the mouth is considered a desired negative space because no light enters when standing. An example of an undesirable negative space is anterior or lateral crowded teeth creating shadows, a diastema, or even a loss of a prominent tooth that stands out from the whiteness of the rest of the teeth. For a long time, clinicians have used **Angle's classification of malocclusion** (Table 20-1) because it has not been adequately replaced by another system. Although Angle's system has many inadequacies, it does serve to initially and simply address malocclusion. Many malocclusions do not fit neatly into Angle's system, but this classification system of malocclusion does give clinicians a starting point in describing a particular case.

TABLE 20-1

Angle's Classification of Malocclusion*

Class	Model	Arch Relationships	Descriptions
Class I		Molar: MB cusp of the maxillary first occluding with the MB groove of the mandibular first Canines: Maxillary occluding with the distal half of the mandibular canine and the mesial half of the mandibular first premolar	Dental malalignment(s) present (see text), such as crowding or spacing; mesognathic profile
Class II	Division I Division II	Molar: MB cusp of the maxillary first occluding (by more than the width of a premolar) mesial to the MB groove of the mandibular first Canines: Distal surface of the mandibular canine distal to the mesial surface of the maxillary canine by at least the width of a premolar	Division I: Maxillary anteriors protruding facially from the mandibular anteriors, with deep overbite; retrognathic profil Division II: Maxillary central incisors either upright or retruded, and lateral incisors either tipped labially or overlapping the central incisors with deep overbite; mesognathic profile.
Class III		Molar: MB cusp of the maxillary first occluding (by more than the width of a premolar) distal to the MB groove of the mandibular first Canines: Distal surface of the mandibular mesial to the mesial surface of the maxillary by at least the width of a premolar	Mandibular incisors in complete crossbite; prognathic profile

*Note that this system deals with the classification of the permanent dentition.
MB = mesiobuccal

Classification of Malocclusion

Angle's classification of malocclusion does *not* describe normal or even ideal occlusion, only malocclusion of the molars and canines. The basis of Angle's classification system was the simple hypothesis that the permanent maxillary first molar was the key to occlusion. Later, the relationship of the opposite arch canines was also evaluated. Therefore Angle's system does not describe lateral or protrusive discrepancies, only those that are mesiodistally placed as related to the molars or canines.

Angle's system also assumes that a patient is occluding in a position of centric occlusion; thus it does not address the functional discrepancies between centric relation and centric occlusion. Additional infor-

mation is needed to fully evaluate a patient's occlusion. Angle also assumed that patients in malocclusion had all their permanent teeth. Thus his classification system does not describe primary or mixed dentition malocclusions (although there are specific ways to classify a primary dentition's relationships of canines and molars, discussed later).

In Angle's classification, most cases of malocclusion are grouped into three main classes, according to the position of the permanent maxillary first molar to the mandibular first molar. Thus this classification system is based on the relationship of the teeth and *not* the skeletal considerations that are due to the disproportionate size or position of the jaws (discussed later). These three main classes are designated by Roman numerals, and they assume that both sides of the

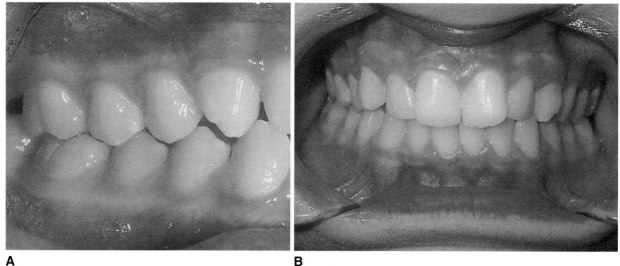

A   B

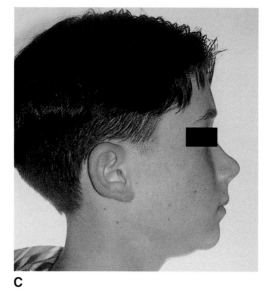

C

FIGURE 20-17 Clinical case of a Class I malocclusion in a permanent dentition. **A:** Buccal view. **B:** Facial view. **C:** Facial profile. The mesiobuccal cusp of the maxillary first molar occludes with the mesiobuccal groove of the mandibular first molar, and the maxillary canine occludes with the distal half of the mandibular canine and the mesial half of the mandibular first premolar. The malocclusion in this case is due to dental malalignments such as anterior crowding (completed orthodontic case is shown in Figure 20-1). The patient has a normal, or mesognathic, profile. (Courtesy of Dr. Dona M. Seely, DDS, MSD, Orthodontic Associates, Bellevue, WA.)

dentition are affected equally. (However, separate classifications can be made, depending on which side is affected.) Placement into Angle's system is only a classification, *not* a diagnosis of occlusal problems.

CLASS I MALOCCLUSION

All cases in a **Class I malocclusion** (neutroclusion) are characterized by an ideal mesiodistal relationship of the jaws and dental arches (Figure 20-17). In these cases in the permanent dentition, the mesiobuccal cusp of the maxillary first molar occludes with the mesiobuccal groove of the mandibular first molar. In

relation to the opposite arch canines, the maxillary canine occludes with the distal half of the mandibular canine and the mesial half of the mandibular first premolar.

Class I malocclusion is due to dental malalignments, such as crowding ("crooked teeth") or spacing within normal jaws (see Figure 20-17). These patients have a normal facial profile, described by many clinicians with the older term **mesognathic.** The facial profile in centric occlusion has slightly protruded jaws, giving the facial outline a relatively flat appearance or straight profile (Figure 20-18).

Problems with crowding in which the teeth are out of line within the dental arch occur because of a disproportion between the size of the teeth and arch size. Spacing problems occur within an arch where the teeth are small in relation to the size of the arch or where teeth are missing. Included in this class of malocclusion is the crowding that occurs because of **mesial drift** as the dentition ages (see Chapter 14; Figure 20-19). Mesial drift, or physiological drift, is a normal, natural movement phenomenon in which all the teeth move slightly toward the midline of the oral cavity over time. This can cause crowding late in life of a once-perfect dentition. It occurs rather slowly, depending mostly on the degree of wear of the contact points between adjacent teeth and on the number of missing teeth. Overall, amounts may total no more than 1 cm over a lifetime. However, this may eventually lead to poor oral hygiene and aesthetics in the area of crowding.

Class I cases frequently have some protrusive or retrusive discrepancies in the anterior teeth (Figure 20-20). Within this grouping may be slight, moderate, or severe overbites. Some cases of Class I have an **open bite,** in which the anterior teeth do not occlude (see also Chapter 16 for clinical view). In addition, Class I cases may have an **end-to-end bite,** or edge-to-edge bite, in which the teeth occlude without the maxillary teeth overlapping the mandibular teeth. With this type of occlusion, the anterior teeth of both jaws meet along their incisal edges when the teeth are in centric occlusion. An end-to-end bite can occur both anteriorly and posteriorly, unilaterally or bilaterally. Within Class I may also be included a **crossbite,** which occurs when a mandibular tooth or teeth are placed facially to the maxillary teeth. A crossbite can occur either anteriorly or posteriorly, unilaterally or bilaterally. Individual teeth may be slightly deviated labially or lingually in regards to the adjoining teeth in the same arch; they may be in labioversion or linguoversion.

CLASS II MALOCCLUSION

All cases in **Class II malocclusion** (distoclusion) in the permanent dentition are characterized by the mesiobuccal cusp of the maxillary first molar occluding (by more than the width of a premolar) mesial to the mesiobuccal groove of the mandibular first molar (Figure 20-21). The distal surface of the mandibular canine is distal to the mesial surface of the maxillary canine by at least the width of a premolar. A tendency to this type of malocclusion (less than the width of a premolar) can be noted. The major group of Class II malocclusion has two subgroups, division I and division II, based on the position of the anteriors, shape of the palate, and resulting facial profile.

In **Class II malocclusion, division I** in the permanent dentition, the maxillary anteriors protrude facially from the mandibular anteriors (Figure 20-22).

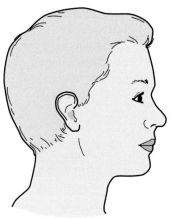

Mesognathic

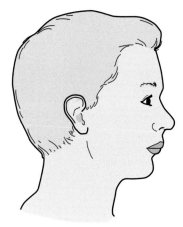

Retrognathic

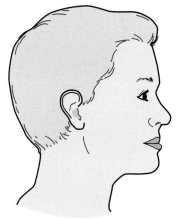

Prognathic

FIGURE 20-18 Three facial profiles: mesognathic, retrognathic, and prognathic. These can be measured by the **gnathic index** (or alveolar index), which is the ratio of the distance from the middle of the nasion to the basion. It gives the degree of prominence of the maxilla as opposed to the mandible jaw. Note that an index below 98 is retrognathic, from 98 to 103 is mesognathic, and above 103 is prognathic.

The mandibular incisors usually overerupt, causing a severe overbite (deep overbite). The palate is often narrow and V-shaped. The facial profile shows a protruding upper lip, or a recessive mandible and chin, or convex profile. The older term for describing the facial

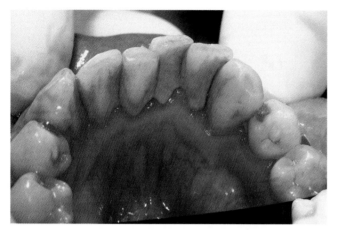

FIGURE 20-19 Mesial drift is a normal, natural movement phenomenon in which all the teeth move slightly toward the midline of the oral cavity over time. It can cause crowding late in life of a once-perfect dentition and may lead to poor oral hygiene in the area of crowding, as the presence of calculus demonstrates.

profile in Class II, division I is **retrognathic** (see Figure 20-18).

In **Class II malocclusion, division II** in a permanent dentition, the molars are in the same position, but rather than having protrusive maxillary anteriors, the maxillary central incisors are either upright or retruded (Figure 20-23). The maxillary lateral incisors are either tipped labially or overlap the central incisors. Overbite is severe (deep overbite), yet the palate is either normal or wide compared with division I. The facial profile for Class II, division II is usually a normal or mesognathic profile, often with a rather prominent chin (see Figure 20-18).

CLASS III MALOCCLUSION

In all cases of a **Class III malocclusion** (mesioclusion) in a permanent dentition, the mesiobuccal cusp of the maxillary first molar occludes (by more than the width of a premolar) distal to the mesiobuccal groove of the mandibular first molar (Figure 20-24). The distal surface of the mandibular canine is mesial to the mesial surface of the maxillary canine by at least the width of a premolar.

In comparison with Class II, division I cases, in which the maxillary incisors are flared mesially, the mandibular incisors are usually in complete crossbite.

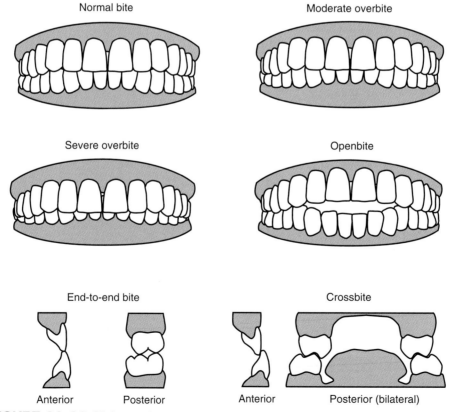

Normal bite

Moderate overbite

Severe overbite

Openbite

End-to-end bite

Anterior   Posterior

Crossbite

Anterior   Posterior (bilateral)

FIGURE 20-20 Slight, moderate, and severe overbites; open bite, end-to-end bites, and crossbites.

In most cases, the mandibular incisors are also inclined lingually despite the crossbite. The facial profile usually shows a rather prominent mandible and possibly a normal or even retrusive maxilla, thus a concave profile. The older term that describes the facial profile with a Class III malocclusion is **prognathic** (see Figure 20-18). A tendency to this type of malocclusion (less than the width of a premolar) can be noted.

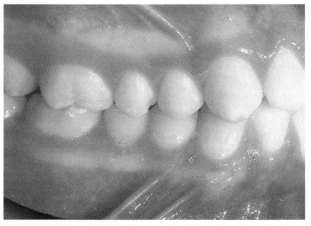

FIGURE 20-21 Clinical case of a Class II malocclusion in a permanent dentition (buccal view). The mesiobuccal cusp of the maxillary first molar is occluding (by more than the width of a premolar) mesial to the mesiobuccal groove of the mandibular first molar, and the distal surface of the mandibular canine is distal to the mesial surface of the maxillary canine by at least the width of a premolar. (Courtesy of Dr. Dona M. Seely, DDS, MSD, Orthodontic Associates, Bellevue, WA.)

SUBDIVISIONS OF MALOCCLUSION

Angle's system recognized that a case of malocclusion did occasionally have differing classifications on each side of the dentition. These asymmetrical cases were labeled *subdivisions* and usually demonstrated the main characteristics of the main class and division.

Thus Angle's classification of malocclusion allows for a Class II malocclusion, division I subdivision in which the patient has both a Class II and Class I, showing a division I anterior pattern. Also possible is a Class II malocclusion, division II subdivision in which a patient has both a Class II and Class I, showing a division II anterior pattern. Finally, also possible is a Class III malocclusion subdivision in which a patient has both a Class III and Class I malocclusion on each side of the dentition.

PRIMARY OCCLUSION

Similar to the permanent dentition, the primary dentition also has an ideal form (Figure 20-25). The canine relationship between the arches in primary teeth is the same as that of the permanent dentition. The ideal molar relationship in the primary dentition when in centric occlusion is referred to as the **terminal plane.** This can involve either a **flush terminal plane,** in which the primary maxillary and mandibular second molars are in an end-to-end relationship, or a **mesial step,** in which the primary mandibular second molar is mesial to the maxillary molar.

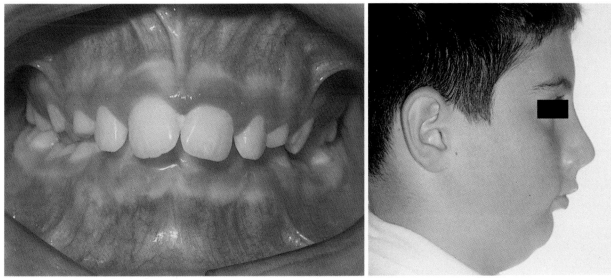

A   **B**

FIGURE 20-22 Clinical case of a Class II malocclusion, division I in a permanent dentition. **A:** Facial view. **B:** Facial profile. The maxillary anteriors also protrude facially from the mandibular anteriors, causing a deep overbite. The facial profile is convex, or retrognathic. (Courtesy of Dr. Dona M. Seely, DDS, MSD, Orthodontic Associates, Bellevue, WA.)

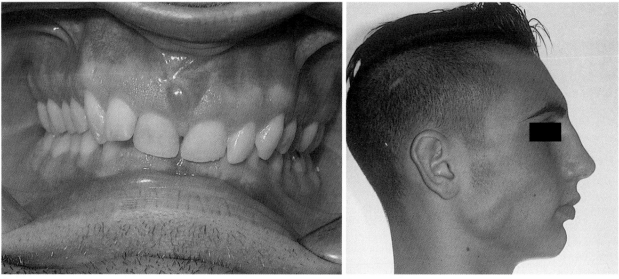

A

B

FIGURE 20-23 Clinical case of a Class II malocclusion, division II in a permanent dentition. **A:** Facial view. **B:** Facial profile. The central incisors are in a retruded position, and the lateral incisors are tipped labially. The patient also has a deep overbite. The facial profile is normal, or mesognathic. (Courtesy of Dr. Dona M. Seely, DDS, MSD, Orthodontic Associates, Bellevue, WA.)

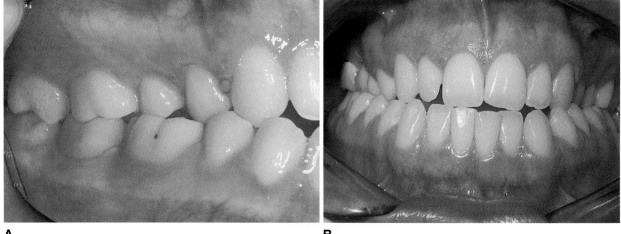

A

B

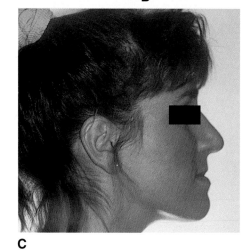

C

FIGURE 20-24 Clinical case of a Class III malocclusion in a permanent dentition. **A:** Buccal view. **B:** Facial view. **C:** Facial profile. The mesiobuccal cusp of the maxillary first molar is occluding (by more than the width of a premolar) distal to the buccal groove of the mandibular first molar, and the distal surface of the mandibular canine is mesial to the mesial surface of the maxillary canine by at least the width of a premolar. The mandibular incisors are also in crossbite, as are other teeth. The facial profile is concave, or prognathic. (Courtesy of Dr. Dona M. Seely, DDS, MSD, Orthodontic Associates, Bellevue, WA.)

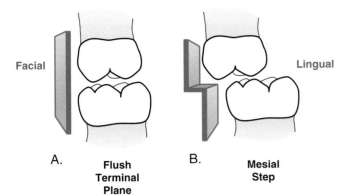

FIGURE 20-25 Evaluation of the primary dentition (buccal view of right side). **A:** A flush terminal plane, in which the primary maxillary and mandibular second molars are in an end-to-end relationship. This may allow a normal molar relationship to occur in the permanent dentition. **B:** A mesial step, in which the mandibular second molar is mesial to the maxillary molar. This will most likely allow a normal molar relationship to occur in the permanent dentition.

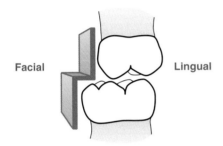

FIGURE 20-26 Primary dentition (buccal view of right side) in which distal step relationship exists with the primary mandibular second molar distal to the maxillary second molar. This is not a beneficial molar relationship because it will not usually result in a normal molar relationship in the permanent dentition when it erupts and the primary teeth are shed.

A **distal step** relationship, in which the primary mandibular second molar is distal to the maxillary second molar, is not an ideal molar relationship in the primary dentition and thus is not a type of terminal plane relationship (Figure 20-26). With the presence of mesial step, an ideal permanent molar relationship most likely occurs after the eruption of the permanent dentition. Ideal molar relationship in the permanent dentition may still occur with a flush terminal plane but rarely with the presence of a distal step relationship.

Within a primary dentition, **primate spaces** may occur between the primary teeth; a space is noted between the maxillary lateral incisor and the canine and between the mandibular first molar and canine (see Chapter 18 for more discussion). If primate spacing exists in the primary mandibular arch, after the eruption of the permanent first molar, the permanent first molar puts pressure on the primary second and first molars, causing forward movement of the primary mandibular canine and first molar (discussed earlier with regard to arch development). Thus this primate space actually allows for this movement,

which then facilitates the development of an ideal permanent molar relationship, along with the presence of a mesial step relationship.

When the child patient enters the mixed dentition period, analysis of space is performed. This analysis can range from a general examination to a specific arch length analysis by radiographs, size of erupted permanent mandibular incisors, and prediction scheme by orthodontists. This analysis is performed during the mixed dentition period because there is no appreciable growth of the jaws anterior to the permanent first molars after age 7 or 8 without intervention.

Parafunctional Habits

Parafunctional habits are those movements of the mandible that are *not* within the normal range of motion associated with mastication, speech, or respiratory movements. Thus these habits occur more commonly and in longer duration than motions associated with normal functioning. The etiology and treatment of these parafunctional habits are somewhat controversial. More studies must be conducted to obtain more information about these habits and their treatment.

Parafunctional habits include **clenching** the teeth in centric occlusion for long periods without a break into a mandibular rest position or interocclusal clearance. Grinding the teeth, or **bruxism,** is also a parafunctional habit. Grinding the teeth involves forceful meshing of the teeth, often causing audible noises. Attrition of the masticatory surfaces of differing levels is evident in cases of grinding, especially in the canines' cusp tips (see Figure 20-8 and Chapters 16 and 17), as well as gingival recession caused by **abfraction** (see Chapters 10 and 12). In addition, in cases of both grinding and clenching, a larger area of the buccal mucosa than just the linea alba becomes hyperkeratinized (see Chapter 9).

These parafunctional habits of clenching and grinding are often subconscious and occur when a person is sleeping or concentrating deeply, such as when driving, reading, watching television, or using the computer. Conscious retraining for adults during waking hours involves placing the tongue between the teeth with the lips closed and mandibular arch positioning (leaning the head forward to prevent teeth from occluding).

A person with these habits may have enlarged masseter muscles and may consider it normal to feel facial and masticatory tension. Directed relaxing of the facial and masticatory muscles, especially the masseter muscles, also helps in some cases. Stress may be a factor in the etiology of these habits, although it is not always present. Parafunctional habits may be linked to the way some individuals process neurological impulses. Whether malocclusion contributes to these two parafunctional habits is controversial.

Patients who clench or grind their teeth can wear a professionally made flat plane nonrepositioning oral splint, or night guard, during waking hours or when sleeping. An oral splint consists of a removable plastic dental appliance that covers the dental arch (or arches). This device can protect the teeth from further damage, such as attrition or recession from abfraction, and can spread the occlusal stress of the habit throughout the dentition.

The parafunctional habit of nonnutritive sucking of the thumb or fingers in children or young adults can cause an excessive anterior overjet, lips irreversibly stretched by protruding teeth, a deep narrow palate, and a callus on the thumb or fingers. Again, this activity, similar to clenching and grinding, is largely unconscious.

The main suggested intervention in prolonged nonnutritive sucking includes gently increasing the child's awareness of the habit by discussing the problem by the time the child is 5 years of age. Similar problems are associated with the prolonged overuse of pacifiers in young children, but a pacifier may be taken away. A myofunctional therapist may be useful in working with and controlling these habits (further involvement of this specialist is discussed later). Contrary to popular belief, research shows that no emotional trauma results from stopping chronic sucking in children.

Skeletal Considerations

Many malocclusions are linked not only to the teeth, such as in Angle's classification of malocclusion, but also to discrepancies between the maxilla and mandible that then affect the occlusion of the teeth. These skeletal abnormalities of the jaws can be corrected by an oral surgeon working with an orthodontist; orthodontic therapy with tooth movement alone is not effective. In many cases, timely orthodontic intervention in young children using certain orthodontic appliances can direct bone growth of the jaws by arch expansion and by increasing arch length and arch level. These interventions may prevent the need for surgical intervention. In adults and those patients whose bone growth is complete, however, orthognathic surgery may be the only remedy for jaw discrepancies because orthodontic appliances do not in themselves produce ideal results.

Generally, orthodontic patients requiring orthognathic surgical intervention undergo an initial period of orthodontic treatment before surgery so that the teeth occlude properly after surgery. Any orthodontic appliances used to align the teeth before surgery are left in place during the surgical procedure to stabilize

the teeth and jaws. After surgery, a period of follow-up orthodontic treatment helps achieve the final alignment of the teeth.

Most commonly corrected problems include a protruding or retruding chin, unsightly display of gingiva above the maxillary anterior teeth, an inability to achieve resting lip closure, and an overall elongation of the face. Temporomandibular joint disorders may also be minimized with surgery in severe cases (see Chapter 19 for more discussion).

Three basic spatial planes are involved in the classification of skeletal malocclusions: horizontal, vertical, and transverse. Horizontal malocclusions are further classified as either Class II or Class III malocclusions, similar to Angle's classification system. Vertical malocclusions include open bites and severe overbites. Transverse malocclusions include crossbites. Most patients undergoing orthognathic surgery have a combination of these types of skeletal malocclusions.

Myofunctional Considerations

One of the most controversial considerations in occlusion is the importance of the surrounding musculature in forming the occlusion. Certified orofacial myologists have been trained to identify, diagnose, and treat myofunctional problems (Figure 20-27). Many dental professionals are beginning to endorse these findings or support any treatment performed by orofacial myologists. Orofacial myologists work with speech therapists and dental professionals, especially orthodontists, who agree with the basis for this specialty.

A specific treatment plan for each patient involves making the patient aware of the problem, producing new muscle functions, toning appropriate muscula-

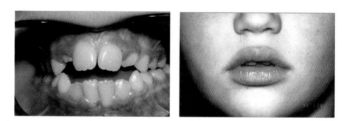
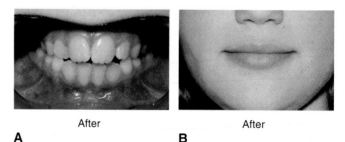

Before   Before

After   After

A   **B**

FIGURE 20-27 Before and after photos with orofacial myology therapy. **A:** Tongue thrust. **B:** Open-mouth breathing. (Courtesy of Sandra R. Coulson, BA, COM, Coulson Institute of Orofacial Myology, Englewood, CO.)

ture, and helping in making the new patterns habitual. Orofacial myologists believe that early identification is an advantage but that young adults and older adults can benefit from therapy. Many dental professionals are expanding into this field. Further studies are necessary to ascertain whether myofunctional considerations are important in malocclusion and whether such therapy has a long-term benefit.

The most common myofunctional problem cited by many orofacial myologists in regard to occlusion is a tongue thrust. During the act of swallowing and during rest posture, the tongue is believed to contribute to the formation of malocclusion by the infantile habit of thrusting the tongue and resting it against or between the anterior teeth to form an oral seal. Many orofacial myologists believe that a tongue thrust may result in an anterior open bite, deformation of the jaws, and abnormal function.

Another myofunctional problem cited by many orofacial myologists is an incorrect resting position of the lips, which can affect the position of the anterior teeth and facial aesthetics. The competency of the lips to maintain a lip seal when at rest can affect the position of the maxillary incisors. Competent lips allow these tooth tips to lie below the lower lip border, helping to maintain normal inclination. Incompetent lips that fail to provide a lip seal do not control this inclination and may even allow the maxillary incisors to lie in front of the lower lip, exaggerating already buccally inclined teeth. A tongue thrust may be associated with this problem, complicating the treatment. In comparison, overactive and tight lips can cause the maxillary incisors to become lingually inclined.

Orofacial myologists believe that the tongue thrust and negative tongue and lip resting positions are due to disharmony between the tongue, lips, cheeks, and teeth. Etiological factors cited by orofacial myologists include nonnutritive sucking habits, habitual mouth breathing, open-lips position, structural problems, developmental problems, or a combination of any of these factors. Speech problems may be associated with these noted myofunctional disorders. The most important of these seems to be the rest posture of the lips and tongue. Habitual open-mouth rest posture does not allow the tongue to provide the valuable pressure into the palate that helps to widen the maxillary arch. Another issue is the length of the lingual frenulum. If it is restricted, it also limits the possibility for the maxillary arch to expand and increases speech and articulation problems. Allergies are an issue for all orofacial myologists. They seem to be increasing in all ages of the population and present a challenge in achieving proper tongue-resting posture.

Bibliography

Ash MM. *Wheeler's Dental Anatomy, Physiology and Occlusion*, ed 8. WB Saunders, Philadelphia, 2002.

Dorland's Illustrated Medical Dictionary, ed 30. WB Saunders, Philadelphia, 2003.

Fehrenbach MJ, Herring SW. *Illustrated Anatomy of the Head and Neck*, ed 2. WB Saunders, Philadelphia, 2002.

Moore KL, Persaud TVN. *The Developing Human*, ed 7. WB Saunders, Philadelphia, 2003.

Mosby. *Mosby's Dental Dictionary*. Mosby, St. Louis, 2004.

Nanci A. *Ten Cate's Oral Histology: Development, Structure, and Function*, ed 6. Mosby, St. Louis, 2003.

Newman MG, Takei HH, Carranza FA. *Carranza's Clinical Periodontology*, ed 9. WB Saunders, Philadelphia, 2001.

Neville BW. *Oral & Maxillofacial Pathology*, ed 2. WB Saunders, Philadelphia, 2001.

Standring S. *Gray's Anatomy*, ed 39. Churchill Livingstone, Edinburgh, 2005.

Stevens A, Lowe J. *Human Histology*, ed 3. Mosby, St. Louis, 2005.

Terminologia Anatomica. Thieme Medical Publishers, New York, ed bilingual, 2000.

Young B, Heath JW. *Wheater's Functional Histology*, ed 4. Churchill Livingstone, Edinburgh, 2000.

Glossary

A

Abfraction (ab-frak-shen) Hard tooth tissue loss, possibly caused by tensile and compressive forces during tooth flexure.

Abrasion (u- brey-zhun) Hard tooth tissue loss caused by friction from toothbrushing and toothpaste (or both).

Accessory canals Extra openings located on the lateral portions of the roots of some teeth.

Accessory root Extra root or roots on a tooth.

Acellular cementum First layers of cementum deposited without many embedded cementocytes.

Acinus (plural, acini) (as-i-nus, as-i-ny) Group of secretory cells of salivary gland.

Active eruption Actual vertical movement of the tooth.

Adipose connective tissue (ad-i-pose) Specialized connective tissue composed of fat, little matrix, and adipocytes.

Afferent vessels (af-er-int) Lymphatic vessels that allow the flow of lymph into the lymph node.

Ala (plural, alae) (a-lah, a-lay) Winglike cartilaginous structures bounding the nares laterally.

Alveolar bone (al-ve-o-lar) Portion of the maxilla or mandible that supports the teeth.

Alveolar bone proper Bone lining the alveolus.

Alveolar crest Most cervical rim of the alveolar bone proper.

Alveolar crest group Portion of the alveodental ligament that originates in the alveolar crest and fans out to insert into the cervical cementum.

Alveolar mucosa Portion of the oral mucosa immediately apical to the mucogingival junction.

Alveolar process Dental arch or tooth-bearing portion of each jawbone that contains the alveoli.

Alveolodental ligament (al-ve-o-lo-den-tl) Main principal fiber group, which consists of five groups: alveolar crest, horizontal, oblique, apical, and interradicular.

Alveolus (plural, alveoli) (al-ve-o-lus, al-ve-o-lie) Socket of the tooth.

Ameloblasts (ah-mel-oh-blasts) Cells that differentiate from preameloblasts and that will form enamel during amelogenesis.

Amelogenesis (ah-mel-oh-jen-i-sis) Apposition of enamel matrix by ameloblasts.

Amelogenesis imperfecta (im-per-fek-tah) Hereditary type of enamel dysplasia in which the teeth have absent or thin enamel.

Amniocentesis (am-nee-o-sen-tee-sis) Prenatal diagnostic procedure in which the amniotic fluid is sampled.

Amniotic cavity (am-nee-ot-ik) Fluid-filled cavity that faces the epiblast layer.

Anaphase (an-ah-faz) Third phase of mitosis, which involves separation of the two chromatids of each chromosome and migration to opposite poles of the cell.

Anatomical crown Portion of crown covered by enamel.

Anatomical root Portion of root covered by cementum.

Anchoring collagen fibers Fibers from the connective tissue involved in the basement membrane.

Angle of the mandible Thickened area on the posterior-inferior border of the mandibular ramus.

Angle's classification of malocclusion System used to initially and simply classify malocclusion.

Ankyloglossia (ang-kel-o-gloss-ee-ah) Lingual frenum that is abnormally short, extends to the tongue apex, and possibly restricts tongue movement.

Anodontia (an-ah-don-she-ah) Absence of a single tooth or multiple teeth owing to lack of initiation.

Anterior teeth Incisors and canines at the front of the oral cavity.

Anterior faucial pillar (faw-shawl) Anterior lateral folds of tissue created by underlying muscle.

Apex of the nose Tip of the nose.

Apical foramen (ay-pi-kl for-ay-men) Opening from the pulp at the apex of the tooth.

Apical group Portion of the alveolodental group of the periodontal ligament that radiates apically from the cementum to insert into the alveolar bone proper.

Apposition (ap-oh-zish-in) Layered formation of a firm or hard tissue such as cartilage, bone, enamel, dentin, and cementum.

Appositional growth (ap-oh-zish-in-al) Growth by the addition of layers to the outside of the tissue mass.

Arrest lines Smooth, stained microscopic lines in cartilage, bone, and cementum caused by apposition occurring in these tissues.

Articular eminence (ar-tik-you-ler) Rounded protuberance on the inferior aspect of the zygomatic process that is part of the articulating area of the temporomandibular joint.

Articular fossa Depression on the inferior aspect of the temporal bone that is part of the articulating area of the temporomandibular joint.

Articulating surface of the condyle (ar-**tik**-you-late-ing kon-dyl) Head of mandibular condyle involved in the temporomandibular joint.

Attached gingiva Gingiva that tightly adheres to the alveolar bone around the roots of the teeth.

Attrition (ah-**trish**-un) Hard tooth tissue loss caused by tooth-to-tooth contact during mastication or parafunctional habits.

Avulsion (ah-**vul**-shin) Complete displacement of the tooth from the socket because of extensive trauma to the area.

B

Balancing interference Situation in which teeth are in contact on the balancing side during lateral occlusion.

Balancing side Other side of the arch from the working side during lateral occlusion.

Basal bone (bay-sal) Portion of the jawbones that forms the body of the maxilla or mandible.

Basal lamina (lam-**i**-nah) Superficial portion of the basement membrane. Within the dentogingival junction, there is an external and internal basal lamina surrounding the junctional epithelium.

Basal layer Single layer of cuboidal epithelial cells overlying the basement membrane.

Basement membrane Extracellular material consisting of a basal and reticular lamina produced by the epithelium and connective tissue, respectively.

Base of the tongue Most posterior portion of the tongue.

Basophil (**bay**-sah-fil) White blood cell that contains granules of histamine and heparin.

Bell stage Fourth stage of odontogenesis, in which differentiation occurs to its furthest extent and the enamel organ assumes a bell shape.

Bicuspid (bi-**kus**-pid) Older dental term for a premolar.

Bifurcated (bi-fer-**kay**-ted) Tooth having two root branches.

Bilaminar embryonic disc (by-**lam**-i-nar) Circular plate of bilayered cells developed from the blastocyst.

Bilateral symmetry The primitive streak causes the disc to divide into a right and left half, so that each half mirrors the other half of the embryo.

Black hairy tongue Tongue lesion marked by buildup of a thick layer of dead cells and keratin that becomes extrinsically stained.

Blastocyst (**blas**-tah-sist) Structure during prenatal development consisting of trophoblast cells and an inner mass of cells that develop into the embryo.

Blood Fluid connective tissue that contains cells and plasma.

Body of the tongue Anterior portion of the tongue.

Bone Rigid connective tissue.

Bone marrow (**mar**-oh) Innermost portion of bone in the medullary cavity.

Branchial apparatus (**brang**-ke-al ap-pah-**ra**-tis) Group of structures that includes the branchial arches, branchial grooves and membranes, and the pharyngeal pouches.

Branchial arches Six stacked bilateral swellings of tissue that appear inferior to the stomodeum and include the mandibular arch.

Branchial grooves Grooves between neighboring branchial arches on each side of the embryo.

Bruxism (**bruk**-sizm) Parafunctional habit of grinding the teeth.

Buccal (buk-al) Describes structures or facial surfaces of a tooth close to the inner cheek.

Buccal developmental depressions Depression on each side of the buccal ridge on certain posterior teeth.

Buccal fat pad Pad of underlying adipose connective tissue at the posterior portion of each vestibule.

Buccal mucosa Mucosa that lines the inner cheek.

Buccal region Region of the face composed of the soft tissues of the cheek.

Buccal ridge Ridge extending vertically in the center of the buccal surface of the crown of certain posterior teeth.

Bud stage of odontogenesis Second stage of tooth development with the growth of the dental lamina or buds into the ectomesenchyme.

C

Calcium hydroxyapatite (hy-drox-see-**ap**-ah-tite) Main inorganic crystal in enamel, bone, dentin, and cementum, with the chemical formula of $Ca_{10}(PO_4)_6(OH)_2$.

Canaliculi (kan-ah-**lik**-u-lie) Tubular canals in bone and cementum.

Cancellous bone (kan-**sel**-us) Spongy bone within the compact bone.

Canine eminence (**kay**-nine **em**-i-nins) Vertically oriented and labially placed bony ridge of alveolar bone evident in the jawbones, especially in the maxilla.

Canine rise Situation in which the canine should be the only tooth in function during lateral occlusion.

Canines (**kay**-nines) Anterior teeth that also are the third teeth from the midline in each quadrant.

Cap stage of odontogenesis Third stage of tooth development, in which the tooth bud of dental lamina grows into a cap shape.

Capillary blood plexus Groups of capillaries between the papillary layer and the deeper layers of the lamina propria.

Capsule (**kap**-sule) Connective tissue that surrounds the outer portion of the entire gland or lesion.

Caries Cavities with hard tooth tissue loss resulting from demineralization of the tooth owing to acid produced by cariogenic bacteria.

Cartilage (**kar**-ti-lij) Firm, noncalcified connective tissue.

Caudal end (**kaw**-dal) Tail end of a structure, such as in the trilaminar embryonic disc.

Cell Smallest unit of organization in the body.

Cell membrane Membrane that completely surrounds a cell.

Cellular cementum Outer layers of cementum, which contain embedded cementocytes.

Cemental spurs Symmetrical spheres of cementum attached to the root surface.

Cementicles (see-**men**-ti-kuls) Calcified bodies of cementum either attached to the root or free in the periodontal ligament.

Cementoblasts (see-**men**-toe-blasts) Cells that form cementoid and are differentiated from the dental sac.

Cementocytes (see-**men**-toe-sites) Cementoblasts entrapped by the cementum they produce.

Cementoenamel junction (CEJ) Portion of the tooth where the enamel of the crown and the cementum of the root meet at the neck or cervix.

Cementogenesis (see-men-toe-**jen**-i-sis) Apposition of cementum in the root area.

Cementoid (see-**men**-toyd) Cementum matrix laid down by cementoblasts.

Cementum (see-**men**-tum) Outermost layer of the root of a tooth.

Central cells of the dental papilla Primordium of the pulp.

Central fossa Fossa located at the convergence of the cusp ridges in a central point on the occlusal surface of posterior teeth.

Central groove Most prominent developmental groove on posterior teeth, which generally travels mesiodistally and separates the occlusal table buccolingually.

Central incisor Incisor that is closest to the midline.

Centric occlusion (CO) Voluntary position of the dentition that allows maximal contact when the teeth occlude.

Centric relation (CR) End point of closure of the mandible in which the mandible is in the most retruded position.

Centrioles (**sen**-tree-ols) Pair of cylindrical structures in the centrosome.

Centromere (**sen**-tro-mere) Clear constricted area where the two chromatids of chromosome are joined.

Centrosome (**sen**-tro-some) Organelle associated with centrioles.

Cephalic end (se-**fal**-ik) Head end of a structure, such as in the trilaminar embryonic disc.

Cervical cysts (**ser**-vi-kal) Developmental cysts formed when branchial grooves do not become obliterated.

Cervical loop Most cervical portion of the enamel organ that is responsible for root development.

Cervical ridge Ridge running mesiodistally in the cervical one third of the buccal crown surface on the entire primary dentition and permanent molars.

Cheek Portion of buccal region that forms the side of the face; broad area of the face between the nose, mouth, and ear.

Chondroblasts (**kon**-dro-blasts) Cells that produce cartilage tissue.

Chondrocytes (**kon**-dro-sites) Mature chondroblasts.

Chromatids (**kro**-mah-tids) Two filamentous daughter chromosomes joined at a centromere during cell division.

Chromatin (**kro**-mah-tin) Chief nucleoprotein in the non-dividing nucleoplasm.

Chromosomes (**kro**-mah-somes) Separate concentrations of chromatin in a dividing nucleus of a cell.

Cingulum (**sin**-gu-lum) Raised and rounded area on the cervical third of the lingual surface on anterior teeth.

Circumpulpal dentin (serk-um-**pul**-pal) Layer of dentin around the outer pulpal wall.

Circumvallate lingual papillae (serk-um-**val**-ate) Large, mushroom-shaped lingual papillae that line up along the anterior side of the sulcus terminalis on the tongue.

Class I malocclusion Type of malocclusion characterized by an ideal mesiodistal relationship of the jaws and dental arches with dental malalignments.

Class II malocclusion Type of malocclusion in which the mesiobuccal cusp of the maxillary first molar occludes by more than the width of a premolar mesial to the mesiobuccal groove of the mandibular first molar.

Class III malocclusion Type of malocclusion in which the mesiobuccal cusp of the maxillary first molar occludes by more than the width of a premolar distal to the mesiobuccal groove of the mandibular first molar.

Class II malocclusion, division I Class II type of malocclusion in which the permanent maxillary anteriors protrude facially from the mandibular anteriors.

Class II malocclusion, division II Type of Class II malocclusion in which the maxillary central incisors are either upright or in a retruded position.

Cleavage (**kleve**-ij) Process during prenatal development when individual cell division or mitosis converts a zygote to a blastocyst.

Cleft lip (kleft) Developmental disturbance of the upper lip owing to failure of fusion of the maxillary processes with the medial nasal process.

Cleft palate Developmental disturbance owing to failure of fusion of the palatal shelves with the primary palate or with each other.

Cleft uvula Mildest form of cleft palate.

Clenching Parafunctional habit in which the teeth are held in centric occlusion for long periods without a break into interocclusal clearance.

Clinical crown Portion of the anatomical crown that is visible in the oral cavity and not covered by the gingiva.

Clinical root Portion of the anatomical root that is visible.

Cloacal membrane (klo-**ay**-kal) Membrane at the caudal end of the embryo that is the location of the future anus.

Col (kohl) Portion of the interdental gingiva apical to the contact area that assumes a nonvisible concave form between the facial and lingual gingival surfaces.

Collagen fibers (**kol**-ah-jen) Main protein fiber type found in the body.

Colloid (**kol**-oid) Material in the follicles of the thyroid gland that is reserved for the production of thyroxine.

Compact bone (**kom**-pak) Type of bone deep to the periosteum.

Concrescence (kahn-**kres**-ens) Union of the root structure of two or more teeth through the cementum only.

Condyle of the mandible (**kon**-dyl) Bony projection off the posterior and superior border of the mandibular ramus.

Congenital malformations (kon-**jen**-i-til mal-for-**may**-shins) Birth defects that are developmental problems evident at birth.

Connective tissue Basic tissue type composed of cells and matrix as well as other components.

Connective tissue papillae (pah-**pil**-ay) Extensions of loose connective tissue into the epithelium as they appear on histological section.

Connective tissue proper Two adjacent layers of both loose and dense connective tissue.

Contact area Portion of a tooth where adjacent tooth crowns in the same arch physically touch on each proximal surface.

Contour lines of Owen Adjoining imbrication lines in dentin that demonstrate a disturbance in body metabolism.

Copula (**kop**-u-lah) Pair of posterior swellings formed from the third and fourth branchial arches, which overgrow the second arches to form the base of the tongue.

Coronal pulp Pulp located in the crown of the tooth.

Coronoid notch (**kor**-ah-noid) Main portion of the anterior border of the mandibular ramus, which forms a forward curve.

Coronoid process Bony projection at the anterior border of the mandibular ramus.

Cortical bone Plates of compact bone on the facial and lingual surfaces of the alveolar bone.

Crossbite Type of malocclusion in which the mandibular tooth or teeth are placed facially to the maxillary teeth.

Crown   Portion of a tooth composed of dentin and pulp covered by enamel.

Curve of Spee   If imaginary planes are placed on the masticatory surfaces of each dental arch, the maxillary arch is convex occlusally, and the mandibular arch is concave, producing an anteroposterior curvature.

Curve of Wilson   Concave curve results when a frontal section is taken through each set of both maxillary and mandibular molars, the firsts, seconds, and then thirds.

Cusp (kusp)   One or more major elevations on the masticatory surface of canines and posterior teeth.

Cuspid (kus-pid)   Older dental term for canine.

Cusp of Carabelli   Small cusp usually seen on a permanent maxillary first molar.

Cusp of Carabelli groove   Groove associated with a cusp of Carabelli.

Cusp ridges   Ridges that descend from each cusp tip on posterior teeth.

Cusp slopes   Two ridges on the incisal edge of canines, which are divided by the cusp tip.

Cusp tip   Tip of the cusp on the incisal surface of canines and the occlusal table of posterior teeth.

Cytodifferentiation (sy-to-dif-er-en-she-ay-shin)   Development of different cell types.

Cytoplasm (sy-to-plazm)   Fluid portion contained within the cell membrane.

Cytoskeleton (sy-to-skel-it-on)   Three-dimensional system of support within the cell.

D

D-A-Q-T System   System to designate teeth: *D* for dentition, *A* for arch, *Q* for quadrant, and *T* for tooth type.

Deciduous dentition (de-sij-you-us)   Older dental term for the primary dentition.

Dens in dente (denz in den-tay)   Developmental disturbance caused by invagination of enamel organ into dental papilla.

Dense connective tissue   Deepest layers of the dermis or lamina propria.

Dental anatomy   Area of dental sciences dealing with the morphology of the teeth.

Dental arch   Alveolar process or tooth-bearing portion of each jawbone, in either maxillary or mandibular arch.

Dental formula   Formula for each dentition that is used when comparing human teeth with those of other mammals.

Dental lamina (lam-i-nah)   Growth from the oral epithelium that gives rise to the tooth buds.

Dental papilla (pah-pil-ah)   Inner mass of ectomesenchyme of the tooth germ that produces the dentin and pulp tissue.

Dental sac   Portion of the tooth germ consisting of ectomesenchyme surrounding the outside of the enamel organ, which produces the periodontium of a tooth.

Dentigerous cyst (den-ti-jer-os)   Odontogenic cyst that forms from the reduced enamel epithelium.

Dentin (den-tin)   Hard inner layer of the crown of a tooth overlying the pulp.

Dentin dysplasia (dis-play-ze-ah)   Faulty development of dentin.

Dentinal fluid   Fluid within the dentinal tubule in dentin.

Dentin hypersensitivity (hi-per-sen-si-tiv-it-ee)   Exposed dentin that is sensitive to various stimuli.

Dentinal tubules   Long tubes in the dentin.

Dentinocemental junction (DCJ)   Junction between the dentin and cementum during the formation of the root of the tooth.

Dentinoenamel junction (DEJ)   Junction between the dentin and enamel formed by the mineralization of the disintegrating basement membrane.

Dentinogenesis (den-tin-oh-jen-i-sis)   Apposition of predentin by the odontoblasts.

Dentition (den-tish-in)   Natural teeth in the jawbones, consisting of primary and permanent.

Dentition periods   Three periods that occur throughout a lifetime: primary, mixed, and permanent dentition periods.

Dentogingival junction (den-to-jin-ji-val)   Junction between the tooth surface and the gingival tissues.

Dentogingival junctional tissues   Tissues that include the sulcular epithelium and junctional epithelium.

Depression of the mandible (de-presh-in)   Lowering of the lower jaw.

Dermis (der-mis)   Connective tissue proper in the skin.

Desmosome (dez-mo-some)   Intercellular junction between cells.

Developmental depression   Depression usually evident in a specific area on a tooth.

Developmental groove   Primary groove that marks the junction among the developmental lobes on the lingual surface of anterior teeth and the occlusal table of posterior teeth.

Developmental pits   Pits on the lingual surface of anterior teeth and on the occlusal table and buccal or lingual surface of posterior teeth.

Diastema (di-ah-ste-mah)   Open contact that can exist between the permanent maxillary central incisors.

Differentiation (dif-er-en-she-ay-shin)   Change in the embryonic cells, which are genetically identical but become quite distinct structurally and functionally.

Dilaceration (di-las-er-ay-shun)   Crown or root(s) showing angular distortion.

Disc of the joint   Disc of the temporomandibular joint that is located between the temporal bone and condyle of the mandible.

Distal (dis-tl)   Surface of the tooth farthest away from the midline.

Distal contact   Contact area on the distal surface of a tooth.

Distal marginal ridge   Marginal ridge on the distal portion of the lingual surface of anterior teeth or the distal portion of the occlusal table on posterior teeth.

Distal step   Not a type of terminal plane relationship because the primary mandibular second molar is distal to the maxillary second molar.

Distolingual marginal groove   Developmental groove that crosses the distal marginal ridge on the lingual surface and extends onto the root on certain anterior teeth.

Dorsal surface of the tongue   Top surface of the tongue.

Down syndrome   Developmental defect, also called trisomy 21, in which an extra copy of chromosome no. 21 is present.

Duct   Passageway that allows a glandular secretion to be emptied directly into the location where the secretion is to be used.

E

Ectoderm (ek-toe-derm**)** Layer in the trilaminar embryonic disc derived from the epiblast layer and lining the stomodeum.

Ectodermal dysplasia (dis-**play**-ze-ah**)** Syndrome involving abnormal development of one or more ectodermal structures, including anodontia.

Ectomesenchyme (ek-toe-mes-eng-kime**)** A type of mesenchyme from the ectoderm, which is influenced by neural crest cells that have migrated to the area.

Ectopic pregnancy (ek-**top**-ik**)** Implantation occurring outside the uterus.

Edentulous (e-**den**-tu-lus**)** Dentition with partial or complete loss of teeth.

Efferent vessel (ef-er-ent**)** Lymphatic vessel in which lymph flows out of the lymph node.

Elastic connective tissue (e-**las**-tik**)** Specialized connective tissue with mostly elastic fibers.

Elastic fibers (e-**las**-tik**)** Type of protein fiber in connective tissue composed of microfilaments.

Elevation of the mandible (el-eh-**vay**-shun**)** Raising of the lower jaw.

Embrasures (em-**bray**-zhers**)** Spaces formed from the curvatures where two teeth in the same arch contact.

Embryo (em-bre-oh**)** Structure derived from the implanted blastocyst.

Embryoblast layer (em-bre-oh-blast**)** Small inner mass of embryonic cells in the blastocyst.

Embryology (em-bre-**ol**-ah-jee**)** Study of prenatal development.

Embryonic cell layers (em-bre-**on**-ik**)** Germ layers derived from the increased number of embryonic cells.

Embryonic folding Folding of the embryo that places the tissues in their proper positions for further embryonic development.

Embryonic period of prenatal development Time period from the beginning of the second week to the end of the eighth week.

Enamel (ih-**nam**-l**)** Hard outer layer of the crown of a tooth.

Enamel dysplasia (dis-**play**-ze-ah**)** Faulty development of enamel resulting from many factors.

Enamel lamellae Partially calcified vertical sheets of enamel matrix.

Enamel matrix Matrix of enamel formed during amelogenesis by the ameloblasts.

Enamel organ Cap or bell-shaped portion of the tooth germ that produces enamel.

Enamel pearls Small spherical enamel projections on the tooth surface.

Enamel rods The crystaline structural unit of enamel.

Enamel spindles Microscopic feature present in mature enamel consisting of short dentinal tubules near the dentinoenamel junction.

Enamel tufts Microscopic feature in mature enamel consisting of small dark brushes with their bases near the dentinoenamel junction.

Endochondral ossification (en-do-**kon**-dril os-i-fi-**kay**-shun**)** Formation of osteoid within a cartilage model.

Endocrine gland (en-dah-krin**)** Ductless gland that secretes directly into the blood.

Endocytosis (en-do-sigh-**toe**-sis**)** Uptake of materials from the extracellular environment into the cell.

Endoderm (en-doe-derm**)** Layer in the trilaminar embryonic disc derived from the hypoblast layer.

Endoplasmic reticulum (ER) (en-do-**plas**-mik rey-**tik**-u-lum**)** Membrane-bound organelle that consists of channels that are either rough or smooth in appearance.

Endosteum (en-**dos**-te-um**)** Lining of the medullary cavity of bone.

Endothelium (en-do-**theel**-ee-um**)** Unstratified squamous epithelium lining vessels and serous cavities.

End-to-end bite Teeth that occlude without the maxillary teeth overlapping the mandibular teeth.

Eosinophil (e-ah-**sin**-ah-fil**)** White blood cell that increases in numbers during an immune response.

Epiblast layer (ep-i-blast**)** Superior layer in the bilaminar disc.

Epidermis (ep-i-**der**-mis**)** Superficial layers of the skin.

Epiglottic swelling (ep-ee-**glot**-ik**)** Posterior swelling that develops from the fourth branchial arches and marks the development of the future epiglottis.

Epithelial attachment (EA) Device that attaches the junctional epithelium to the tooth surface.

Epithelial rests of Malassez (mal-ah-**say**)** Groups of epithelial cells in the periodontal ligament after the disintegration of Hertwig's epithelial root sheath that can become cystic.

Epithelium (ep-ee-**thee**-lee-um**)** Basic tissue type that covers and lines the external and internal body surfaces.

Erectile tissue (e-**rek**-tile**)** Thin-walled vessels in the nasal cavity that are capable of considerable engorgement.

Erosion (e-**ro**-zhun**)** Hard tooth tissue loss through chemical means (acid), not involving bacteria.

Excretory duct (ex-**kreh**-tor-ee**)** Duct of a salivary gland through which saliva exits into the oral cavity.

Exocrine gland (ek-sah-krin**)** Gland having a duct associated with it.

Exocytosis (ek-so-sigh-**toe**-sis**)** Active transport of material from a vesicle out into the extracellular environment.

Exostoses (ek-sos-**toe**-sese**)** Normal variation in bone growths noted usually on the facial surface of the alveolar process of the maxilla.

F

Facial (fay-shal**)** Describes structures or tooth surfaces closest to the facial surface.

Fauces (faw-seez**)** Opening posteriorly from the oral cavity proper into the pharynx.

Fertilization (fur-til-uh-**zay**-shun**)** Process by which the sperm penetrates the ovum during the preimplantation period.

Fetal alcohol syndrome Syndrome occurring in an infant that is a result of ethanol ingested by a pregnant woman during the embryonic period.

Fetal period of prenatal development (fete-il**)** Period of prenatal development from the beginning of the third month to the ninth month.

Fetus (fete-is**)** Structure of the fetal period of prenatal development derived from the enlarged embryo.

Fibroblast (fi-bro-blast**)** Cell that synthesizes certain types of protein fibers and intercellular substance.

Fifth branchial arches (brang-ke-al**)** Rudimentary branchial arches in the embryo that are sometimes absent or included with the fourth branchial arches.

Filiform lingual papillae (fil-i-form) Slender, threadlike lingual papillae that give the dorsal surface of the tongue its velvety texture.

First branchial arch (brang-ke-al) Mandibular arch in the embryo.

First molar Type of molar closest to the midline, at the sixth position from it.

First premolar Type of premolar closer to the midline, at the fourth position from it.

Flush terminal plane Type of terminal plane relationship in which the primary maxillary and mandibular second molars are in an end-to-end relationship in centric occlusion.

Fluting Elongated developmental depression that can occur on the surface of the root branches of certain teeth.

Foliate lingual papillae (fo-le-ate) Vertical ridges of lingual papillae on the lateral surface of the tongue.

Follicles (fol-i-kls) Masses that are embedded in a meshwork of reticular fibers within the lobules of the thyroid gland.

Foramen cecum (for-ay-men **se**-kum) Small pitlike depression located where the sulcus terminalis points backward toward the pharynx.

Fordyce's spots (for-die-seez) Small yellowish elevations on the mucosa resulting from deeper deposits of sebum from trapped or misplaced sebaceous glands.

Foregut (fore-gut) Anterior portion of the future digestive tract or primitive pharynx that forms the oropharynx.

Fossa (plural, fossae) (fos-ah, **fos**-ay) Shallow, wide depressions on the lingual surface of anterior teeth or on the occlusal table of posterior teeth.

Fourth branchial arch (brang-ke-al) Branchial arch in the embryo that participates in the formation of most of the laryngeal cartilages.

Free gingival crest Most superficial portion of the marginal gingiva.

Free gingival groove Groove that separates the attached gingiva from the marginal gingiva.

Frontal region (frunt-il) Region of the face that includes the forehead area and the area above the eyes.

Frontonasal process (frun-to-**na**-zil) Prominence in the upper facial area at the most cephalic end of the embryo.

Fungiform lingual papillae (fun-ji-form) Smaller mushroom-shaped lingual papillae on the dorsal surface of the tongue.

Furcation (fer-kay-shin) Area between two or more root branches before they divide from the root trunk.

Furcation crotches Spaces between the roots at the furcation.

Fusion (fu-zhin) During prenatal development, the joining of embryonic tissues of two separate surfaces, the elimination of a groove between two adjacent swellings, or a dental developmental disturbance in which two adjacent tooth germs unite to form a large tooth.

G

Gemination (jem-i-**nay**-shin) Developmental disturbance that occurs because the single tooth germ tries unsuccessfully to divide, resulting in a large single-rooted tooth.

Generalized resorption Resorption of a hard tissue or the entire skeleton of bone in varying amounts as a result of endocrine activity.

Geographic tongue Lesion that appears as red and then paler pink to white patches on the body of the tongue and that changes shape with time.

Germinal center (jurm-i-nil) Center region of the lymphatic nodule of a lymph node where the lymphocytes mature.

Gingiva (jin-**ji**-vah) Gum tissue composed of mucosa surrounding the maxillary and mandibular teeth in their alveoli and covering the alveolar processes.

Gingival fiber group Fiber groups within the gingiva that have no bony attachments.

Gingival fluid Fluid in the gingival sulcus.

Gingival hyperplasia (hi-per-**play**-ze-ah) Overgrowth of the interproximal gingiva.

Gingival recession (re-**sesh**-un) Teeth associated with a lower margin of the free gingival crest.

Gingival sulcus (sul-kus) Space facing the sulcular gingiva.

Gland Structure that produces a chemical secretion necessary for normal body functioning.

Globular dentin Areas of both primary and secondary mineralization in dentin.

Gnathic index (nath-ick) Measurement that gives the degree of prominence of the maxillary arch.

Goblet cells Cells in respiratory mucosa that produce mucus that keeps the mucosa moist.

Goiter (goy-ter) Enlarged thyroid gland.

Golden Proportions The golden rule is an ancient principle used in mathematics, art, and architecture to provide a guide for aesthetically pleasing proportion.

Golgi complex (gol-jee) Organelle of the cells that is involved in protein segregation, packaging, and transport.

Granular layer Layer superficial to the prickle layer in some forms of keratinized epithelium.

Granulation tissue (gran-yoo-**lay**-shin) Immature connective tissue formed during initial repair.

Group function Situation in which the entire posterior quadrant functions during lateral occlusion.

H

Hard palate Anterior portion of the palate.

Haversian canal (hah-**ver**-zi-an) Vascular tissue space in an osteon.

Haversian system Organized arrangement of lamellae and canals in compact bone.

Height of contour Crest of curvature, which is the greatest elevation of the tooth either incisocervically or occlusocervically on a specific surface of the crown.

Hemidesmosome (hem-eye-**des**-mah-some) Type of intercellular junction that involves an attachment of a cell to a nearby noncellular surface.

Hertwig's epithelial root sheath (HERS) (hirt-**wigz**) Portion of the cervical loop that functions to shape the root(s) and induce dentin formation in the root area.

Hilus (hi-lus) Depression on one side of the lymph node.

Hindgut (hind-gut) Posterior portion of the future digestive tract.

Histodifferentiation (his-toe-dif-er-en-she-**ay**-shin) Development of different tissues.

Histology (his-**tol**-oh-je)   Study of the microscopic structure and function of tissues.

Horizontal group   Portion of the alveodental ligament that originates in the alveolar bone proper and inserts horizontally into the cementum.

Howship's lacuna (**how**-ships)   Large shallow pit in bone created by the resorptive process of an osteoclast.

Hutchinson's incisors (**hutch**-in-suns)   Developmental disturbance in permanent incisors caused by congenital syphilis, which leaves the incisors with screwdriver-shaped crowns.

Hyoid arch (**hi**-oid)   Second branchial arch that lies inferiorly to the mandibular arch in the embryo.

Hyoid bone   Bone suspended in the anterior midline of the neck that has many muscle attachments.

Hypercementosis (hi-per-see-men-**toe**-sis)   Excessive production of cellular cementum.

Hyperkeratinized (hi-per-**ker**-ah-tin-izd)   Epithelial tissue with excessive production of keratin.

I

Imbrication lines (im-bri-**kay**-shun)   Slight ridges that extend mesiodistally in the cervical third on certain teeth and associated with the lines of Retzius in enamel.

Imbrication lines of von Ebner (von **eeb**-ner)   Incremental lines or bands in mature dentin.

Immature bone   First bone to be produced by either method of ossification.

Immunogen (**im**-un-ah-jen)   An antigen treated as foreign by the body that is capable of triggering an immune response.

Immunoglobulin (Ig) (im-u-no-**glob**-u-lin)   A protein in the blood or antibody produced by plasma cells during an immune response.

Impacted (im-**pak**-ted)   Unerupted or partially erupted tooth that is positioned against another tooth, bone, or even soft tissue so that complete eruption becomes unlikely.

Implantation (im-plan-**ta**-shin)   Embedding of a blastocyst in the endometrium.

Incisal angles (in-**sigh**-zl)   Two angles on the permanent incisors formed from the incisal ridge (or incisal edge) and each proximal surface.

Incisal edge   Incisal ridge on permanent incisors that appears flattened from its labial, lingual, or incisal views after eruption.

Incisal ridge   Linear elevation on the incisal or masticatory surface of permanent incisors when newly erupted.

Incisal surface   Masticatory surface for anterior teeth.

Incisive papilla (in-**sy**-ziv pah-**pil**-ah)   Small bulge of tissue at the most anterior portion of the hard palate, lingual to the anterior teeth.

Incisors (in-**sigh**-zers)   Anterior teeth that are the first and second from the midline and consist of both centrals and laterals, respectively.

Inclined cuspal planes   Sloping planes located between these cusp ridges on posterior teeth.

Inclusions (in-**kloo**-zhins)   Metabolically inert substances or transient structures within the cell.

Induction (in-**duk**-shin)   Process by which the action of one group of cells on another leads to the establishment of the developmental pathway in the responding tissue.

Infraorbital region (in-frah-**or**-bit-al)   Region of the face located both inferior to the orbital region and lateral to the nasal region.

Initiation stage   First stage of tooth development.

Inner enamel epithelium (IEE)   Innermost cells of the enamel organ, which form ameloblasts.

Intercalated duct (in-**tur**-kah-lay-ted)   Duct associated with an acinus or terminal portion of the salivary gland.

Intercellular junctions   Mechanical attachments between cells and possibly between cells and nearby noncellular surfaces.

Intercellular substance   Transparent substance that fills in the spaces between cells in a tissue.

Interdental gingiva (in-ter-**den**-tal)   Gingiva between adjacent teeth that is an extension of attached gingiva.

Interdental ligament   Principal fiber group that inserts interdentally into the cervical cementum of neighboring teeth.

Interdental septum   Alveolar bone between two neighboring teeth.

Interglobular dentin   Areas in dentin where only primary mineralization has occurred.

Intermaxillary segment (in-ter-**mak**-si-lare-ee)   Fused internal and inferior growth from the paired medial nasal processes on the inside of the stomodeum of the embryo.

Intermediate filaments (**fil**-ah-ments)   Components of the cytoskeleton that are composed of various types of thicker, threadlike microscopic structures.

Intermediate layer   Layer of epithelium superficial to the basal layer in nonkeratinized epithelium.

International Standards Organization Designation System for Teeth (ISO System)   International system for tooth designation using a two-digit code.

Interocclusal clearance (in-ter-ah-**kloo**-zhal)   Space between the arches when the mandible is at rest.

Interphase (**in**-ter-faz)   Period when the cell is between divisions.

Interprismatic region (in-ter-**priz**-mat-ik)   Outer region surrounding each enamel rod, also called *interred enamel*.

Interproximal space (in-ter-**prok**-si-mal)   Area between adjacent tooth surfaces.

Interradicular group   Portion of the alveolodental group on multirooted teeth that is inserted on the cementum of one root to the cementum of the other root(s).

Interradicular septum (in-ter-rah-**dik**-u-lar)   Alveolar bone between the roots of the same tooth.

Interstitial growth (in-ter-**stish**-il)   Growth that occurs from deep within a tissue or organ.

Intertubular dentin (in-ter-**tube**-u-lar)   Type of dentin that is found between the dentinal tubules.

Intramembranous ossification (in-trah-**mem**-bran-us os-i-fi-**kay**-shun)   Formation of osteoid within dense connective tissue.

J

Joint capsule   Two-layered connective tissue that completely encloses the temporomandibular joint.

Junctional epithelium (JE) (**jungk**-shun-al)   Epithelium that is a deeper extension of the sulcular epithelium of the marginal gingiva.

K

Karyotype (kare-e-oh-tipe) Photographic analysis of a person's chromosomes.

Keratin (ker-ah-tin) Type of intermediate protein filament that is found in calloused epithelial tissues and consists of an opaque waterproof substance.

Keratin layer Most superficial layer in keratinized epithelium.

Keratohyaline granules (ker-ah-toe-hi-ah-lin) Prominent granules in the cytoplasm of certain epithelial cells that form a chemical precursor for the keratin.

L

Labial (lay-be-al) Structures or facial surfaces of the teeth close to the lips.

Labial commissures (kom-i-shoors) Corners of the mouth where the upper and lower lips meet.

Labial developmental depressions Depressions that extend the length of the crown cervicoincisally and that show the division of the surface into labial developmental lobes.

Labial frenum (free-num) Fold of tissue located at the midline between the labial mucosa and the alveolar mucosa.

Labial mucosa Mucosal lining of the inner portions of the lips.

Labial ridge Central ridge on the labial surface of canines owing to a greater development of the middle labial developmental lobe.

Lacuna (plural, lacunae) (lah-ku-nah, lah-ku-nay) Small space that surrounds the chondrocyte or osteocyte within the cartilage matrix or bone, respectively.

Lamellae (lah-mel-ay) Closely apposed sheets of bone tissue in compact bone.

Lamina dura (lam-i-nah dur-ah) Radiopaque line representing the alveolar bone proper.

Lamina propria (lam-i-nah pro-pree-ah) Connective tissue proper region of oral mucosa.

Laryngopharynx (lah-ring-gah-fare-inks) Most inferior part of the pharynx, close to the laryngeal opening.

Larynx (lare-inks) Voice box in the midline of neck, composed of cartilages.

Lateral deviation of the mandible (de-vee-ay-shun) Shifting the lower jaw to one side.

Lateral incisor Incisor second from the midline.

Lateral lingual swellings Portions of the developing tongue that form on each side of the tuberculum impar.

Lateral nasal processes Tissue on the outer portion of the nasal pits that forms the nasal alae.

Lateral occlusion Type of occlusal movement that occurs when the mandible moves to either the right or the left until the canines on that side are in a cusp-to-cusp relationship.

Lateral surface of the tongue Side of the tongue.

Leeway space Space created when the primary molars are shed to make room for the much smaller mesiodistal permanent premolars.

Lens placodes Placodes in the embryo that form the eyes and related tissues.

Line angle Imaginary line formed by the junction of two crown surfaces.

Linea alba (lin-ee-ah al-bah) White ridge of raised keratinized epithelial tissue on the buccal mucosa that extends horizontally at the level where the teeth occlude.

Lines of Retzius (ret-zee-us) Incremental lines in preparations of mature enamel.

Lingual (ling-gwal) Describes structures or tooth surfaces closest to the tongue.

Lingual fossa Fossa on the lingual surface of certain anterior teeth.

Lingual frenum (free-num) Midline fold of tissue between the ventral surface of the tongue and the floor of the mouth.

Lingual groove Groove on the lingual surface of certain anterior teeth.

Lingual papillae (pah-pil-ay) Small elevated structures of specialized mucosa on the tongue.

Lingual pit Developmental pit on the lingual surface of anterior teeth and the lingual surface of certain maxillary posterior teeth.

Lingual ridge Vertically oriented and centrally placed ridge that extends from the cusp tip to the cingulum on the lingual surface of certain canines.

Lingual tonsil (ton-sil) Irregular mass of tonsillar tissue located posteriorly on the dorsal surface of the tongue.

Linguogingival groove Vertically placed groove on the lingual surface of certain anterior teeth that originates in the lingual pit and extends cervically and slightly distally onto the cingulum.

Linguoincisal edge Raised edge on the incisal border of the lingual fossa of a maxillary central incisor.

Lining mucosa Mucosa associated with nonkeratinized stratified squamous epithelium.

Lobes Large inner portions of certain glands or controversal regions of a tooth during development.

Lobules (lob-ules) Smaller inner portions of certain glands.

Localized resorption Resorption of bone or other hard tissue that occurs in a specific area.

Loose connective tissue Tissue that forms the superficial layer of the dermis of the skin and lamina propria of the oral mucosa.

Lumen (loo-men) In a salivary gland, a central opening where the saliva is deposited into a duct after being produced by the secretory cells.

Lymph (limf) Tissue fluid that drains from the surrounding region into the lymphatic vessels.

Lymph nodes (limf) Bean-shaped bodies grouped in clusters along the connecting lymphatic vessels, positioned to filter toxic products from the lymph.

Lymphadenopathy (lim-fad-uh-nop-ah-thee) Enlarged and palpable lymph nodes.

Lymphatic ducts (lim-fat-ik) Ducts that the smaller lymphatic vessels containing lymph converge into and that then empty into the venous system.

Lymphatic nodules (nah-jools) Masses of lymphocytes in a lymph node.

Lymphatic vessels (lim-fat-ik) System of endothelium-lined channels that carry lymph.

Lymphatics Network of lymphatic vessels that collect and transport lymph, linking lymph nodes throughout most of the body.

Lymphocyte (lim-fo-site) Second most common white blood cell in the blood, involved in the immune response.

Lysosomes (li-sah-somes) Organelles of the cell that function in both intracellular and extracellular digestion of materials.

M

Macrodontia (mak-roe-don-she-ah) Abnormally large teeth.

Macrophage (mak-rah-faje) Most common white blood cell in the connective tissue proper; termed *monocyte* before it migrated from the blood into the tissues.

Major salivary glands Large paired glands that have named ducts associated with them.

Malocclusion (mal-ah-kloo-zhun) Failure to have an overall ideal form to the dentition while in centric occlusion.

Mamelons (mam-ah-lons) Rounded enamel extensions on the incisal ridge from the labial or lingual views of certain anterior teeth.

Mandible (man-di-bl) Lower jawbone.

Mandibular arch (man-dib-you-lar) Lower dental arch with mandibular teeth or the first branchial arch inferior to the stomodeum in the embryo.

Mandibular processes Processes of the first branchial arch that fuse at the midline to form the mandibular arch.

Mandibular symphysis (sim-fi-sis) Midline area of the mandible where the bone formed by fusion of right and left mandibular processes.

Mandibular teeth Teeth in mandibular arch of the lower jawbone or mandible.

Mandibular torus (plural, tori) (tore-us, tore-eye) Normal variation of bone growth noted on the lingual aspect of the mandibular arch.

Mantle dentin Outermost layer of dentin found in the crown region, adjacent to the dentinoenamel junction.

Marginal gingiva Gingiva at the gingival margin of each tooth.

Marginal grooves Developmental grooves that cross either marginal ridge.

Marginal ridges Rounded raised borders on the mesial and distal portions of the lingual surface of anterior teeth and the occlusal table of posterior teeth.

Mast cell White blood cell that is similar to the basophil because it is also involved in allergic responses.

Mastication (mass-ti-kay-shin) Chewing process.

Masticatory mucosa (mass-ti-ka-tor-ee) Mucosa associated with keratinized stratified squamous epithelium.

Masticatory surface Chewing surface on the crown.

Matrix (may-triks) Substance in connective tissue composed of intercellular substance and fibers or extracellular substance that is partially calcified and serves as a framework for later calcification.

Maturation (ma-cher-ray-shin) Attainment of the correct adult size as well as the correct adult form and function, such as that which occurs with the hard dental tissues when they are fully calcified or when the embryo becomes a fetus.

Maxilla (mak-sil-ah) Upper jaw.

Maxillary arch (mak-si-lar-ee) Upper dental arch with maxillary teeth.

Maxillary process Prominence from the mandibular arch that grows superiorly and anteriorly on each side of the stomodeum of the embryo.

Maxillary teeth Teeth in the maxillary arch or upper jawbone or maxilla.

Maxillary tuberosity (too-beh-ros-i-tee) Tissue-covered elevation of the bone just distal to the last tooth of the maxillary arch.

Meckel's cartilage (mek-els kar-ti-lij)) Cartilage that forms within each side of the mandibular arch and that disappears as the bony mandible is formed.

Medial nasal processes Middle portion of the tissue growing around the nasal placodes located between the nasal pit on the embryo.

Median lingual sulcus Midline depression on the dorsal surface of the tongue.

Median palatine raphe (pal-ah-tine ra-fe) Midline ridge of tissue on the hard palate that overlies the bony fusion of the palate.

Meiosis (my-oh-sis) Process of reproductive cell production that ensures the correct number of chromosomes for the future embryo.

Melanin pigmentation (mel-a-nin) Localized macules of pigmentation caused by the presence of melanin.

Mental region (ment-il) Region of the face where the chin is the major feature.

Mesenchyme (mes-eng-kime) Embryonic connective tissue.

Mesial (me-ze-il) Surface of a tooth closest to the midline.

Mesial contact Contact area on the mesial surface of the tooth.

Mesial drift Natural movement of all the teeth over time toward the midline of the oral cavity.

Mesial marginal ridge Marginal ridge on the mesial portion of the lingual surface of anterior teeth or the mesial portion of the occlusal table of posterior teeth.

Mesial step Type of terminal plane relationship in which the primary mandibular second molar is mesial to the maxillary molar.

Mesiodens (me-ze-oh-denz) Supernumerary tooth between the two permanent maxillary central incisors.

Mesoderm (mes-oh-derm) Embryonic layer located between the ectoderm and endoderm.

Mesognathic (me-so-nath-ik) Facial profile in centric occlusion with slightly protruded jaws, giving the facial outline a relatively flat appearance or straight profile.

Metaphase (met-ah-faz) Second phase of mitosis, in which the chromosomes are aligned into equatorial position.

Microdontia (mi-kro-don-she-ah) Abnormally small teeth.

Microfilaments (my-kroh-fil-ah-ments) Delicate, thread-like microscopic structures that are components of the cytoskeleton.

Microtubules (my-kroh-too-bules) Components of the cytoskeleton that are slender tubular microscopic structures.

Midgut (mid-gut) Middle portion of the future digestive tract.

Minor salivary glands Numerous small salivary glands with short unnamed ducts.

Mitochondria (mite-ah-kon-dree-ah) Organelles associated with manufacture of ATP.

Mitosis (my-toe-sis) Portion of cell division that occurs in phases and results in two daughter cells that are identical to the parent cell.

Mixed dentition period (den-tish-in) Dentition period that occurs between 6 and 12 years of age and has both primary and permanent teeth present.

Molars (mo-lerz) Most posterior teeth, including firsts, seconds, and thirds.

Monocyte (mon-ah-site) White blood cell that becomes a macrophage after it migrates from the blood into the tissues.

Morphodifferentiation (mor-foe-dif-er-en-she-ay-shin) Development of the differing form that will create a specific structure.

Morphogenesis (mor-fo-jen-is-is) Process of development of specific tissue morphology.

Morphology (mor-fol-ah-je) Form of a structure.

Mucobuccal fold (mu-ko-buk-al) Area within the vestibule where the labial mucosa or buccal mucosa meets the alveolar mucosa.

Mucocele (mu-kah-sele) Lesion due to retention of saliva in a minor salivary gland.

Mucogingival junction (mu-ko-jin-ji-val) Line of demarcation between the attached gingiva and the alveolar mucosa.

Mucoperiosteum (mu-ko-per-ee-os-te-im) Loose connective tissue acting as a periosteum to the underlying bone.

Mucosa (mu-ko-sah) Mucous membrane lining.

Mucoserous acinus (mu-ko-sere-us) Group of mucous cells surrounding the lumen with a serous demilune producing a mixed secretory product.

Mucous acinus (mu-kis) Group of mucous cells producing a mucous secretory product.

Mucous cells Secretory cells that produce mucous secretory product.

Mulberry molars (mull-bare-ee) Developmental disturbance that occurs as a result of congenital syphilis, in which enamel nodules are present on the occlusal surface of the molars.

Multirooted Teeth that have two or more root branches.

Myoepithelial cells (my-oh-ep-ee-thee-lee-al) Contractile epithelial cells that are located on the surface of some of the acini to facilitate the flow of saliva out of each lumen into the connecting ducts.

N

Naris (plural, nares) (nay-ris, nay-rees) Nostril of the nose.

Nasal ala (plural, alae) (a-lah, a-lay) Winglike cartilaginous structures of the nose that bound the nares laterally.

Nasal cavity (nay-zil kav-it-ee) Inner space of the nose.

Nasal conchae (kong-kay) Projecting structures that extend inward from each lateral wall of the nasal cavity.

Nasal pits Depressions in the center of each nasal placode that evolve into the nasal cavities.

Nasal placodes Placodes that develop into olfactory organ for the sensation of smell located in the mature nose.

Nasal region Region of the face occupied by the external nose.

Nasal septum (sep-tum) Midline portion of the nose that separates the nares.

Nasmyth's membrane (nas-miths) Residue on newly erupted teeth that may become extrinsically stained.

Nasolacrimal duct (nay-zo-lak-ri-mal) Duct that drains the tears or lacrimal fluid from the eye.

Nasolacrimal groove Groove that extends from the medial corner of the eye to the nasal cavity.

Nasopharynx (nay-zo-fare-inks) Division of the pharynx that is superior to the level of soft palate.

Neonatal line (ne-oh-nate-l) Accentuated incremental line of Retzius in enamel or contour line of Owen in dentin that results from birth process.

Nerve Bundle of neural processes outside the central nervous system.

Neural crest cells (noor-al) Specialized group of cells developed from neuroectoderm that migrate from the crests of the neural folds and disperse to specific sites within the mesenchyme. They also influence a special type of mesenchyme, the ectomesenchyme, to form dental tissues.

Neural folds Raised ridges in the neural plate that surround the deepening neural groove.

Neural groove Groove resulting from further growth and thickening of the neural plate.

Neural plate Centralized band of cells that extends the length of the embryo.

Neural tube Tube formed when the neural folds meet and fuse superior to the neural groove.

Neuroectoderm (noor-oh-ek-toe-derm) Specialized group of cells that differentiates from the ectoderm.

Neuron (noor-on) Functional cellular component of the nervous system.

Neutrophil (noo-trah-fil) Most common white blood cell, which is also called a *polymorphonuclear leukocyte (PMN)* and is involved in the inflammatory response.

Nicotinic stomatitis (nik-ah-tin-ik sto-mah-ti-tis) Whitish lesion on the hard palate caused by the heat from smoking or hot liquid consumption.

Nonkeratinized stratified squamous epithelium (non-ker-ah-tin-izd) Epithelium in the superficial layers of lining mucosa.

Nonsuccedaneous (non-suk-seh-dane-ee-us) Permanent teeth without primary predecessors, namely the molars.

Nuclear envelope (noo-kle-er) Double membrane completely surrounding the nucleus.

Nuclear pores Avenues of communication between the inner nucleoplasm and the outer cytoplasm.

Nucleolus (noo-kle-ah-lis) Rounded nuclear organelle that is often centrally placed in the nucleoplasm.

Nucleoplasm (noo-kle-ah-plazm) Semifluid portion within the nucleus.

Nucleus (plural, nuclei) (noo-kle-eye) Largest, densest, and most conspicuous organelle in the cell.

O

Oblique group Portion of the alveolodental ligament that originates in the alveolar bone proper and extends apically and obliquely to insert into the cementum.

Oblique ridge (o-bleek) Type of transverse ridge that crosses the occlusal table obliquely on most maxillary molars, from mesiolingual to distobuccal.

Occlusal developmental pits (ah-kloo-zl) Pits in the deepest portions of the fossae on the occlusal table of posterior teeth.

Occlusal surface Masticatory surface of posterior teeth.

Occlusal table Portion of the occlusal surface of posterior teeth that is bordered by the marginal ridges.

Occlusal trauma Trauma to the periodontium resulting from occlusal disharmony.

Occlusion (ah-kloo-zhun) Anatomical alignment of the teeth and their relationship to the rest of the masticatory system.

Odontoblastic process (oh-don-toe-blast-ik) Attached cellular extension of the odontoblast within the dentinal tubule through the entire width of the dentin.

Odontoblasts (oh-don-toe-blasts) Cells that produce dentin and differentiate from the outer cells of the dental papilla.

Odontoclasts (oh-don-toe-klasts) Cells that resorb dentin, cementum, and enamel.

Open bite Type of malocclusion in which the anterior teeth do not occlude.

Oral cavity proper Inside of the mouth.

Oral epithelium (ep-ee-theel-ee-um) Embryonic lining of the oral cavity derived from ectoderm, which along with underlying tissues gives rise to the teeth and associated tissues.

Oral mucosa (mu-ko-sah) Mucosa or mucous membrane lining the oral cavity.

Oral region Region of the face that contains the lips and oral cavity.

Orbit Bony socket that contains the eyeball and all its supporting structures.

Orbital region (or-bit-al) Region of the face that includes the bony orbit and the eyeball and all its supporting structures.

Organ Somewhat independent body part that performs a specific function or functions and that is formed from tissues.

Organelles (or-gah-nels) Specialized structures within the cell that are permanent and metabolically active.

Oronasal membrane (or-oh-nay-zil) Embryonic membrane that disintegrates, bringing the nasal and oral cavities into communication.

Oropharyngeal membrane (or-oh-fah-rin-je-al) Membrane at the cephalic end of the embryo that is the location of the future primitive mouth.

Oropharynx (or-o-fare-inks) Oral division of the pharynx that is located between the soft palate and the opening of the larynx.

Orthokeratinized stratified squamous epithelium (or-tho-ker-ah-tin-izd) Keratinized epithelial tissue that demonstrates keratinization of the epithelial cells throughout its most superficial layers.

Ossification (os-i-fi-kay-shun) Bone formation.

Osteoblasts (os-te-oh-blasts) Bone-forming cells.

Osteoclast (os-te-oh-klast) Cell that functions in resorption of bone.

Osteocytes (os-tee-oh-sites) Mature osteoblasts entrapped in bone matrix.

Osteoid (os-te-oid) Initially formed bone matrix.

Osteons (os-te-onz) Concentric layers of lamellae in compact bone.

Otic placodes (o-tik) Placodes in the embryo that form the future internal ear and related tissues.

Outer cells of the dental papilla Cells of dental papilla tissue that differentiate into odontoblasts.

Outer enamel epithelium (OEE) Outer cells of the enamel organ that serve as a protective barrier during enamel production.

Overbite Situation in which the maxillary incisors overlap the mandibular incisors.

Overjet Situation in which the maxillary dental arch overhangs the mandibular arch facially.

Ovum (oh-vum) Female reproductive cell or egg, which can be fertilized.

P

Palatal (pal-ah-tal) Describes lingual structures or tooth surfaces closest to the palate on the maxillary arch.

Palatal shelves Two processes derived from the maxillary processes during prenatal development.

Palatal torus (tore-us) Normal variation of bone growth noted on the midline of the hard palate.

Palate (pal-it) Roof of the mouth.

Palatine rugae (ru-ge) Firm, irregular ridges of tissue directly posterior to this incisive papilla.

Palatine tonsils (pal-ah-tine **ton-**sils) Tonsillar tissue located between the faucial pillars.

Palmer method System of tooth designation commonly used in orthodontics.

Papillary layer (pap-i-lar-ee) Layer of loose connective tissue of the dermis or lamina propria.

Parafunctional habits (pare-ah-funk-shun-al) Movements of the mandible that are not within the normal motions associated with mastication, speech, or respiratory movements.

Parakeratinized stratified squamous epithelium (pare-ah-ker-ah-tin-izd) Keratinized epithelium associated with the masticatory mucosa of the attached gingiva; may be an immature form of orthokeratinized epithelium.

Paranasal sinuses (pare-ah-na-zil **sy-**nus-es) Paired air-filled cavities in bone.

Parathyroid glands (par-ah-thy-roid) Endocrine glands that are close to or even inside the posterior aspects of the thyroid gland.

Parotid duct (pah-rot-id) Duct associated with the parotid gland.

Parotid papilla (pah-pil-ah) Small elevation of tissue on the inner portion of the buccal mucosa, just opposite the maxillary second molar, that protects the parotid duct.

Parotid salivary gland Two major salivary glands located irregularly from the zygomatic arch down to the posterior border of the lower jaw.

Passive eruption Eruption that takes place that occurs as we age, when the gingiva recedes and no actual tooth movement takes place.

Peg lateral A lateral incisor crown that is especially small because of the developmental disturbance partial microdontia.

Peg third molar A small molar crown with one cusp resulting from the developmental disturbance partial microdontia.

Perichondrium (per-ee-kon-dre-im) Outermost connective tissue layer surrounding most cartilage.

Perikymata (per-ee-**ki**-mot-ah) Grooves evident on some teeth in the oral cavity, associated with the lines of Retzius in enamel.

Periodontal ligament (PDL) (pare-ee-o-**don**-tal) Ligament surrounding the teeth that supports and attaches the teeth to the bony surface of the alveoli.

Periodontal space Radiolucent area representing the periodontal ligament on radiographs.

Periodontium (per-e-o-**don**-she-um) Supporting hard and soft dental tissues between and including portions of the tooth and the alveolar bone.

Periosteum (per-ee-**os**-te-im) Dense connective tissue layer on the outer portion of bone.

Peripheral cells of the dental papilla Outer cells of the dental papilla that become odontoblasts.

Peritubular dentin (pare-i-**tube**-u-lar) Type of dentin that creates the wall of the dentinal tubule.

Permanent dentition or teeth (den-**tish**-in) The second dentition.

Permanent dentition period Dentition period that begins just after 12 years of age and includes all the permanent teeth.

Phagocytosis (fag-oh-sigh-**toe**-sis) Engulfing and then digesting of solid waste or foreign material by the cell.

Pharyngeal pouches (fah-**rin**-je-il) Four pairs of evaginations from the lateral walls lining the pharynx between the branchial arches.

Pharyngeal tonsils Located on the superior and posterior walls of the nasopharynx and forming an incomplete ring, Waldeyer's ring.

Pharynx (**fare**-inks) Muscular tube of the throat.

Philtrum (**fil**-trum) Vertical groove on the midline of the upper lip, extending downward from the nasal septum to the tubercle of the upper lip.

Pit and groove patterns Patterns formed from pits and grooves on the occlusal surface of permanent posterior teeth.

Placenta (pla-**sen**-tah) Temporary prenatal organ that provides nutrition and oxygen to the developing embryo, removes wastes, and produces the hormones related to pregnancy.

Placodes (**plak**-odz) Areas of ectoderm found at the location of developing special sense organs on the embryo.

Plasma (**plaz**-mah) Fluid substance in the blood vessels that carries the blood cells and metabolites.

Plasma cells White blood cells that are derived when B-cell lymphocytes divide during the immune response and that later form immunoglobulins.

Platelets (**plate**-lits) Blood cell fragments that function in the clotting mechanism.

Plica fimbriata (plural, **plicae fimbriatae**) (**pli**-kah fim-bree-**ay**-tah, **pli**-kay fim-bree-**ay**-tay) Fold with fringelike projections on the ventral surface of the tongue.

Point angle Imaginary line formed by the junction of three crown surfaces.

Polymorphonuclear leukocyte (PMN) (pol-ee-mor-fah-**noo**-klee-er **loo**-ko-site) Most common white blood cell involved in the inflammatory response; also called a *neutrophil*.

Posterior teeth Molars, and premolars if present, because these teeth are in the back of the mouth.

Posterior faucial pillar (**faw**-shawl) Posterior lateral folds of tissue created by underlying muscle that help form the fauces.

Preameloblasts (pre-ah-**mel**-oh-blasts) Cells formed from the inner enamel epithelium of the enamel organ that differentiate into ameloblasts.

Preimplantation period of prenatal development (pre-im-plan-**ta**-shin) Period of the unattached conceptus that takes place during the first week of prenatal development.

Predentin Dentin matrix laid down by apposition by the odontoblasts.

Premature contacts Situation in which one or two teeth initially contact before the other teeth.

Premolars (pre-**mo**-lerz) Posterior teeth that are the fourth and fifth teeth from the midline in the permanent dentition and that include firsts and seconds, respectively.

Prenatal development (pre-**nay**-tal) Processes that occur from the start of pregnancy to birth of the child.

Prepubertal periodontitis Severe periodontal disease within the primary dentition.

Prickle layer Layer that is superficial to the basal layer in keratinized epithelium.

Primary dentin Dentin formed in a tooth before the completion of the apical foramen.

Primary dentition or teeth (den-**tish**-in) First dentition present, also called the *deciduous dentition*.

Primary dentition period Dentition period that occurs between 6 months and 6 years of age during which all the teeth present are primary teeth.

Primary palate Anterior portion of the final palate derived from the intermaxillary segment during prenatal development.

Primate spaces Spaces between certain primary teeth.

Primitive pharynx Cranial portion of the foregut that forms the oropharynx.

Primitive streak Furrowed, rod-shaped thickening in the middle of the embryonic disc.

Primordium (pry-**more**-de-um) Earliest indication of a part or an organ during prenatal development.

Principal fibers Collagen fibers organized into groups on the basis of their orientation to the tooth and related function.

Prognathic (prog-**nath**-ik) Facial profile that usually shows a rather prominent mandible and possibly a normal or even retrusive maxilla or concave profile.

Proliferation (pro-lif-er-**ay**-shin) Controlled cellular growth.

Prophase (**pro**-faz) First phase of mitosis, in which the chromatin condenses into chromosomes.

Protrusion of the mandible (pro-**troo**-zhin) Moving the lower jaw forward.

Protrusive occlusion Occlusion in which the mandible undergoes protrusion.

Proximal root concavities Depressions on the proximal root surfaces of certain teeth.

Proximal surfaces (**prok**-si-mal) Both the mesial and distal surfaces between adjacent teeth.

Pseudostratified epithelium (soo-doh-**strat**-i-fide) Simple epithelium that falsely appears as multiple cell layers.

Pterygomandibular fold (teh-ri-go-man-**dib**-yu-lar) Fold of tissue that extends from the junction of the hard and soft palates down to the mandible and is just behind the most distal mandibular tooth.

Pulp   Soft innermost connective tissue in both the crown and root of the tooth.

Pulp cavity   Portion of the tooth composed of pulp tissue and covered by dentin.

Pulp chamber   Portion of the tooth that contains the mass of pulp.

Pulp horns   Extensions of coronal pulp into the cusps of posterior teeth.

Pulp stones   Masses of calcified dentin in the pulp tissue.

Pulpitis   Inflammation of the pulp.

Q

Quadrants (kwod-rints)   Division of each dental arch into two parts, with four quadrants in the entire oral cavity.

R

Radicular pulp (rah-**dik-**u-lar)   Portion of the pulp located in the root area of the tooth.

Ramus (ray-**mus)**   Plate of mandible that extends upward and backward from the body of the mandible on each side.

Ranula (ran-u-lah)   Lesion that results from retention of saliva in the submandibular salivary gland.

Red blood cell (RBC)   Blood cell whose cytoplasm contains hemoglobin, which binds and then transports the oxygen.

Reduced enamel epithelium (REE)   Layers of flattened cells overlying the enamel surface resulting from a compression of the enamel organ.

Regions of the face   Areas of the facial surface including the frontal, orbital, nasal, infraorbital, zygomatic, buccal, oral, and mental regions.

Regions of the neck   Areas of the neck that extend from the skull and lower jaw down to the clavicles and sternum and are based on different cervical triangles.

Reichert's cartilage (rike-erts)   Cartilage in the second branchial arch that eventually disappears, although parts of it form a middle ear bone and other bones.

Remodeling   Process by which bone is replaced over time.

Repolarization (re-po-ler-i-**za-**shun)   Process that occurs in a cell in which the nucleus moves away from the center to a position farthest away from the basement membrane.

Resorption (re-**sorp-**shun)   Removal of a hard tissue such as bone, enamel, dentin, or cementum.

Respiratory mucosa   Mucosa that consists of pseudostratified ciliated columnar epithelium.

Rete ridges (ree-tee)   Extensions of the epithelium into the connective tissue as they appear on histological section.

Reticular connective tissue (re-**tik-**u-ler)   Delicate network of interwoven reticular fibers.

Reticular fibers   Fibers that are found in relation to an embryonic tissue.

Reticular lamina (lam-i-nah)   Deeper portion of the basement membrane.

Reticular layer   Dense connective tissue in the dermis and lamina propria.

Retraction of the mandible (re-**trak-**shun)   Moving the lower jaw backward.

Retrognathic (re-tro-**nath-**ik)   Facial profile with a protruding upper lip or the appearance of a recessive mandible and chin or convex profile.

Retromolar pad (re-tro-**mo-**ler)   Dense pad of tissue just distal to the last tooth of the mandibular arch.

Reversal lines   Stained, scalloped microscopic lines caused by resorption in cartilage, bone, and cementum.

Ribosomes (ry-bo-somes)   Organelles of the cell that are associated with protein production.

Ridges   Linear elevations on the masticatory surface of both anterior and posterior teeth.

Root   Portion of a tooth composed of dentin covered by cementum.

Root axis line (RAL)   Imaginary line representing the long axis line of a tooth, drawn to bisect cervical line.

Root concavities   Indentations on the surface of the root(s).

Root fusion   Developmental disturbance that creates deep developmental grooves when the roots fuse.

Root of the nose   Portion of the nose located between the eyes.

Root trunk   Portion of the root of multirooted teeth where the root originates from the crown.

Rubella virus (roo-**bell-**ah)   Infective teratogen transmitted by way of the placenta to the embryo from the pregnant woman.

S

Saliva (sah-**li-**vah)   Secretion from salivary glands that lubricates and cleanses the oral cavity and helps in digestion.

Salivary glands (sal-i-ver-ee)   Glands that produce saliva.

Second branchial arch (brang-ke-al)   Branchial arch inferior to the mandibular arch, also called the *hyoid arch* in the embryo.

Second molar   Type of molar distal to the first molar and in the seventh position from the midline.

Second premolar   Type of premolar in the fifth position from the midline.

Secondary bone   Mature bone tissue that replaces immature bone.

Secondary dentin   Dentin that is formed after the completion of the apical foramen.

Secondary palate   Posterior portion of the final palate formed by the fusion of the two palatal shelves.

Secretory cells (sek-**kre-**tory)   Epithelial cells that produce saliva.

Septum (plural, **septa) (**sep-tum, sep-tah)   Connective tissue that helps divide the inner portion of certain glands.

Serous acinus (sere-us)   Group of serous cells producing serous secretory product.

Serous cells   Secretory cells that produce serous secretory product.

Serous demilune (dem-ee-lune)   Serous cells superficial to the mucous secretory cells in a mucoserous acinus.

Sextants (sex-tants)   Division of each dental arch into three portions based on the relationship to the midline.

Sharpey's fibers (shar-peez)   The collagen fibers from the periodontal ligament that are partially inserted into the cementum and bone.

Simple epithelium (un-strat-i-fide)   Epithelium that consists of a single layer of cells.

Simple squamous epithelium (skway-mus)   Lining of the blood and lymphatic vessels, heart, and serous cavities and important interfaces in the lungs and kidneys.

Sinusitis (sy-nu-si-tis) Inflamed mucosal tissues in the paranasal sinuses.

Sixth branchial arch (brang-ke-al) Branchial arch in the embryo that fuses with the fourth branchial arch and then participates in the formation of most of the laryngeal cartilages.

Skeletal muscles Voluntary muscles that are under the voluntary control of the central and peripheral nervous systems and that appear striated.

Soft palate Posterior portion of the palate.

Somites (so-mites) Paired cuboidal aggregates of cells differentiated from the mesoderm.

Specialized mucosa Mucosa found on the dorsal and lateral surface of the tongue in the form of the lingual papillae.

Sperm Cell containing the male contribution of chromosomal information that fertilizes the female ovum during the preimplantation period.

Spina bifida (spi-nah bif-ah-dah) Neural tube defect affecting the vertebral arches and causing varying degrees of disability.

Squames (skwaymz) Flattened platelike epithelial cells.

Stellate reticulum (stel-ate reh-tik-u-lum) One of the two layers between the outer and inner enamel epithelium of the enamel organ; consists of star-shaped cells.

Sternocleidomastoid muscle (stir-no-klii-do-mass-toid) Large strap muscle of the neck.

Stippling Pin-point depressions present on the surface of the attached gingiva.

Stomodeum (sto-mo-de-um) Primitive mouth, which initially appears as a shallow depression in the embryonic surface.

Stratified epithelium (strat-i-fide) Epithelium that consists of two or more layers.

Stratified squamous epithelium (skway-mus) Epithelium that includes the superficial layers of the skin and oral mucosa.

Stratum intermedium (stra-tum in-ter-mede-ee-um) One of the two layers between the outer and inner enamel epithelium of the enamel organ, consisting of a compressed layer of flat to cuboidal cells.

Striated duct (stri-ate-ed) Larger duct to which intercalated ducts connect in the lobules of a salivary gland.

Sublingual caruncle (sub-ling-gwal kar-unk-kl) Small papilla at the anterior end of each sublingual fold, containing openings of the submandibular and sublingual ducts.

Sublingual duct Short duct associated with a sublingual gland.

Sublingual fold Ridge of tissue on each side of the floor of the mouth.

Sublingual salivary glands Two major salivary glands located in the neck.

Subluxation (sub-luk-say-shun) Partial dislocation of both temporomandibular joints.

Submandibular duct (sub-man-dib-you-lar) Duct associated with the submandibular gland.

Submandibular salivary gland Major salivary gland located in the neck.

Submucosa (sub-mu-ko-sah) Tissue deep to the oral mucosa, composed of loose connective tissue.

Succedaneous (suk-seh-dane-ee-us) Permanent teeth with primary predecessors; include the anterior teeth and premolars.

Successional dental lamina (suk-sesh-shun-al) Extension of the dental lamina into the ectomesenchyme lingual to the developing primary tooth germs that will form the succedaneous permanent teeth.

Sulcular epithelium (sul-ku-lar) Epithelium that stands away from the tooth, creating a gingival sulcus.

Sulcus terminalis (sul-kus ter-mi-nal-is) V-shaped groove located posteriorly on the dorsal surface of the tongue.

Superficial layer Most superficial layer in nonkeratinized epithelium.

Supernumerary teeth (soo-per-nu-mer-air-ee) Developmental disturbance characterized by one or more extra teeth.

Supplemental groove Secondary groove that is a shallower, more irregular linear depression and that branches from the developmental grooves on the lingual surface of anterior teeth and the occlusal table on posterior teeth.

Supporting cusps Cusps that function during centric occlusion and include the lingual cusps of the maxillary posterior teeth and the buccal cusps of the mandibular posterior teeth, as well as the incisal edges of the mandibular anterior teeth.

Synapse (sin-aps) Junction between two neurons or between a neuron and an effector organ where neural impulses are transmitted.

Synovial cavities (sy-no-vee-al) Upper and lower compartments divided by the disc of the temporomandibular joint.

Synovial fluid Fluid in the joint capsule that fills and lubricates the temporomandibular joint.

Synovial membrane Inner layer of the joint capsule that produces synovial fluid.

Syphilis spirochete (sif-i-lis spi-ro-keet) *Treponema pallidum*, which is an infective teratogen for an embryo because it produces defects in the incisors and molars, as well as other generalized defects.

System Group of organs functioning together.

T

Taste buds Barrel-shaped organs of taste associated with certain lingual papillae of the tongue.

Taste pore Opening in the most superficial portion of the taste bud.

Telophase (tel-oh-faz) Final phase of mitosis, in which the division into two daughter cells occurs, with the reappearance of the nuclear membrane.

Temporomandibular disorder (TMD) (tem-poh-ro-mandib-you-lar) Disorder associated with one or both temporomandibular joints.

Temporomandibular joint (TMJ) Joint where the temporal bone of the skull articulates with the mandible.

Teratogens (ter-ah-to-jens) Environmental agents or factors such as infections, drugs, and radiation that can cause malformations.

Terminal plane Ideal molar relationship in the primary dentition when in centric occlusion.

Tertiary dentin Dentin formed in response to a localized injury to the exposed dentin.

Tetracycline staining (tet-rah-si-kleen) Intrinsic staining of the teeth resulting from ingestion of the antibiotic tetracycline during the time of enamel and dentin development.

Third branchial arch (brang-ke-al) Branchial arch in the embryo that is responsible for the formation of portions of the hyoid bone.

Third molar Type of molar distal to the second molar and in the eighth position from the midline.

Thirds Division of a crown surface or root into three portions: the crown horizontally and vertically and root horizontally.

Thyroid cartilage (thy-roid) Includes the midline prominence of the larynx.

Thyroid gland Endocrine gland in the neck.

Thyroglossal duct (thy-ro-gloss-al) Tube that connects the thyroid gland with the base of the tongue during prenatal development and later is obliterated.

Tissue Structure formed by the grouping of cells with similar characteristics of shape and function.

Tissue fluid Interstitial body fluid.

Tomes' granular layer (tomes) Portion of dentin beneath the cementum and adjacent to the dentinocemental junction that looks granular.

Tomes' process Secretory surface of each ameloblast.

Tonofilaments (ton-oh-fil-ah-ments) Type of intermediate filament that has a major role in intercellular junctions.

Tonsillar tissue Nonencapsulated masses of lymphoid tissue.

Tooth fairy Mythological creature who at night takes children's shed primary teeth from under their pillows and leaves a sum of cash.

Tooth germ Primordium of the tooth, which consists of the enamel organ, dental papilla, and dental sac.

Trabeculae (trah-bek-u-lay) Joined matrix pieces forming a lattice in cancellous bone or bands of connective tissue in a lymph node that separate the node into lymphatic nodules.

Trabecular bone (trah-bek-u-lar) Cancellous bone that is located between the alveolar bone proper and the plates of cortical bone.

Transverse ridge (trans-vers) Ridge formed by the joining of two triangular ridges crossing the occlusal table transversely or from the labial to the lingual outline.

Triangular fossa Fossa that has a triangular shape where triangular grooves terminate.

Triangular grooves Grooves that separate a marginal ridge from the triangular ridge of a cusp and which at the termination of the ridges form the triangular fossae.

Triangular ridges Cusp ridges that descend from the cusp tips toward the central portion of the occlusal table.

Trifurcated (try-fer-kay-ted) Tooth having three root branches.

Trilaminar embryonic disc (try-lam-i-ner) Embryonic disc with three distinct layers: ectoderm, mesoderm, and endoderm.

Trophoblast layer (trof-oh-blast) Layer of peripheral cells of the blastocyst.

Tubercle of the upper lip (too-ber-kl) Midline thickening of the upper lip.

Tubercles (too-ber-kls) Accessory cusps on the cingulum of certain anterior teeth or occlusal tables of permanent molars.

Tuberculum impar (too-ber-ku-lum im-par) One of the initial portions of the developing tongue, located in the midline.

Turnover time Time that it takes for the newly divided cells to be completely replaced throughout the entire tissue.

U

Universal Tooth Designation System System for numbering permanent teeth in consecutive arrangement by using Arabic numerals #1 through #32 and for primary teeth by using capital letters *A* through *T*.

Uvula of the palate (u-vu-lah) Midline muscular structure that hangs down from the posterior margin of the soft palate.

V

Vacuoles (vak-you-oles) Spaces or cavities within the cytoplasm.

Ventral surface of the tongue Underside of the tongue.

Vermilion border (ver-mil-yon) Transition zone where the lips are outlined from the surrounding skin.

Vermilion zone Darker appearance of the lips compared with the surrounding skin.

Vertical dimension of the face Dividing the face into three horizontal portions.

Vestibular fornix (ves-ti-bu-lar fore-niks) Deepest recess of each vestibule.

Vestibules (ves-ti-bules) Maxillary and mandibular spaces in the oral cavity between the lips and cheeks anteriorly and laterally and the teeth and gums medially and posteriorly.

Volkmann's canals (volk-manz) Vascular canals other than the Haversian canals for transport of nutrients in compact bone.

von Ebner's salivary glands (von eeb-ners) Serous type of minor salivary glands associated with the circumvallate lingual papillae.

W

White blood cell (WBC) Blood cells that form from the bone marrow's stem cells and mature there or in lymphatic tissue.

Working side Side to which the mandible has been moved during lateral occlusion.

X

Xerostomia (zer-oh-sto-me-ah) Dry mouth caused by a decreased production of saliva.

Y

Yolk sac Fluid-filled cavity that faces the hypoblast layer.

Z

Zygomatic arch (zy-go-mat-ik) Bony support for the cheek.

Zygomatic region Region of the face that overlies the zygomatic arch.

Zygote (zy-gote) The fertilized egg resulting from the union of ovum and sperm.

Anatomical Position

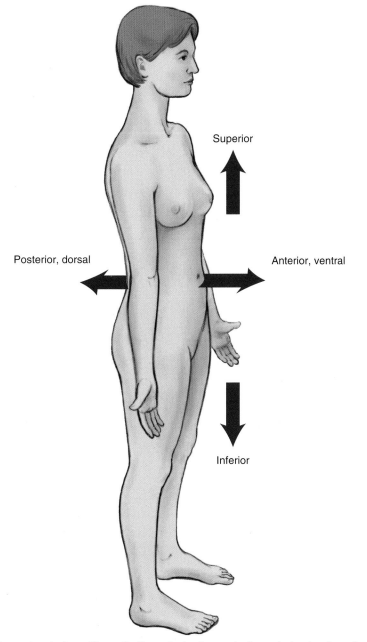

A-1 Body in anatomical position with the anterior (or ventral), posterior (or dorsal), superior, and inferior areas noted. (From Fehrenbach MJ, Herring SW. *Illustrated Anatomy of the Head and Neck,* ed 2. WB Saunders, Philadelphia, 2002.)

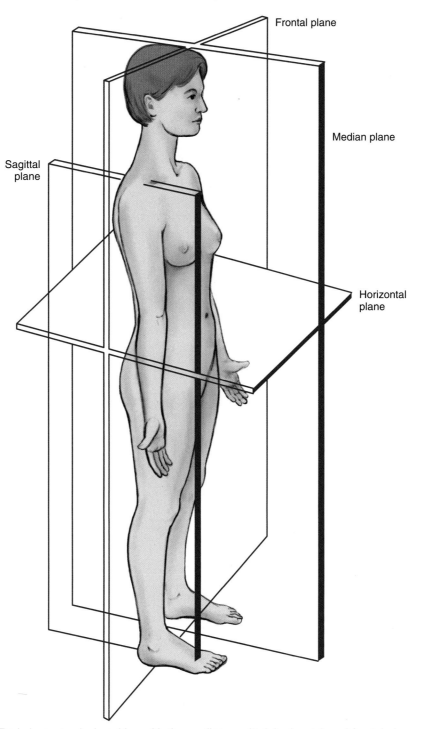

Frontal plane

Median plane

Sagittal
plane

Horizontal
plane

A-2 Body in anatomical position with the median, sagittal, horizontal, and frontal planes noted. (From Fehrenbach MJ, Herring SW. *Illustrated Anatomy of the Head and Neck,* ed 2. WB Saunders, Philadelphia, 2002.)

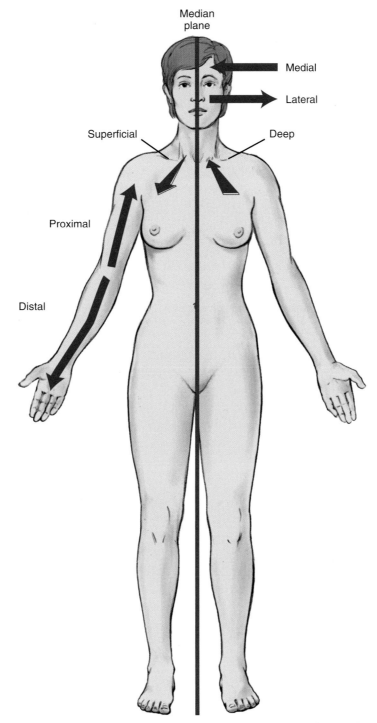

Median
plane

Medial

Lateral

Superficial

Deep

Proximal

Distal

A-3 Body in anatomical position with the medial (or proximal), lateral (or distal), and superficial (or deep) areas noted. (From Fehrenbach MJ, Herring SW. *Illustrated Anatomy of the Head and Neck,* ed 2. WB Saunders, Philadelphia, 2002.)

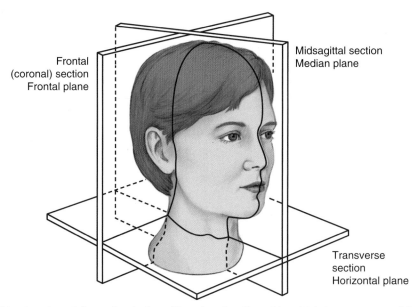

Frontal
(coronal) section
Frontal plane

Midsagittal section
Median plane

Transverse
section
Horizontal plane

A-4 Head and neck in anatomical position showing the midsagittal, transverse, and frontal sections. (Fehrenbach MJ, Herring SW. *Illustrated Anatomy of the Head and Neck,* ed 2. WB Saunders, Philadelphia, 2002.)

Units of Measure

Unit	Abbreviation	Equivalent	Measurement Application
Centimeter	cm	0.4 inch	Naked eye: pathological lesions
Millimeter	mm	0.1 cm	Naked eye: extremely large human cells (muscle, liver), periodontal pockets
Micrometer	mm	0.001 mm	Light microscopy: most human cells; large organelles and bacteria, ameloblasts
Nanometer	nm	0.001 μm	Electron microscopy: smaller organelles, largest of macromolecules, dental tissue units

Tooth Measurements

TABLE 1

Measurements of the Permanent Incisors (in Millimeters)

	Cervicoincisal Length of Crown	Length of Root	Mesiodistal Diameter of Crown	Mesiodistal Diameter Crown at Cervix	Labiolingual Diameter of Crown	Labiolingual Diameter of Crown at Cervix	Curvature of Cervical Line: Mesial	Curvature of Cervical Line: Distal
Maxillary central incisor	10.5	13.0	8.5	7.0	7.0	6.0	3.5	2.5
Maxillary lateral incisor	9.0	13.0	6.5	5.0	6.0	5.0	3.0	2.0
Mandibular central incisor	9.0	12.5	5.0	3.5	6.0	5.3	3.0	2.0
Mandibular lateral incisor	9.5	14.0	5.5	4.0	6.5	5.8	3.0	2.0

(All adapted from Ash MM. *Wheeler's Dental Anatomy, Physiology and Occlusion,* ed 8. WB Saunders, Philadelphia, 2002.)

TABLE 2

Measurements of the Permanent Canines (in Millimeters)

	Cervicoincisal Length of Crown	Length of Root	Mesiodistal Diameter of Crown	Mesiodistal Diameter of Crown at Cervix	Labiolingual Diameter of Crown	Labiolingual Diameter of Crown at Cervix	Curvature of Cervical Line: Mesial	Curvature of Cervical Line: Distal
Maxillary canine	10.0	17.0	7.5	5.5	8.0	7.0	2.5	1.5
Mandibular canine	11.0	16.0	7.0	5.5	7.5	7.0	2.5	1.0

TABLE 3

Measurements of the Permanent Premolar Teeth (in Millimeters)

	Cervico-Occlusal Length of Crown	Length of Root	Mesiodistal Diameter of Crown	Mesiodistal Diameter of Crown at Cervix	Buccolingual Diameter of Crown	Buccolingual Diameter at Cervix	Curvature of Cervical Line: Mesial	Curvature of Cervical Line: Distal
Maxillary first premolar	8.5	14.0	7.0	5.0	9.0	8.0	1.0	0.0
Maxillary second premolar	8.5	14.0	7.0	5.0	9.0	8.0	1.0	0.0
Mandibular first premolar	8.5	14.0	7.0	5.0	7.5	6.5	1.0	0.0
Mandibular second premolar	8.0	14.5	7.0	5.0	8.0	7.0	1.0	0.0

TABLE 4

Measurements of the Permanent Maxillary Molars (in Millimeters)

	Cervico-Occlusal Length of Crown	Length of Root	Mesiodistal Diameter of Crown	Mesiodistal Diameter of Crown at Cervix	Buccolingual Diameter of Crown	Buccolingual Diameter at Cervix	Curvature of Cervical Line: Mesial	Curvature of Cervical Line: Distal
Maxillary first molar	7.5	buccal = 12 lingual = 13	10.0	8.0	11.0	10.0	1.0	0.0
Maxillary second molar	7.0	buccal = 11 lingual = 12	9.0	7.0	11.0	10.0	1.0	0.0
Maxillary third molar	6.5	11.0	8.5	6.5	10.0	9.5	1.0	0.0

TABLE 5

Measurements of the Permanent Mandibular Molar (in Millimeters)

	Cervico-Occlusal Length of Crown	Length of Root	Mesiodistal Diameter of Crown	Mesiodistal Diameter of Crown at Cervix	Buccolingual Diameter of Crown	Buccolingual Diameter at Cervix	Curvature of Cervical Line: Mesial	Curvature of Cervical Line: Distal
Mandibular first molar	7.5	14.0	11.0	9.0	10.5	9.0	1.0	0.0
Mandibular second molar	7.0	13.0	10.5	8.0	10.0	9.0	1.0	0.0
Mandibular third molar	7.0	11.0	10.0	7.5	9.5	9.0	1.0	0.0

TABLE 6

Measurements of the Primary Teeth (in Millimeters)

	Length Overall	Length of Crown	Length of Root	Mesiodistal Diameter of Crown	Mesiodistal Diameter at Cervix	Facial-Lingual Diameter of Crown	Facial-Lingual Diameter at Cervix
Maxillary Teeth							
Central incisor	16.0	6.0	10.0	6.5	4.5	5.0	4.0
Lateral incisor	15.8	5.6	11.4	5.1	3.7	4.8	3.7
Canine	19.0	6.5	13.5	7.0	5.1	7.0	5.5
First molar	15.2	5.1	10.0	7.3	5.2	8.5	6.9
Second molar	17.5	5.7	11.7	8.2	6.4	10.0	8.3
Mandibular Teeth							
Central incisor	14.0	5.0	9.0	4.2	3.0	4.0	3.5
Lateral incisor	15.0	5.2	10.0	4.1	3.0	4.0	3.5
Canine	17.0	6.0	11.5	5.0	3.7	4.8	4.0
First molar	15.8	6.0	9.8	7.7	6.5	7.0	5.3
Second molar	18.8	5.5	11.3	9.9	7.2	8.7	6.4

Tooth Development

TABLE 1

Development of Permanent Incisors

	Maxillary Central Incisor	Maxillary Lateral Incisor	Mandibular Central Incisor	Mandibular Lateral Incisor
Number of lobes		4 lobes		
First evidence of calcification	3–4 months	1 year	3–4 months	3–4 months
Completion of enamel	4–5 years	4–5 years	4–5 years	4–5 years
Eruption date	7–8 years	8–9 years	6–7 years	7–8 years
Completion of root	10 years	11 years	9 years	10 years

TABLE 2

Development of Permanent Canines

	Maxillary Canine	Mandibular Canine
Number of lobes		4 lobes
First evidence of calcification	4–5 months	4–5 months
Completion of enamel	6–7 years	6–7 years
Eruption date	11–12 years	9–10 years
Completion of root	13–15 years	12-14 years

(All adapted from Ash MM. *Wheeler's Dental Anatomy, Physiology and Occlusion*, ed 8. WB Saunders, Philadelphia, 2002.)

TABLE 3

Development of Permanent Premolars

Specific Teeth	Maxillary First Premolar	Maxillary Second Premolar	Mandibular First Premolar	Mandibular Second Premolar
Number of lobes		4 lobes		4 or 5 lobes
First evidence of calcification	$1\frac{1}{2}$–$1\frac{3}{4}$ years	2–$2\frac{1}{2}$ years	$1\frac{3}{4}$–2 years	$2\frac{1}{4}$–$2\frac{1}{2}$ years
Completion of enamel	5–6 years	6–7 years	5–6 years	6–7 years
Eruption date	10–11 years	10–12 years	10–12 years	11–12 years
Completion of root(s)	12–13 years	12–14 years	12–13 years	13–14 years

TABLE 4

Development of Permanent Maxillary Molars

	Maxillary First Molar	Maxillary Second Molar	Maxillary Third Molar
Number of lobes	5 lobes	4 lobes	
First evidence of calcification	Birth	$2\frac{1}{2}$ years	7–9 years
Completion of enamel	3–4 years	7–8 years	12–16 years
Eruption date	6–7 years	12–13 years	17–21 years
Completion of root(s)	9–10 years	14–16 years	18–25 years

TABLE 5

Development of Permanent Mandibular Molars

	Mandibular First Molar	Mandibular Second Molar	Mandibular Third Molar
Number of lobes	5 lobes	4 lobes	
First evidence of calcification	Birth	$2\frac{1}{2}$–3 years	8–10 years
Completion of enamel	$2\frac{1}{2}$–3 years	7–8 years	12–16 years
Eruption date	6–7 years	11–13 years	17–21 years
Completion of root(s)	9–10 years	14–15 years	18–25 years

Index

Note: Index entries followed by b indicate boxes; f, figures; t, tables.

Anatomy, embryology, and histology topics *(Continued)*
  orofacial embryology topics, 23–92
    developmental data, 383–384
    face and neck development, 39–50
    orofacial structures development, 51–60
    prenatal development, 25–38
    tooth development and eruption, 61–92
  overview and summary topics. *See* Overviews and summaries.
  reference resources, 355
  structures fundamentals, 1–22
    face and neck regions, 3–12
    oral cavity and pharynx, 13–22
  terminology and definitions, 357–372
Anatomy-specific topics, 231–354, 373–376. *See also under individual topics.*
  anatomical positions, 231–354, 373–376
  dentition, 233–246, 313–324
    fundamentals, 233–246
    primary, 313–324
  eruption and shedding ages (approximate), 313–315, 314t
  occlusion, 335–354
  permanent teeth, 247–272, 273–312
    anterior, 247–272
    posterior, 273–312
  TMJ (temporomandibular joint), 325–334
Anchoring collagen fibers, 110–111, 357
Androgen effects, 27t
Angle's classification (malocclusion), 344–349, 345t, 357
Angulations and curvatures, 339–342, 339f–342f
Ankyloglossia, 59, 59f, 357
Anodontia, 65t, 224, 357
Anterior arch forms, 338–339
Anterior faucial pillars, 357
Anterior permanent teeth, 247–272
  canines, 263–271, 264t, 265f–267f
    general features, 263–266, 264t
    incisors, 248, 248f, 251t
    mandibular (22 and 27), 264t, 269–271, 270f–271f
    maxillary (6 and 11), 264t, 266–269, 266f–268f
  clinical considerations, 249–250, 253, 256, 259–260, 266, 269
  defined, 357
  developmental disturbances, 252, 256, 259, 261, 263, 269, 271
  incisors, 248–263, 248f–250f, 251t, 252f–263f
    anatomical data, 251t
    canine, 248, 248f, 251t
    central *vs.* lateral, 250, 251t
    general features, 252–253
    mandibular, 251t, 259–263, 259f–263f
    mandibular (central 24 and 25), 251t, 260–262, 260f–262f
    mandibular (general features), 259–260
    mandibular (lateral 23 and 26), 251t, 262–263, 262f–263f
    maxillary, 248, 248f, 251f–259f, 251t, 252–259
    maxillary (central 8 and 9), 251t, 253–256, 253f–256f
    maxillary (general features), 252–253
    maxillary (lateral 7 and 10), 251t, 256–259, 256f–259f
  objectives, 247
  overviews and summaries, 247–250, 248f–249f, 357
  terminology and definitions, 247, 357
Apex, nose, 357
Apical fiber groups, 226–230, 226t, 357
Apical foramen, 201, 357
Apparatus, branchial, 47–49, 358
Apposition and apposition stage, 63t, 75–78, 76f–78f, 192, 193, 357
Appositional growth, 117–118, 357
Arch forms, 338–339
Arches. *See also under individual topics.*
  branchial, 42–43, 43t, 47–49, 57, 258

Arches *(Continued)*
  defined, 365
  dental, 17–18, 360
  mandibular, 42–44, 43f–44f, 365
  maxillary, 234–245, 365
  zygomatic, 371
Arrest lines, 211–212, 357
Articular eminances, 357
Articular fossae, 326–327, 357
Articulating surfaces, condyle, 7, 327, 357
ATP (adenosine triphosphate), 98–99
Attached gingiva, 135t, 137–138, 357
Attrition, 192, 250, 260, 357
Avulsion, 256, 357

B

B and I molars (first maxillary), 320–321, 321f
Baby bottle mouth, 316, 317f
Balancing interferences, 343, 358
Balancing sides, 343, 358
Basal bones, 215, 358
Basal lamina, 110, 358
Basal layers, 132–133, 358
Basement membranes, 64, 76–78, 110–111, 110f, 358
Bases, tongue, 358
Basic topics. *See* Overviews and summaries.
Basophils, 121t, 122, 358
Bell stage, 63t, 73–74, 74f, 75t, 358
  defined, 358
  description, 63t, 73–74, 74f, 75t
Bibliography, 355
Bicuspids, 276, 358. *See also* Premolars.
Bifurcated teeth, 278, 358
Bilaminar embryonic discs, 31, 32f, 358
Bilateral symmetry, 31, 32f
Black hairy tongue, 145, 358
Blastocysts, 28–31, 29f, 31f, 358
Blastocytes, 28, 29t, 358
Blood, 119–123, 120f, 120t–122t, 122f, 358
  defined, 358
  description, 119–123, 120f, 120t–122t, 122f
Body, tongue, 358
Bone marrow, 115, 358
Bones. *See also under individual topics.*
  basal, 215, 358
  cancellous, 115, 358
  colloid, 359
  compact, 115, 359
  cortical, 218, 359
  defined, 358
  development, 82
  hyoid, 11, 363
  immature, 118, 363
  marrow. *See* Bone marrow.
  secondary, 118, 369
  temporal, 326–327
  trabecular, 218, 371
Branchial apparatus, 47–49, 358
Branchial arches, 42–43, 43t, 47–49, 57, 258, 358
  defined, 358
  descriptions, 42–43, 43t, 47–49, 57, 258
Branchial grooves, 49, 358
Bruxism (grinding), 351, 358
Buccal cervical ridges, 320–322, 358
Buccal cusps, 280, 286
  defined, 280
  tips, 286
Buccal developmental depressions, 286

Grooves *(Continued)*
  distal marginal, 281
  free gingival, 153, 362
  lingual, 255, 364
  linguogingival, 253, 255, 259, 364
  marginal, 281, 365
  mesiolingual, 286
  nasolacrimal, 366
  supplemental, 249, 249f, 275, 370
  triangular, 275, 371
Group functions, 343, 362

H

H and C canines (maxillary), 319–320, 319f–320f
Hard palates, 135t, 138–141, 362
Haversian canals, 116, 362
Haversian system, 116, 362
Head and neck structures, 161–178. *See also* Face and neck;
    Neck.
  clinical considerations, 168, 171, 173, 177
  glands, 162–171, 163–165f, 163t, 167f, 169f–171f
    parathyroid, 169
    salivary, 162–171, 163f–165f, 163t, 167f, 169f–171f
    thyroid, 169–171, 170f–171f
  lymphatics, 171–174, 173f–174f
    intraoral tonsillar tissues, 172–174
    lymph nodes, 172
  nasal cavities, 174–175, 175f
  objectives, 161
  overviews and summaries, 161–162
  paranasal sinuses, 176–177, 176f
  terminology and definitions, 161–162
Heart-shaped molars, 301
Heights, contour, 248, 249f, 362
Hemidesmosomes, 102–103, 110, 362
Herpes simplex virus effects, 27t
HERS (Hertwig's epithelial root sheath), 80–84, 362
Hilus, 172, 362
Hindguts, 362
Histodifferentiation, 362
Histology, defined, 363
Histology, embryology, and anatomy topics. *See also under*
    individual topics.
  anatomy-specific topics, 231–354, 373–376
    anatomical positions, 231–354, 373–376
    dentition (fundamentals), 233–246
    dentition (primary), 313–324
    occlusion, 335–354
    permanent teeth (anterior), 247–272
    permanent teeth (posterior), 273–312
    TMJ (temporomandibular joint), 325–334
  clinical considerations. *See* Clinical considerations.
  developmental disturbances. *See* Developmental disturbances.
  measurement-related topics, 377–382
    tooth measurements, 379–382
    units of measure, 377–378
  objectives (learning). *See* Objectives.
  oral histology topics, 93–230
    cell fundamentals, 95–104
    dentin and pulp, 191–206
    enamel, 179–190
    gingival and dentogingival junctional tissues, 151–160
    head and neck structures, 161–178
    oral mucosa, 127–150
    periodontium (cementum, alveolar bone, periodontal
        ligament), 207–230
    tissue fundamentals, 105–126
  orofacial embryology topics, 23–92

Histology, embryology, and anatomy topics *(Continued)*
    developmental data, 383–384
    face and neck development, 39–50
    orofacial structures development, 51–60
    prenatal development, 25–38
    tooth development and eruption, 61–92
  overview and summary topics. *See* Overviews and summaries.
  reference resources, 355
  structures fundamentals, 1–22
    face and neck regions, 3–12
    oral cavity and pharynx, 3–12, 13–22
    terminology and definitions, 356–372
Histology, oral. *See* Oral histology topics.
HIV (human immunodeficiency virus) effects, 27t
Horizontal fiber groups, 226–230, 226t, 363
Horns, pulp, 317f, 369
Hyoid arches, 43t, 47–49, 363
Hyoid bones, 11, 363
Hypercementosis, 214, 363
Hyperkeratinization, 133
Hyperkeratinized tissues, 363
Hyperplasia, gingival, 154, 362
Hypersensitivity, dentin, 196, 360
Hypoblast layers, 32f

I

I and B molars (first maxillary), 320–321, 321f
IEE (inner enamel epithelium), 75–78, 75t, 363
Imbrication lines of von Ebner, 199–200, 255–257, 363
  defined, 363
  descriptions, 199–200, 255–257
Immature bones, 118, 363
Immunogens, 121–122, 363
Immunoglobulin, 121–122, 122t, 363
Impacted teeth, 269, 363
Implantation, 29, 363
Incisal angles, 255, 317, 363
Incisal edges, 250, 256, 317, 319, 363
Incisal surfaces, 248, 248f, 363
Incisors, 248–263, 248f–250f, 251t, 252f–263f, 363
  anatomical data, 251t
  anatomy, 234–245, 234f
  canine, 248, 248f, 251t. *See also* Canines.
  central *vs.* lateral, 250, 251t
  defined, 363
  general features, 317–318
  mandibular, 251t, 259–263, 318–319
    central (O and P), 318–319, 318f–319f
    general features, 259–260
    lateral (23 and 26), 251t, 262–263, 262f–263f
    lateral (Q and N), 319, 319f
  maxillary, 248, 251t, 252–259, 317–318
    central 8 and 9, 251t, 253–256, 253f–256f
    central (E and F), 317, 317f
    general features, 252–253
    lateral (7 and 10), 251t, 256–259, 256f–259f
    lateral (D and G), 317–318, 318f
Inclined cuspal planes, 274, 281, 363
Inclusions, 100, 363
Induction and induction processes, 30–31, 30t, 63–64, 64t, 70–76,
    363
  defined, 363
  descriptions, 30–31, 30t, 63–64, 64t, 70–76
Infection-induced effects, 27t
Infraorbital regions, 363
Initiation stage, 63–65, 63t, 65t, 363
Inner enamel epithelium. *See* IEE (inner enamel epithelium).
Intercalated ducts, 363

evolve

To access your Student Learning Resources, visit:

http://evolve.elsevier.com/Bath-Balogh/illustrated/

Evolve® Student Learning Resources for *Bath-Balogh/Fehrenbach: Illustrated Dental Embryology, Histology, and Anatomy,* **2**nd **edition** offers the following features:

- **Supplemental Considerations**
  The Supplemental Considerations provide the students with additional areas of study, expanding upon the material found in the book.

- **Discussion Questions**
  Discussion Questions are provided for each chapter in the text. They can be used to stimulate classroom discussion and for group or self-study and review.

- **Update Section**
  Content Updates will be posted periodically to help keep students informed of new and exciting developments in the field as well as address additional concepts and information that may not be covered in the text.

- **Weblinks**
  A variety of weblinks are provided so students can pursue further study.

ILLUSTRATED

Dental Embryology, Histology, AND Anatomy

W9-CDX-663